PROGRESS IN BRAIN MAPPING RESEARCH

PROGRESS IN BRAIN MAPPING RESEARCH

F.J. CHEN
EDITOR

Nova Science Publishers, Inc.
New York

Library of Congress Cataloging-in-Publication Data
Available upon request

ISBN 1-59454-580-4

Published by Nova Science Publishers, Inc. ✢ New York

Contents

Preface

This outstanding book includes research derived from non-invasive brain imaging modalities used to explore the spatial and temporal organization of the neural systems supporting human behavior. Imaging modalities of interest include positron emission tomography, event-related potentials, electro-and magnetoencephalography, magnetic resonance imaging, and single-photon emission tomography. Coverage includes novel brain imaging methods, analyses for detecting or localizing neural activity, synergistic uses of multiple imaging modalities, and strategies for the design of behavioral paradigms and neural-systems modeling.

Chapter 1 reviews the most important applications of DT-MRI. The fundamentals of DT-MRI encoding and data acquisition methodologies will be first outlined. Some DT-MRI processing and computational steps will be discussed and summarized. The chapter concludes by providing some example applications from on-going research that the author is involved in on both 1.5 T and 3.0 T MRI clinical scanners. A special focus on the DTI of the aging human corpus callosum (CC) and its use as a marker of the brain pathology is also provided.

Chapter 2 starts with an anatomical description of the auditory cortices derived from recent cytoarchitectonic and histochemical experiments. Next, a definition and description of each of the acoustic parameters to be reviewed are provided. The research intended to establish auditory cortical maps for each of these parameters is then analyzed. An integration of the current knowledge in this field of research is presented at the end.

The aim of chapter 3 is to introduce the key models used in imaging neuroscience, focussing on functional magnetic resonance imaging (fMRI) and electroencephalography (EEG), and how they relate to each other. In particular, the authors consider how the analysis of neuronal dynamics can be used to infer functional segregation and integration. They start with anatomical models of functional brain architectures, which motivate some of the fundaments of neuroimaging. They then turn to basic statistical models (*e.g.* the general linear model) used for making classical and Bayesian inferences about *where* neuronal responses are expressed (regionally specific responses). By incorporating biophysical constraints, these basic models can be finessed and, in a dynamic setting, rendered causal. This allows us to infer *how* interactions among brain regions are mediated. The latter models afford mechanistic inferences about how evoked responses are caused, at the level of neuronal subpopulations and the coupling among them.

Positron emission tomography (PET) enables human brain functions to be investigated *in vivo*. The technique has greatly enhanced our understanding of central nervous system diseases by measuring changes in neurochemical levels, activation patterns and cerebral metabolism. Chapter 4 studies how the ability of PET for quantitative and dynamic assessments is particularly pertinent in the investigation of movement disorders such as Parkinson's disease, which are characterised by disturbances and fluctuations in the level of neurotransmitters in the basal ganglia neuronal circuits. The subjects may be examined in a resting state, whilst performing certain tasks, or after external interventions such as pharmacological challenges or electromagnetic stimulations. This chapter describes recent advances in the study of underlying biochemical abnormalities in Parkinson's disease using PET, and how these have enhanced our understanding of disease pathogenesis and progression.

The objective of chapter 5 was to evaluate the feasibility of using an eigensystem-based study in EEG data in order to validate brain functional mappings associated with the characterization effects of an Auditory/Comprehension paradigm. The study associates key parameters, which relate the correlation between electrodes and the EEG activity and also analyzes key frequency bands (Alpha, Beta, Delta, and Theta) in order to corroborate findings that associate brain activity with specific auditory/comprehension tasks. The theoretical perspective for this research is established to set course for the elaboration of topographical analysis in order to distinguish the areas of the brain displaying prominent activities while specific events are taking place.

Chapter 6 focuses on free-motion neuroimaging studies, a novel neuroimaging study, with the wearable NIRS system. The authors also describe the basic theory, techniques, problems, and future prospects of NIRS. Near-infrared spectroscopy (NIRS) is a completely non-invasive neuroimaging technique, which does not require strict motion restriction and can be used in a daily life environment. Especially, a portable NIRS instrument combined with a wireless telemetry system (the wearable NIRS system) allows subjects to move during measurements like with portable ECG and EEG instruments. Thus, NIRS enables neuroimaging studies on children, the elderly, and patients with psychoneurological problems, who have not been fully examined until now. Yet several challenges that the NIRS field has spent more than 25 years attempting to overcome remain unsolved. These limiting factors in advancement of NIRS are addressed in this chapter.

Neuroimaging studies seek to determine 'when' and/or 'where' activation occurs in the brain. Different techniques have the ability to adequately measure either one or the other type of information. Electrophysiological recordings have excellent time resolution (i.e., they can accurately assess the 'when'), of the order of milliseconds, but the information on localization is poor. Conversely, using metabolic or hemodynamic measurements, such as PET or fMRI, accurate localization (i.e., the 'where') is possible but the time resolution of such measurements is intrinsically limited. Thus, in order to better understand brain function, integration of these different modalities is desirable. In chapter 7, the authors have developed an approach to integration that uses parametric studies wherein the amplitude of a particular ERP is modulated by varying some aspect of a task. These varying amplitudes are then applied as regressors to find activations in a corresponding fMRI data set. The resultant data reveal regions whose activities covary with the ERP. In recent studies, they have applied this method to an oddball (P300) paradigm and a face-detection (N170) paradigm, obtaining a more refined set of activations than with traditional fMRI analyses alone. These are examples of how ERP information may be used synergistically in fMRI analyses, and vice versa. fMRI parametric designs with correlational analysis may provide some timing information on fMRI activity and help identify the generators of ERP signals.

In: Progress in Brain Mapping Research
Editor: F. J. Chen, pp. 1-80 ISBN 1-59454-580-4

Chapter 1

Fundamentals of Diffusion Tensor Imaging of the Entire Human Brain: Review of Basic Theory, Data Acquisition, Processing and Potential Applications at 1.5 T and 3.0 T

Khader M. Hasan*
Department of Diagnostic and Interventional Imaging
The University of Texas Health Science Center at Houston

"As long as our brain is a mystery, the universe, the reflection of the structure of the brain will also be a mystery"
Santiago Ramon y Cajal

Abstract

Water molecular random translational self-diffusion tensor imaging using magnetic resonance (DT-MRI) is a promising quantitative modality for in vivo *and* non-invasive mapping of the organization of soft deep fibrous tissues in both health and disease. The applications of the technique include fetal cortical maturation, brain development and plasticity in response to trauma, neurotoxins, normal aging, psychiatric and neurological conditions. Specific clinical potential applications include multiple sclerosis (MS), Alzheimer's disease (AD), schizophrenia, developmental disorders such as autism, and learning disabilities such as dyslexia and attention deficit disorders (ADHD). The technique is promising in providing objective surrogates in multi-center therapeutic clinical trials to prevent irreversible tissue damage, and in monitoring novel surgical and pharmaceutical approaches to white matter (WM) and gray matter (GM) protection, regeneration and transplantation. Recent advances in Modern hardware, sampling and

* Corresponding Author: Khader M. Hasan, Ph.D.Tel: (713) 500-7690 Fax: (713) 500-7684 Email: Khader.M.Hasan@uth.tmc.edu

computation have enabled the completion of the DT-MRI scan in less than 10 minutes, thus making DT-MRI an important complement to conventional MRI methods. Accurate and reproducible DT-MRI entire brain mapping protocols involve the optimization of an immense parameter space and requires a signal-to-noise ratio (SNR) of at least 20. DT-MRI encoded data are acquired by applying fast-switching spatially dependent magnetic field pulses which may generate image distortions due to parasitic eddy currents. DT-MRI involves large data sets and requires intensive computation and visualization to reduce the information.
In this chapter, we review the most important applications of DT-MRI. The fundamentals of DT-MRI encoding and data acquisition methodologies will be first outlined. Some DT-MRI processing and computational steps will be discussed and summarized. The chapter concludes by providing some example applications from on-going research that the author is involved in on both 1.5 T and 3.0 T MRI clinical scanners. A special focus on the DTI of the aging human corpus callosum (CC) and its use as a marker of the brain pathology is also provided.

Key Words: Diffusion Tensor Imaging, Parameter Space Optimization, Icosahedral Schemes, DTI applications, Fractional Anisotropy, Mean Diffusivity, Tensor Diagonalization

Introduction

Diffusion-based MRI (DW-MRI) of random water molecular translational motion has become an increasingly important modality in the last two decades for understanding tissue injury and repair models such as Wallerian degeneration (Bieulieu et al. 1995; stroke (Sotak 2002; Hoehn-Berlage 1996; Le Bihan 1995; Luypaert et al. 2001), trauma, and epilepsy (Helpern and Huang 1995). Diffusion tensor imaging --which is an extension of DWI technology-- has been used to help understand the organization of normal (Le Bihan 2003; Melhem et al. 2002; Wakana et al. 2003; Dong et al. 2004; Sundgren et al. 2004; Maas 2003) and developing brain structures (Neil 2002; Moseley 2002; Mckinstry et al. 2002; Gupta et al. 2005), as well as neurological and psychiatric disorders (Sotak 2002; Horsfield and Jones 2002; Moseley et al. 2002; Lim and Helpern 2002; Thomalla et al. 2004; Concha et al. 2005). There are many technical and scientific challenges that limit the interpretation, validation, and assignment of the true contributors to the DT-MRI signal in complex living biological systems (Beaulieu 2002; Norris 2001). However, DT-MRI (DTI for short) is a promising non-invasive tool to map the connectivity of fibrous structure of white deep matter (Le Bihan 2003; Basser 1995; Le Bihan 1995; Mori and Van Zijl 2002; Lee et al. 2003).

Overview of this Chapter

The purpose of this chapter is to motivate and introduce the basic principles and applications of DTI technology. The chapter starts by providing a useful window on different aspects of active DTI research and clinical applications. Since DTI seeks to elucidate white matter structure and organization in both health and disease, it is important to understand the physical sources of the DTI signal. The chapter highlights the author's experience with the DTI of the human corpus callosum as a working model to understand the contribution of axonal packing and myelination to the measured signal. The mathematical underpinnings of DTI encoding theory, processing, and computation of large DTI data sets are also underscored. The chapter concludes by providing a host of applications that the author is currently pursuing with other researchers. The interpretation, major limitations, and challenges of DTI are also presented.

Table 1. A collection of useful resources on diffusion tensor imaging that covers background, diffusion principles, mathematics, imaging techniques, challenges, applications, processing and visualization software

Resource	Citation and Comments
For beginners (An excellent introductory but general review by Dr. Mathias Hoehn with focus on Diffusion of Stroke)	• http://www.ujf.grenoble.fr/ismrm/Diffusion/diffusion_outline.htm • Filley 2001 (a treatise on the importance of white matter)
Classical Books on Diffusion	• Einstein 1956 • Berg 1993 • Crank 2002
Relevant diffusion imaging and tensor Books	• Callaghan 1994 • LeBihan et *al.* 1995
Review Special Volumes on DTI	• NMR Biomed Dec 2002 (ed. Le Bihan D) • Neuro Clin North Am. Nov 2002 (ed. Melhem E)
General Review Technical Articles	• Torrey 1956; Karger 1989 • Price 1997; 1998 • Taylor et al. 1985
DTI ISMRM Workshops and Study Groups (Diffusion and Perfusion Study Group)	• http://www.ujf-grenoble.fr/ismrm/ • http://www.ismrm.org/ Has links to past and current DTI workshops and some DTI data sets.
National Institute of Health Section on Tissue Biophysics and Biomimetics (DTI patent is filed by NIH)	• http://dir2.nichd.nih.gov/nichd/stbb/publications.html PJ Basser NIH DTI relevant publications (Free to the public)
DTI Encoding and Uniform Distribution Problem	• http://dti-directions.org/ • http://www.math.niu.edu/~rusin/known-math/95/sphere.faq • http://www.research.att.com/~njas/electrons/ (most encoding sets are *not* isotropic)
Additional Resources	• http://web1.iop.kcl.ac.uk/IoP/Departments/Neurology • /NeurImg/derek/introduction.htm • http://www.uth.tmc.edu/radiology/faculty/hasan.html
DTI Journal Club.	• http://noodle.med.yale.edu/~mjack/dijc.html • http://noodle.med.yale.edu/%7Emjack/dijc-2004.html • http://www.mit.edu/~dtuch/thesis/main.pdf
DTI software (search for) (BrainVoyager, brainvisa, Analyze, SPM99, MEDx, AIR, AFNI, mricro)	• http://noodle.med.yale.edu/~mjack/develop.html • http://www.utradiology.umin.jp/people/masutani/dTV/dTVframe-e.htm • http://neuroimage.yonsei.ac.kr/dodti/ • http://cmrm.med.jhmi.edu/

DTI Examples and Resources

Figure 1 provides an example of the quantitative and qualitative information provided by DTI from an entire brain data set acquired at 1.5 T in 10 minutes with a spatial resolution of ~ 2x2x3 mm^3. Figure 2 provides an illustration of the potential utility of DTI in localizing gray and white matter structures and mapping the entire human brain compact fiber bundles at 3.0 T in about five minutes. Further advances in DTI technology will enable the entire brain exam to be conducted in less than two minutes and thus making DTI a routine choice for clinicians and neuroscientists. Readers with diverse backgrounds and who are interested in different aspects of DTI are advised to browse Table 1 which provides an up-to-date collection of useful resources (in the author's current view) on diffusion tensor imaging that covers background, diffusion principles, mathematics, imaging techniques, challenges, applications, processing and visualization software.

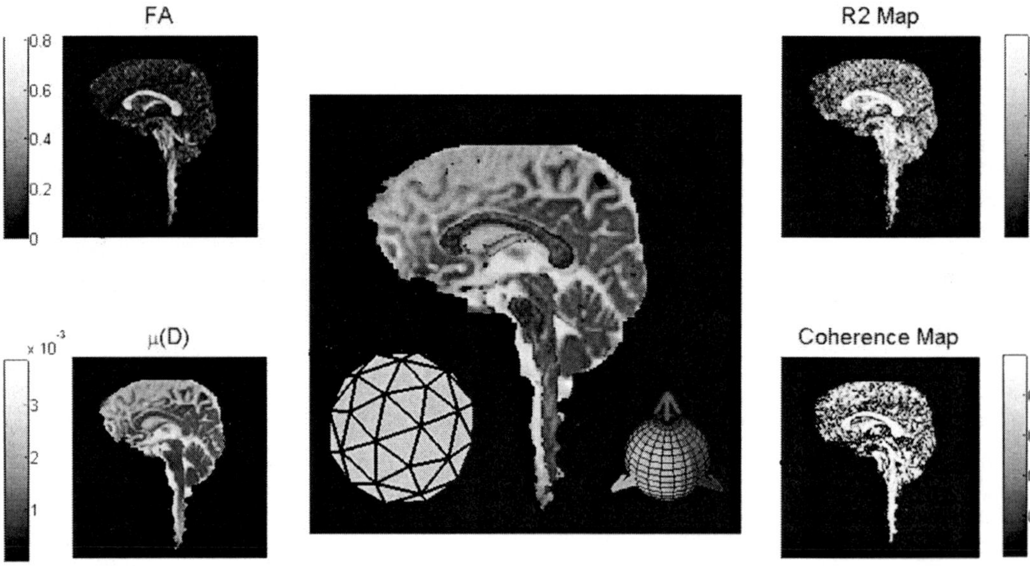

Figure 1. Illustration of the DTI quantitative and qualitative information. DTI estimation provides scalar (fractional anisotropy (FA) $0 \leq FA \leq 1$, mean diffusivity $\mu(\mathbf{D})$, R2 goodness-of-fit) and vector maps (principal vector e_1, coherence) that can provide additional contrast mechanisms to conventional MRI. The coherence map is obtained from the dot product of a reference voxel principal vector with its corresponding neighbors. The central image is an overlay of the mean diffusivity and the FA modulated principal vector $[D_{av}+|e_1*FA|]$. The directional color map is also shown in addition to the tessellated tensor icosahedral encoding scheme (icosa21b). Notice the three major types of white matter bundles: inter-hemispheric or commissural corpus callosum that run right-to-left (red), association or intra-hemispheric (fornix) that run anterior-to-posterior (green) and projection fibers that run inferior-to-superior or head-to-foot such as the corticospinal tract (**blue**).

White Matter in the Human Brain

The human adult intracranial volume (~1700 cm^3: 1400 cm^3 brain, 150 cm^3 blood, 150 cm^3 cerebrospinal fluid or CSF) consists of ~ 40% (volume) of myelinated white matter

(WM), ~ 50 % of gray matter (GM) that includes cell bodies and about 10% of CSF. Since we are interested in magnetic resonance imaging of the human brain using water, it is informative to provide some basic information about the water and tissue distribution (Chudler 2005). The water in the human brain is approximately 77% of its mass, with 10-12% lipids and ~ 8% proteins. The water in the brain is compartmentalized or simply can be located in the intravascular (~5%) or extravascular space. The extravascular space is divided further into intracellular (75%) and extracellular (20%). Thus, at body temperature the thermally agitated and tumbling water molecules can vibrate, rotate, translate and interact with barriers and exchange spins. These motional degrees of freedom and interactions form the basis for the different contrast mechanisms manipulated in MRI (Koenig 1990; Yang 1996; Callaghan 1994; Le Bihan 1995). The volume of the human brain WM, GM, and CSF vary with age and gender (Sowell et al. 2003) and can be affected regionally or globally by diseases or acquired conditions such as trauma, malnutrition, chronic alcoholism, and neurotoxins (Filley 2001). It is estimated that the human brain loses one axon per second due to normal gain axonal elimination from a pool of 100 billion axons that serve all complex tasks the brain is optimized to handle (Marner et al. 2003; Peters and Rosene 2003). Neurodegenerative diseases (multiple sclerosis, Alzheimer's, etc), environmental conditions (malnutrition, abuse, alcohol, neurotoxins, etc) and acquired insults (brain trauma, stroke, etc) to the brain will increase this rate and result in clinical dysfunction. The pathogenesis of many of these diseases are not yet fully understood and may affect different regions to variant extent depending on the insult severity and proximity, the axonal diameter, thickness and connectivity, and the density of channels and the repair mechanisms available (Filley 2001; Trapp et al. 1998; Teipel et al. 1999). It is clear that noninvasive methods to map the developing and aging brain may shed light onto the regional neuronal and functional substrates of such mechanisms and on methods of avoiding and repairing accelerated loss of neuronal communication (Barker and Dunnett 1999). The brain white matter is composed of densely packed myelinated fibers or ''lipids''. The role of myelin is important to facilitate electrical signal conduction and propagation (Waxman et al. 1995; Kandel et al. 1991). Myelin provides the axons with a low capacitance and high resistance protection which prevents electrical shunting and dissipation of electrical signals that are usually initiated at the nodes of Ranvier and propagated through the axons (Waxman et al. 1995; Kandel et al. 1991). Myelin sheaths in the central nervous system are generated by specialized progenitor cells called oligodendrocytes which have become the target of intensive research (Barker and Dunnett 1999). In general, the larger the diameter the fiber, the thicker the myelin sheath, the faster the conduction velocity (Waxman et al. 1995; Kandel et al. 1991; Basser 2004). The presence of myelin in the brain, combined with constraints of limited space and energy, has set limits on its size, functional specialization and efficiency. Myelin and axonal integrity is crucial to the normal function of the brain and its adaptation to acquired conditions and pathologies (Waxman et al. 1995). An interesting quote by G. Lemke (1992) is appropriate here: "If we assume that 10% of the human brain is taken up by myelinated axons, then in the absence of myelin our brains would need to be ten times larger simply to maintain conduction velocity." Classic examples demonstrating the motor dysfunction as a result of genetic or acquired dys or de-myelination include the jimby, shaker, and shiverer mice. The study of rare human genetic dysmyelination diseases such as Krabbe disease, Pelizaeus-Merzbacher disease, adrenoleukodystrophy (Lorenzo's oil) neurodegenerative diseases such as amyotrophic lateral sclerosis (ALS), epilepsy, stroke, autism, dyslexia, and autoimmune inflammatory disease such as multiple sclerosis (MS) and others would benefit tremendously from the development of non-invasive modalities for localization and monitoring of the disease activity and its response to therapy (Le Bihan 2003; Filley 2001; Barker and Dunnett 1999; Waxman 1998; Axer et al. 2000).

White Matter Specialization

The human brain is composed of two hemispheres that can communicate through compact white matter bundles such as the corpus callosum (CC), anterior and posterior commisures. The brain can be divided into functionally specialized regions which can communicate through a network of white matter circuits. The subjects of functional and structural connectivity and macroscopic anatomy are still being debated by neuroscientists (Lee 2003). White matter in the human brain form bundles that facilitate between (inter) and within (intra) hemispheric communication. White matter fiber bundles in the human brain can be grouped as association, projection and commissural fibers (Filley 2001). The study of normal human white matter organization, functional specialization, plasticity and repair is an area of active research and diffusion tensor imaging is expected to be an important non-invasive complement to currently available invasive histology (Heimer and Robard 1981; Axer et al. 2000), functional or metabolic imaging tools such as positron emission tomography (PET) (Buchsbaum et al. 1998), magnetoencephalography (MEG), evoked potential, transmagneto stimulation (TMS) and functional MRI (Crick and Jones 1993; Le Bihan 2003; Filley 2001).

White Matter Complexity and the Corpus Callosum

The human CC is the largest inter-hemispheric commissural fiber network (~ 200-300 million fibers crossing a 500-700 mm^2 area; 3-5 mm thickness) (Cook 1986). The CC is involved in integrating the cortico-cortical communication (Cook 1986; Pandya and Seltzer 1986; Filley 2001; Lamantia and Rakic 1990). The functional specialization of the subdivisions of human CC has been implicated in normal aging (Sullivan et al. 2001; Peters and 2003), handedness (Witelson 1985;1989), neurodegenerative, neurodevelopmental (Barkovich and Norman 1988) and acquired pathologies (de Lacoste et al. 1985) such as closed head traumatic brain injuries (TBI) (Levin et al. 2000; Arfanakis et al. 2000a), multiple sclerosis (Barnard and Triggs 1974; Barkhoff et al. 1998; Evangelou et al. 2000a,b; Georgy et al. 1993; Dietmann et al. 1988), Alzheimer's disease (Rose et al. 2000; Teipel et al. 1999; Hampel et al. 1998; Hanyu et al. 1999; Takahashi et al. 2002), Schizophrenia (Highley et al. 1999; Foong et al. 2000), learning disorders (Giedd et al. 1994), autism (Hardan et al. 2000; Barnea-Goraly et al. 2004) and epilepsy (Arfanakis et al. 2000b; Rugg-Gunn et al. 2002; Concha et al. 2005), environmental neurotoxins such as alcoholism (Lim and Helpern 2002; Sullivan and Pffeferbaum 2003; Pffeferbaum et al. 2002) and cocaine addiction (Ojima et al. 1996; Moeller et al. 2005). There have been some reports that the size of the CC is genetically determined (Scamvougeras et al. 2003; Pfefferbaum et al. 2001), and that the size is larger in left-handed subjects compared to age-matched right-handed subjects (Witelson 1985). There is some controversy on the gender dependence of the CC cross-sectional area (Bishop and Wahlsten 1997). The CC has been subdivided based on functional specialization using different paradigms. The most common CC subdivision approach is that of Witelson's (1989) and Aboitiz's (1992) or the seven subdivisions convention (Levin et al. 2000; Giedd et al. 1994): CC1-Rostrum, CC2-Genu, CC3-Rostral Midbody, CC4-Anterior Midbody, CC5-Posterior Midbody, CC6-Isthmus, and CC7-Splenium (see Figure 2). The midbody, isthmus and splenium are associated with their respective parcellation units (sensorimotor, midtemporal, and occipital); the rostrum and genu are associated with the units comprising frontal lobe structures (Pandya and Seltzer 1986; Aboitiz et al. 1992). Aboitiz et al. (1992) also showed that the area of the corpus callosum correlated most with the number of axons in the genu (less myelinated < 3 microns) and splenium (more myelinated) and showed the least correlation in the mid-body where larger fibers and Oligodendrocytes are densely populated.

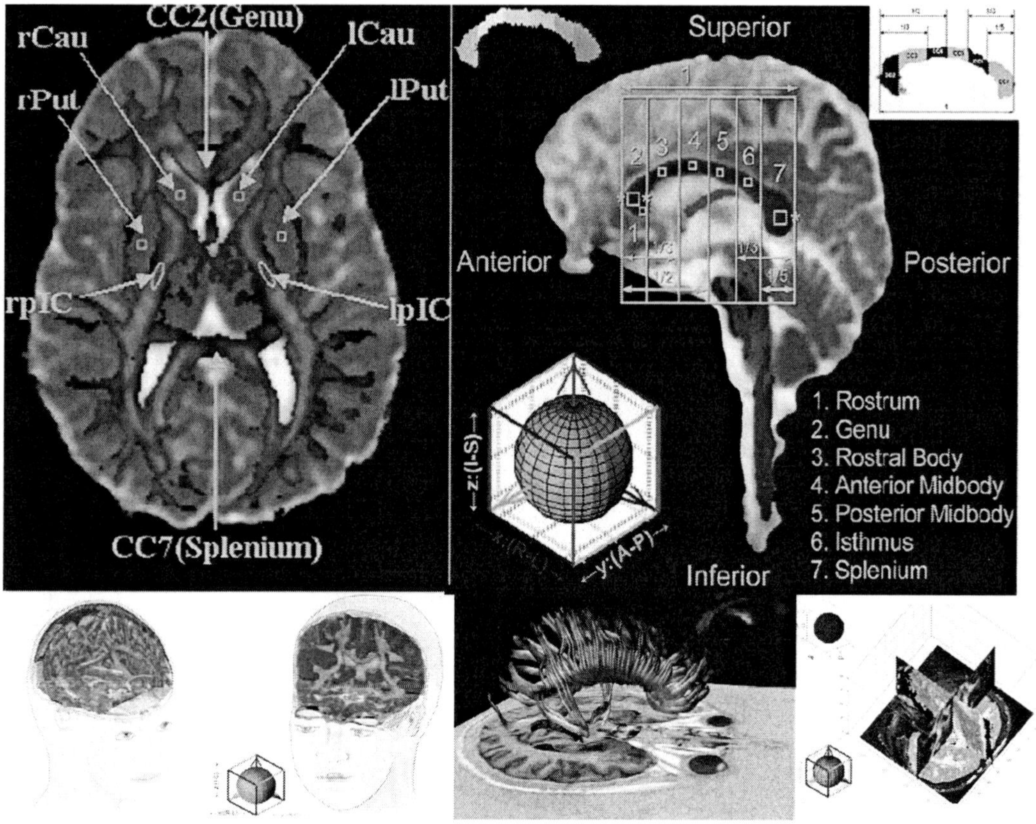

Figure 2. An illustration of the DTI utility in noninvasive digital mapping of the human brain and in quantitative region-of-interest placement in different gray matter such right and left caudate head and putamen and white matter structures such as the right and left posterior limbs of the internal capsule (plIC) and the corpus callosum. The corpus callosum is further subdivided using a DTI guided implementation of the Witelson subdivision procedure. The corpus callosum is also shown using different 3D DTI overlays and views according to the directional-contrast convention in Figure 1.

Due to its unique appearance on DTI images (Chepuri et al. 2002; Xu et al. 2002), the CC can provide an important non-invasive working model to relate the computed diffusion tensor anisotropy with the axonal geometry, distribution and myelination level (Pierpaoli et al. 1996; Beaulieu 2002; Takahashi et al. 2002; Schwartz et al. 2005). There have been different quantitative reports, sometimes conflicting, on the different subregions of the CC and the age-gender variation of this structure (compare Chepuri et al. 2002; Westerhausen et al. 2003; Abe et al. 2002; Arfanakis et al. 2002; Helenius et al. 2000; Nusbaum et al. 2001; Hasan et al. 2005). Quantification of brain atrophy and DTI metrics in the subdivisions of CC and examination of regional brain volumes of areas that project through the callosal subregions can be examined in relation to behavioral and clinical measures (Schmierer et al. 2000; Levin et al. 2000; Giedd et al. 1994). This approach should allow more precise examination of brain-behavior relations and allow characterization of damage to regional components of related neural networks. The CC is often used in MRI or histology brain studies as a marker of brain atrophy or disease activity in the normal appearing white matter (Evangelou et al. 2000). The human corpus callosum cross sectional area has been shown to scale with the forebrain volume (FBV) in an allometric relation: $FBV \sim k * CC_{area}{}^{3/2}$; this simple relation has been validated on children and adult males and females of different age groups (Jancke et al. 1997). It has also been noted that human female adult brains follow this relationship more closely than males of equal age, possibly due to less lateralization and more bilateral inter-hemispheric communication. The male adult brain lateralization may be a result of increased volume, which necessitated reduced dependency on inter-hemispheric communication and, hence, corpus callosum involvement (Zaidel et al. 2003; Bermudez and Zatorre 2001). These old but interesting neuroscience questions of gender-age-handedness-pathology relations are expected to be revisited and scrutinized with the availability of entire brain mapping using DTI. In summary, the CC has been used as a sensitive marker of normal aging and as a disease marker of a host of pathologies such as Alzheimer's disease, MS, schizophrenia, Tourette syndrome, epilepsy, traumatic brain injuries, ADHD and other conditions (Filley 2001). The CC atrophy (loss of area, thickness) can result from proximal lesions or distal cortical connectivity loss. Due to its topology and heterogeneity, the CC has been used by many researchers as a window on human brain development, neuroplasticity, pathogenesis (Zaidel et al. 2003). The CC continues to motivate many researchers (*search pubmed*). In later sections, it will be shown that understanding of the DTI results of the CC will be an important step towards understanding the role of axonal packing, morphology (caliber) and myelin on the signal sources.

Overview of DT-MRI Applications

Conventional magnetic resonance imaging (cMRI) provides several contrast mechanisms to localize and quantify *in vivo* soft and deep tissue pathology with exquisite sensitivity However, its specificity is somewhat limited especially in neurovascular and neurodegenerative diseases such as acute stroke (Le Bihan 1995; Hoehn-Berlage 1995; Sotak 2002) and multiple sclerosis (Wolinsky and Narayana 2002; Barkhoff 2002; Horsfield and Jones 2002). A number of advanced MR-based techniques have been implemented to improve the specificity of cMRI (Le Bihan 2003). Among these techniques, diffusion tensor imaging (DTI) is unique in its ability to provide information about tissue organization at the microscopic level (Le Bihan 1995; Basser 1995). DTI probes the diffusion properties (magnitude, direction and anisotropy) of water molecules in tissues (Figure 1-2) (Le Bihan 2003; Beaulieu 2002; Basser and Pierpaoli 1996; Pierpaoli et al. 1996). The diffusion magnitude and anisotropy reflect the state of the cellular membrane permeability, myelination and axonal integrity, compartmentalization, and hindrance—both intrinsic and geometric—to mobility of water molecules (Le Bihan 1995; 2003; Norris 2001; Beaulieu 2002). Diffusion anisotropy has been shown to be altered by changes in neuronal migration (Mckinstry et al. 2002; Gupta et al. 2005), cellular membrane, white cell polarization (Beppu et al. 2003), fiber straightness (Takahashi et al. 2000), axonal packing and myelination (Suzuki et al. 2003; Guo et al. 2001; Gulani et al. 2001).

Anisotropy has been shown to precede myelination in white matter (Wimberger et al. 1995; Ono et al. 1995; Klingberg et al. 1999) which has been shown to affect the anisotropy (Gulani et al. 2001; Beaulieu 2002).The DT-MRI technique is quantitative and has been compared with anatomical and histochemical findings (Hsu et al. 1998; Axer et al. 2000). The DT-MRI information is important in mapping deep white matter architecture (Mori and Van Zijl 2002; Wakana et al. 2003) and could be useful in linking the geometric contributions to tissue ionic conductance (Haueisen et al. 2002). Recently DTI has been applied to many neuroscience, neurovascular, neurooncology (Beppu et al. 2003; Field and Alexander 2004; Jellison et al. 2004; Nimsky et al. 2005), neurodevelopment, neurodegenerative, and neuropsychiatric studies to monitor white matter microstructural integrity and to provide objective surrogate markers for tissue characterization, disease activity and the efficacy of therapeutic intervention (Bammer and Fazekas 2002; Huisman et al. 2004; Table 2).

Major DTI Clinical Applications

DTI-MRI provides an orientation-based contrast mechanism for compact fibrous tissues (myelinated and unmyelinated) that is not available by conventional MRI methods which are based on spin-spin (T_2) and spin-lattice (T_1) relaxation, time-of-flight, or blood flow, intrinsic or extrinsic contrast mechanisms such as blood oxygen level or Gadolinium. For example, diffusion of water is a sensitive probe for the effect of cellular swelling, those results from the reduced perfusion of cells in the aftermath of stroke incident. Multiple sclerosis (MS) is another challenging application of diffusion imaging as eloquent MS plaques can involve edema, demyelination, active remyelination, axonal loss and reactive gliosis (proliferation of glia). DTI may add a complementary contrast mechanism in the efforts to understand the pathogenesis and design therapy for this complex disease (Trapp et al. 1998; Wolinksy and Narayana 2002; Rudick 1999; Compston 2004; Steinman et al. 2002) (see Figures 3-4). DTI provides a host of scalar and vector co-registered maps that can be used and fused with almost any modality (see Figures 5-6). The major applications of entire brain DTI(summarized in Table 2) have been in (1) understanding the normal brain organization (Makris et al. 1997; Catani 2002; 2003; Wiegell et al. 2003; Behrens et al. 2002; Lehericy et al. 2004), tissue maturation and development of WM, GM (deep and cortical) (2) clinical applications that include neurovascular, neurodegenerative, tumor dissection and surgical

Table 2. Sample publications of the major DTI applications to the human brain

Group	Specific	Sample Citations
General Review Papers	• Concepts • Clinical • Brain Development • Neuropsychiatry • Aging • Ischemic Brain Injury	• LeBihan 2003 • Maas 2003; Dong et al. 2004; Sundgren et al. 2004; Horsfield and Jones 2002 • Neil et al. 2002 • Lim et al. 2002 • Moseley et al. 2002. • Sotak et al. 2002
Normal Brain Mapping	• Fiber Tracking • Language WM Networks • CST localization • Somatosensory area and pre SMA • thalamo-cortical connections • Thalamic Nuclei • Callosal, association Networks	• Bammer et al. 2002, Mori et al. 2002, Melhem 2001, Wakana et al. 2004. • Catani et al. 2005, 2004, 2005 • Holodny et al 2005 • Lehericy et al. 2004 • Wiegell et al. 2003 • Behrens et al. 2002 • Xu et al 2002, Mori et al. 2002, Chepuri et al 2002
Cortical Maturation, Neurodevelopment normal aging and Anomalies	• Cortical Development • Child brain development • Developmental Anomalies • Aging of the Adult Brain	• Mckinstry et al 2002 • Gilmore et al. 2004, Mukherjee et al. 2001 • Schneider et al. 2004 • Lee et al. 2005 • Sullivan et al. 2003, Abe et al. 2002, Suzuki 2003
Neurodegenerative Autoimmune and Genetic Diseases	• Multiple Sclerosis • Amytrophic Lateral Sclerosis • Alzheimer's • Epilepsy • Dysmyelination • Genetic Diseases: X-linked and Krabbe disease	• Horsfield et al 2002. Werring et 1999, Filippi et al. 2001, Cecignani et al. 2003, Hasan et al. 2005 • Head 2004, Rose 2000 • Choi et al 2005 • Song et al 2001; 2002 • Guo et al 2002
Neuropsychiatric, developmental, Cognition and Acquired Diseases	• Schizophrenia • Learning Disorders: Dyslexia, ADHD, Autism • Neurotoxins • Alcoholism • Traumatic Brain Injuries • HIV-AIDS	• Foong et al. 2001, Agartz et al. 2001 • Huppi et al. 1998 • Moseley et al. 2002 • Barnea-Goraly et al. 2004. • Moeller et al. 2005 • Sullivan et al. 2002 Pfeufferbaum et al. 2001 • Huisman et al. 2004 Arfanakis et al 2002 • Pomara et al. 2001
Neurooncology	• Surgical Planning • Tumors	• Holodny et al. 2001 • Jellison et al. 2004
Medication, transplantation, recovery	• Anipsychotic Drugs • Stroke Recovery • Phenytoin and Epilepsy • Stem Cell transplantation	• Minami et al. 2003 • Yamda et al. 2004 • Lee et al. 2003 • Guo et al. 2002

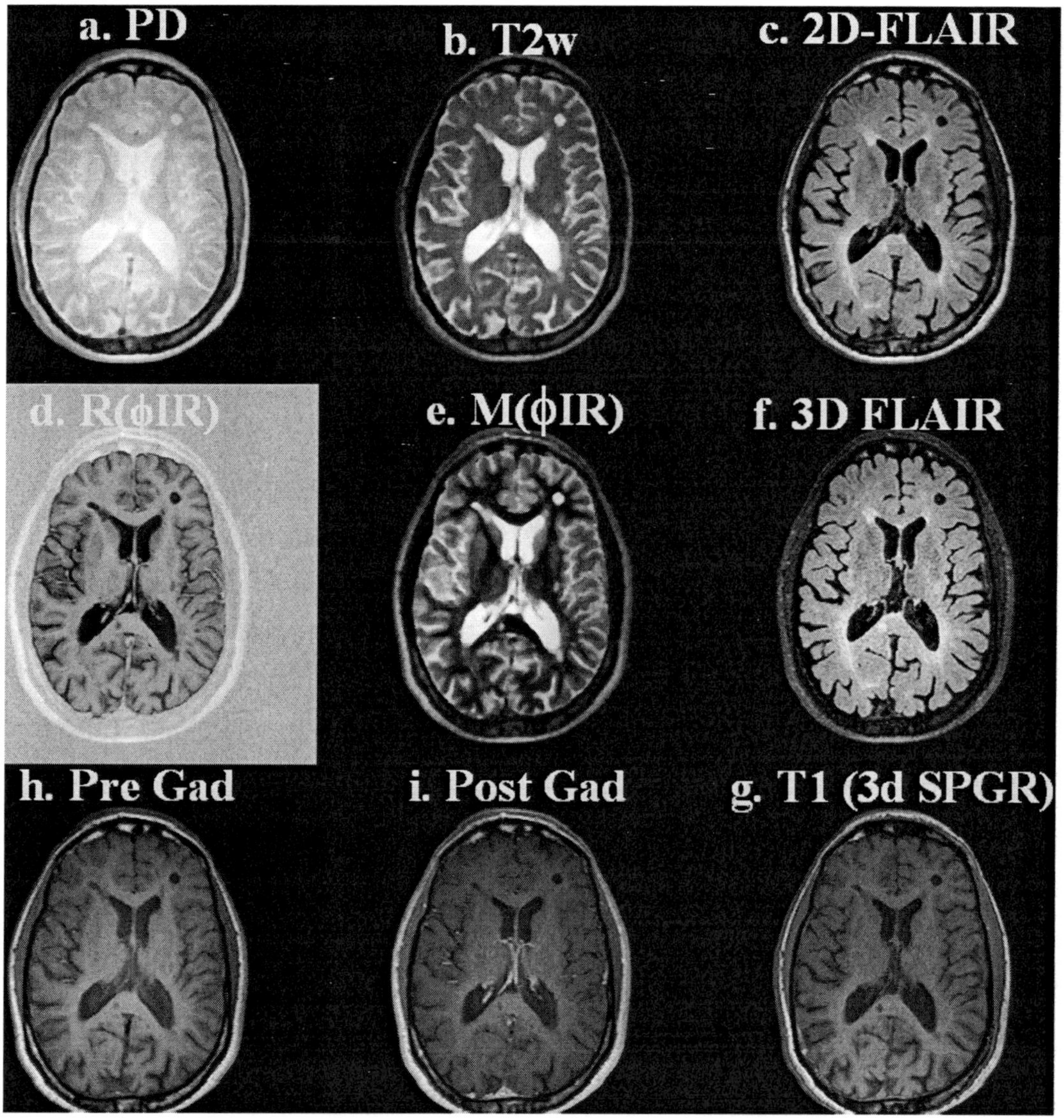

Figure 3. Illustration of a host of conventional MRI modalities that are being used to localize and quantify the MS lesions in on-ongoing multi-center clinical trials in search of MRI disease surrogates in the study of the pathogenesis and therapy of MS (a) PD map (b) T2w (c) 2d-FLAIR (d) the real and (e) magnitude components from a phase sensitive IR acquisition (f) 3d-FLAIR (h) Pre, (i) Post Gadolinium maps and (g) a 3d spoiled gradient acquisition. Notice the sensitivity, contrast appearance of white, gray matter, lesions, edema, and cerebrospinal fluid on these maps.

planning (Field and Alexander 2005; Nimsky et al. 2005), neurooncology (Wieshmann et al. 2000; Holodny et al. 2001) and neuropsychiatry (Lim and Helpern 2002; Hoptman et al. 2002; Moeller et al. 2005). Detailed reviews of many of these applications are beyond the scope of this chapter but some of the most important advances are summarized (Table 2). One of the major and potential applications of DTI on the human brain in modern medicine involves its ability to non-invasively monitor therapy (surgical planning, transplantation,

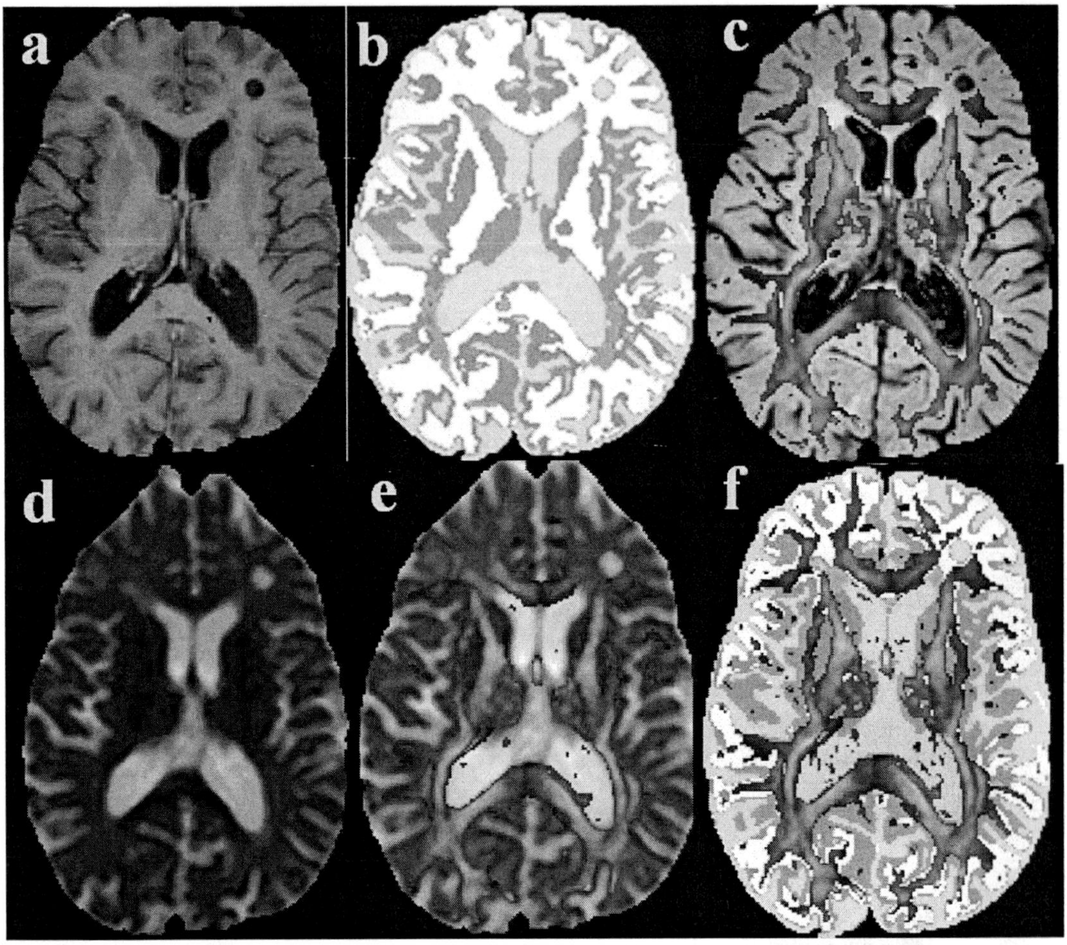

Figure 4. Illustration of data fusion of cMRI and DTI at 3.0 T. DTI matched with conventional MRI (same patient as in Fig. 10) provides fiber connectivity of the FLAIR highlighted lesions. (a) RGB fusion (FLAIR, phase sensitive inversion recovery ps-T1IR, post Gadolinium) (b) cMRI tissue segmentation (PD,T2w, FLAIR) (c) $|FA*e_1|$ over FLAIR (d) RGB (DTI Eigenvalue Map) (e) $|FA*e_1|$ over mean diffusivity D_{av} (f) $|\mathbf{FA*e_1}|$ segmented map in b. Notice the loss of connectivity in the vicinity of the frontal lesion and the sustained tractability of the posterior callosal areas indicating possibly lesion activity, severity and duration

rehabilitation) and provide surrogate markers to disease activity, therapy and recovery (Werring et al. 1998; Guo et al. 2001; Field and Alexander 2004; Alexopoulos et al. 2002; Huisman et al. 2004; Rugg-Gunn 2001; 2002; Munoz et al. 2004). For example, Guo et al. (2001) have presented an important application of DTI anisotropy measures in monitoring white matter progenitor stem cell transplantation efficacy in eight children with a genetic deficit of myelin basic protein (Krabbe disease). Minami et al. (2003) have shown that DTI can be useful in monitoring the effect of antipsychotics on white matter microstructure in Schizophrenia (Buchsbaum et al. 1998; Agartz et al. 2001; Ardekani et al. 2003). Moeller et al. (2005) have used DTI and behavioral data to detect subtle changes in the frontal lobe white matter organization due to addictive neurotoxins such as cocaine. In animal models of demyelination, dysmyelination of optic nerve and acquired spinal spinal cord injury, Nevo

(2001), Song et al. (2001), Gulani et al. (2001) and Schwartz et al. (2005) have shown that DTI-and-DWI metrics (eigenvalues and anisotropy) be able to provide sensitive markers of myelination, axonal integrity and induced repair and functional recovery. DTI measures of white matter integrity have also been shown to correlate with learning disability (Klingberg et al. 1999; Huppi et al. 1998), cognitive scores in preterms (Nagy et al. 2003), normal cortical maturation in extremely premature infants (Mckinstry et al. 2002; Maas et al. 2004; Gupta et al. 2005), development, and normal aging (Moseley et al. 2002; Mukherjee et al. 2001; Abe et al. 2002). The alteration of WM anisotropy with conditions such as focal epilepsy (Arfanakis et al. 2002a), HIV-AIDS (Pomara et al. 2001), Alzheimer's disease (Bozzali et al. 2003; Takahashi et al. 2002; Choi et al. 2005), alcoholism, traumatic brain injuries, multiple sclerosis (Werring et al. 1999; Filippi et al. 2001), autism, and attention deficit disorders (Ashtari et al. 2005) have also been correlated with clinical (extended disability, mini mental status) and psychometric batteries (Table 2) that quantify attention, memory, visual-spatial processing, aggression (Hoptman et al. 2002) or impulsivity (Moeller et al. 2005).

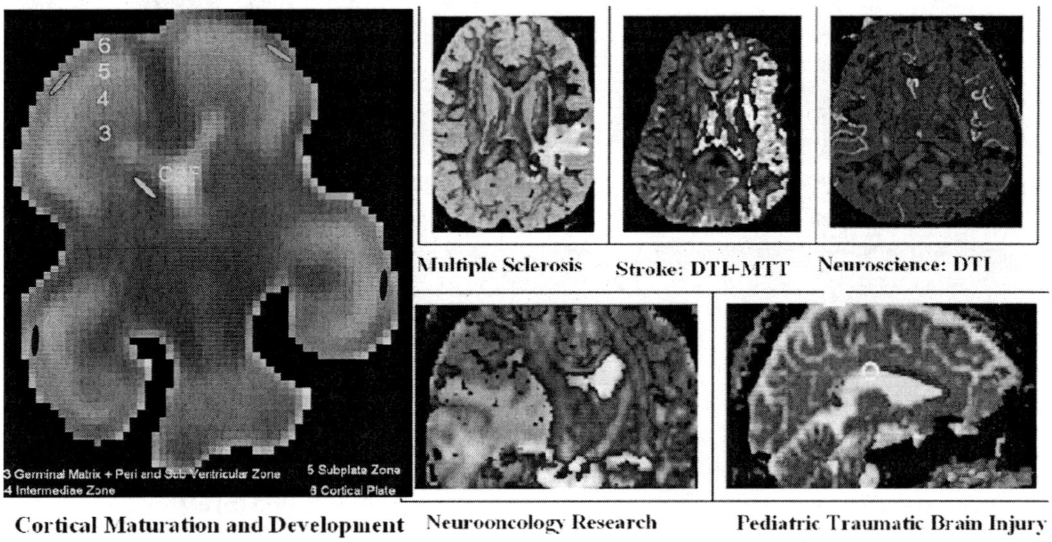

Figure 5. Illustration of different applications of DTI and the ability to fuse DTI orientation maps maps with different DTI scalar maps or information obtained from other modalities (from left-to-right). A fused eigenvalue map demonstrating the ability of DTI to identify cortical regions from a human fetus at 21 weeks post gestation. The application DTI maps fused with FLAIR in MS research, the fusion of DTI orientation maps with mean transit time obtained using blood perfusion on stroke patients. The ability to fuse DTI with high resolution MRI-angiography maximum intensity projection and the utility in tumor and traumatic brain injury research respectively.

It is important to mention that many of the published reports have used different technical acquisition and processing paradigms (slice thickness, region-of-interest placement, encoding scheme, and total scan time) and may have used few samples. Population demographic confounders such as gender, age, and handedness have not been thoroughly examined even on healthy controls. Contradictory quantitative DTI reports are not uncommon as this is a new and rapidly expanding modality, even on simple but compact white matter structures such as the corpus callosum (see Hasan et al. 2005 for a recent review) and posterior limb of the internal capsule.

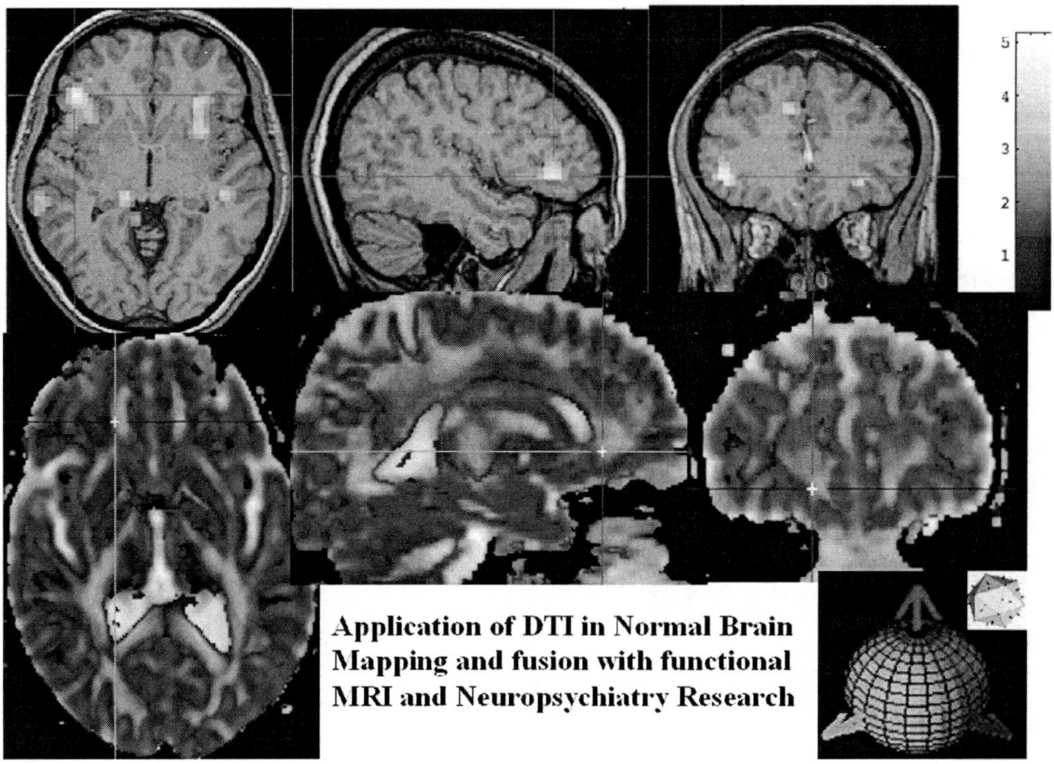

Figure 6. An illustration of the utility and potential of structural DTI fusion with functional MRI. The figure shows a functional MRI activation map overlayed on an anatomical same-subject data set. The DTI multi views provide a 3D structural connectivity template for the gray matter regions that are activated in the fMRI experiment.

Theory: Mathematical and Physical Foundations of DTI

Fundamental Principles behind Diffusion Tensor Imaging

Diffusion MRI is based on the observation that water molecular motion is not the same in all directions. Molecules diffusing along the axons of compact bundles or between the axonal spaces find minimal obstacles compared to motion perpendicular to the axons. Thus, the medium is referred to be anisotropic. The magnitude and orientation information obtained from DTI is represented for each volume element in the field-of-view geometrically by an ellipsoid with three eigenvalues and three orthogonal eigenvectors (Figure 7).

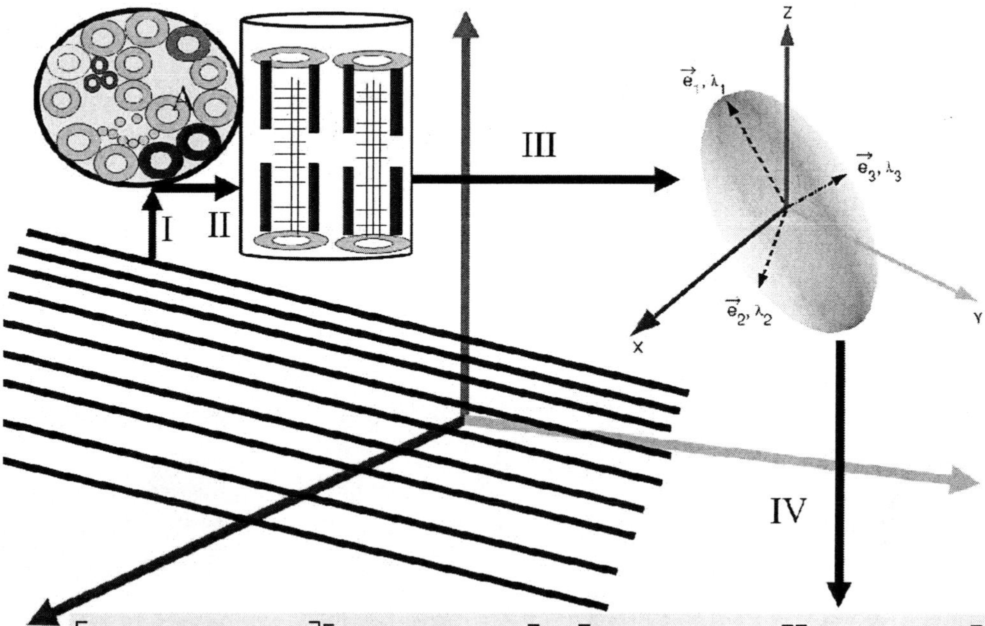

$$\begin{bmatrix} D_{xx} & D_{xy} & D_{xz} \\ D_{xy} & D_{yy} & D_{yz} \\ D_{xz} & D_{yz} & D_{zz} \end{bmatrix} \begin{bmatrix} e_{1x} & e_{2x} & e_{3x} \\ e_{1y} & e_{2y} & e_{3y} \\ e_{1z} & e_{2z} & e_{3z} \end{bmatrix} = \begin{bmatrix} e_{1x} & e_{2x} & e_{3x} \\ e_{1y} & e_{2y} & e_{3y} \\ e_{1z} & e_{2z} & e_{3z} \end{bmatrix} \begin{bmatrix} \lambda_1 & 0 & 0 \\ 0 & \lambda_2 & 0 \\ 0 & 0 & \lambda_3 \end{bmatrix}$$

Figure 7. Illustration of the different water compartments and contributors to the water diffusion signal attenuation from compact fiber bundles. A fiber bundle is viewed as a stack of myelinated cylinders and water can diffuse between the myelin sheaths, inter (between) or intra (within) axons. The axons are viewed as thin cylindrical filaments with myelin and internal cytoskeletal structure. The local diffusion tensor (**D**) is represented as an ellipsoid with three eigenvalues and three eigenvectors. Note that the positive definite and symmetric diffusion tensor can be diagonalized (*DE*=*ΛE*) into three eigenvalues and three eigenvectors (**D**e_i=$\lambda_i e_i$).

The Concept and Mathematical Construction of a Tensor

A Cartesian tensor of rank n has 3^n independent quantities, thus a scalar is a tensor of rank 0, a vector is tensor of rank 1 and a second rank tensor has 9 independent elements which can be represented by a 3x3 matrix (Figure 7). A medium with second rank tensorial physical properties such as thermal expansivity, electrical and thermal conductivity, diffusion, refractive index, etc. implies that vectorial input (cause) and output (effect) may not be directionally commensurate. In general, the medium atomic makeup, interactions and geometric configuration will result in direction-dependent response to the input; hence, the medium is said to have anisotropic properties (Lovet 1989; Nye 1957). An important fundamental requirement of physical laws is the equivalence principle which states that the mathematical form of physical laws should be invariant under coordinate system rotations. For example, Ohm's law relates the cause (electric field E vector) and the effect (electric flux J vector) in an electrical medium with conductivity tensor (σ) and can be written in one coordinate system as $\vec{J} = \sigma\vec{E}$. If the coordinate system is subjected to an orthogonal rotation carried out by a rotation matrix R ($R^{-1}=R^t$, where -1 and t are the matrix inverse and transpose operators respectively), the vectorial quantities such as E and J are expected to be rotated according to: $E_R= R^t E$ and $J_R=R J$. Since, in this case, Ohm's law is required to be form-independent in the rotated frame of reference, we must have:

$$\vec{J}_R = \sigma_R \vec{E}_R = \sigma_R R\vec{E} = R\vec{J} = R\sigma\vec{E} \qquad [1a]$$

which implies that in the rotated frame of reference, the tensor is transformed as:

$$\sigma_R = R\sigma R^t \qquad [1b]$$

This equation implies that the tensor components in the original system are transformed differently from the measured vectorial quantities which transform as simple rotations (i.e. $\boldsymbol{E_R= R^t E}$ and $\boldsymbol{J_R =R J}$). Notice that a special rotation matrix can always be found in which the original tensor is represented as a diagonal matrix. This procedure is called tensor diagonalization which decomposes the tensor into a set of local orthonormal eigenvectors each associated with an eigenvalue.

Transport Translational Diffusion

In an isotropic dilute medium or solution in which the solute molecules can diffuse freely in the solvent in all directions with a translational diffusion coefficient $\boldsymbol{D_{zz}}$, the root mean squared distance traveled over a diffusion time τ and N random and uncorrelated steps, each with a duration δt and random increment δz, is given by the Einstein-Stokes equation (Einstein 1956):

$$Z_{rms} = \sqrt{\langle (z - z_0)^2 \rangle} = \sqrt{\sum_{n=1}^{N} \left(z(n) - z(0)\right)^2} = \sqrt{N[\delta z]^2} = \sqrt{2D_{zz}\tau} \qquad [2]$$

For an assembly of many particles, this quantity can also be interpreted as the standard deviation of a Gaussian distribution with probability of finding a particle between z and $z+dz$:

$$P(z)dz = \frac{1}{(4\pi D_{zz}T)^{\frac{1}{2}}} \exp(-\frac{z^2}{4D_{zz}\tau}) \qquad [3]$$

Notice that the diffusivity (D_{zz}) has units of flux (area per unit time) or equally the velocity autocorrelation integral over time (Berg 1993; Callaghan 1994).

$$D_{zz} \propto \int_0^\infty \langle \vec{v}(0) \bullet \vec{v}(t) \rangle dt = \frac{Z_{rms}{}^2}{2\tau} \qquad [4a]$$

The absence of dependence on the original location and the peculiar dependence of the root mean squared distance, Z_{rms} , on the diffusion time is a characteristic of random Brownian translational motion and the random molecular interactions that each molecule encounters (Einstein 1956). From kinetic transport theory, the diffusion coefficient is expected to increase with the steady state medium temperature (T), decrease with the solution viscosity η and hydrodynamic radius (a_h) according to the Einstein-Smoluchowski relation (Berg 1993):

$$D_{zz} \propto \frac{T}{\eta a_h} \qquad [4b]$$

The factors in the denominator of this equation represent the physical and geometric variables (resistive frictional force) that reduce the effective distance through interactions and bindings with barriers and obstacles. This type of diffusion can be generalized in a medium in which the diffusion is no longer the same in all directions. This transport diffusion results in a net migration of molecules along the concentration gradient given by Fick's first law:

$$\vec{J} = -D\vec{\nabla}c \qquad [5a]$$

The diffusion process is governed by Fick's second law, which is analogous to the conservation of mass:

$$\frac{\partial c}{\partial t} + \vec{\nabla} \bullet \vec{J} = 0 \qquad [5b]$$

Combining the last two equations provides the random diffusion partial differential equation or:

$$\frac{\partial c}{\partial t} = \vec{\nabla} \bullet (D\vec{\nabla}c) \qquad [5c]$$

which can be solved along with initial and boundary conditions both numerically and analytically (Berg 1993; Crank 2002).

MRI Measurement of Diffusion

The water molecules are used as the probe to the tissue microstructural organization. The dependence of diffusion on time and space are crucial for estimating or encoding the diffusivity using MRI phase based spin-tagging methods. By furnishing space-dependent diffusion encoding and symmetric magnetic pulses, through a uniform diffusion gradient, G_d, (Callaghan 1994; Hinshaw and Lent 1983; see Figure 8)

$$\vec{B}(r,t) = (B_{z0} + (\vec{G}_d(t) \bullet \vec{r}))\hat{z}, \qquad [6a]$$

the resonant frequency of a diffusing spin becomes space-dependent according to the Larmor's golden equation of MRI

$$\vec{\omega}(r,t) = \gamma\vec{B}(r,t) \qquad [6b]$$

(where B_{z0} and γ are the main magnetic field and spin gyromagnetic ratio respectively).

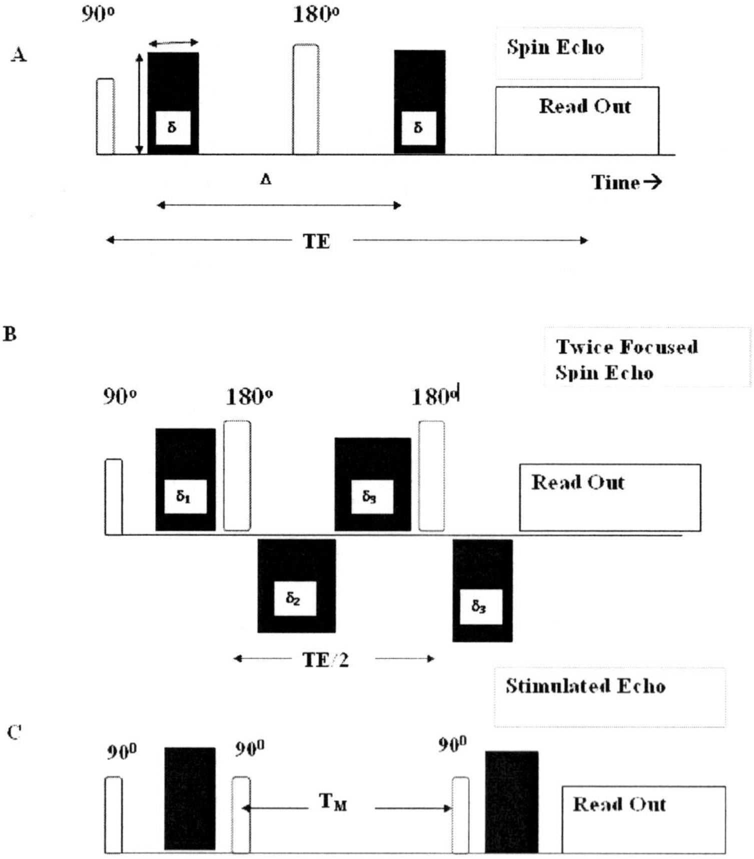

Figure 8. A schematic of the different diffusion sensitization sequences used to encode local random diffusion. (A) The spin-echo, (B) twice-focused and (C) stimulated echo prepared sequences used for DTI and the parameters involved. The conventional spin-echo sequence in A uses a Stejskal-Tanner bipolar magnetic gradient diffusion pulses of equal area and known separation, order, number and orientation sandwiched around the 180° focusing pulse

The accumulated net phase over the diffusion time becomes location-geometry-dependent

$$\delta\phi(\vec{r},\tau) = \int \delta\omega dt = \int \gamma\left(\vec{G}_d(t) \bullet \vec{r}\right)dt \qquad [6c]$$

The MRI coil receives a superposition of random phases from all sensitized molecular spins and, hence, the measured additional signal attenuation is attributable to irreversible translational diffusion (Hinshaw and Lint 1983; Callaghan 1994; Price 1997; 1998; Karger et al. 1989).

$$\left\langle \exp\left(i\delta\phi\right)\right\rangle = \int_{-\infty}^{\infty} P(\delta\phi)\exp(i\delta\phi)d\delta\phi = \exp(-\frac{\phi_{rms}{}^{2}}{2}) = \exp(-bD_{zz}) \qquad [6d]$$

Thus, MRI hardware and software designers control the image diffusion pulse parameters and the measured attenuated signal is decoded to infer the translational diffusivity (Taylor and Bushel 1985; Stejskal and Tanner 1965; Torrey 1956; Callaghan 1994; 1996; LeBihan 1995). Notice that water translational diffusion also sets the ultimate spatial resolution measured by water magnetic resonance (Ahn and Cho 1985). Random translational diffusion has been always described as a nuisance to high resolution magnetic resonance and parasitic phenomenon (Hahn 1950) that motivated the development of specialized sequences to reduce its effect (Carr and Purcell 1954; Callaghan et al. 1994; Price 1997; 1998; Karger et al. 1988). The Stejskal-Tanner introduction of the magnetic pulse sandwich in the Hahn spin-echo sequence (Hahn 1950) is the most widely used approach to quantify and measure diffusion. Variants of this approach (Figure 8) seek to reduce diffusion-external gradient couplings or minimize eddy current generation due to fast switching of large gradients (Stejskal and Tanner 1965; Le Bihan 1995). Notice that relaxation mechanisms and flow have different signal signatures than translational random diffusion and the latter can be modulated and quantified if a separate reference map is acquired. The rotational random diffusion, which is incorporated in the spin-spin (T_2) and spin-lattice relaxation (T_1), will also modulate the measured signal in a predictable manner. The diffusion pulses also encode coherent flow, but, since the latter results in a net phase modulation, the diffusion signal magnitude decouples linear phase fluctuations. Diffusion estimation and quantification artifacts due to mismatches in pulse duration, areas, and spatial uniformity calibration are usually minimized by MRI clinical scanner design specifications. Since DWI uses large duty cycle diffusion gradients for encoding, the main challenges to diffusion encoded imaging are parasitic eddy currents and motion artifacts (Price 1997; 1998; Jones and Basser 2002; Alexander et al. 1996). A detailed discussion of these issues and specialized methods for minimizing DTI artifacts is beyond the scope of this chapter, but reviews are available elsewhere (See Table 1; Callaghan 1994; Price 1997; 1998; Basser and Jones 2002).

Water Apparent Self-Diffusion Tensor in Soft Brain Tissue

In a solvent medium like water, random translation of the solvent molecules in the same solvent medium is referred to as self-diffusion and is governed by analogous laws, but results in no net transport. For example, at a temperature of 37^0 C, in a large spherical container at steady state, water molecules diffuse the same distance in all directions (isotropic diffusion) and cover at the rate $D_{xx}=D_{yy}=D_{zz} \sim 3.2 \times 10^{-3}$ mm^2 sec^{-1} (Le Bihan 1995) and will be able to traverse in $\tau=30$ ms a root-mean-squared distance of 15 μm. In soft brain tissue, the presence of cellular membranes, organized and packed myelinated axons provide directional hindrance; hence, the diffusion distance is expected to be dependent on the organization of the tissue and diffusion is referred to as anisotropic over the measurement time (Beaulieu 2002). A complete interpretation of the true contributors to diffusion anisotropy in living tissues turns out to be a challenging endeavor, but here it is assumed that translational diffusion can be used as a probe of the tissue microstructural organization (Beaulieu 2002; Table 1). The computed diffusivity of water in tissue at body temperature is about 1/3 that of free water, and hence the distance traversed over a 30 ms diffusion time span will be about 10 μm. This distance is important in designing experimental paradigms to sample the geometric barriers encountered by water molecules in different tissue compartments (Le Bihan 2003). This distance scale is also an important reminder that translational diffusion will set the ultimate spatial resolution for imaging water using "fundamentally phase sensitive" magnetic resonance principles. Early papers and workers in magnetic resonance have recognized the parasitic nature of diffusion (Hahn 1950; Carr and Purcell 1954; Torrey 1956; Le Bihan 1995; Callaghan 1994; Price 1997; 1998). In modern industrial and clinical applications, translational random diffusion is used as a contrast mechanism that is quantified and controlled by encoding via magnetic pulse pairs of controlled duration, orientation, strength and separation (Callaghan 1996; 1994; Stejskal and Tanner 1965). Since our measurement is an ensemble average over a large number of randomly diffusing molecules that attained an irreversible random phase, the estimated local diffusivity along all directions in space has been named the bulk or apparent self-diffusion tensor, D, which is a second rank positive definite tensor that can be represented by a 3x3 matrix for each volume element (Le Bihan 1995; Basser 1994; Basser and Jones 2002).

Diffusion Tensor Properties

The diffusion tensor for each voxel can be represented by the 3x3 matrix (Figure 7):

$$D = \begin{bmatrix} D_{xx} & D_{xy} & D_{xz} \\ D_{yx} & D_{yy} & D_{yz} \\ D_{zx} & D_{zy} & D_{zz} \end{bmatrix} \qquad [7]$$

The tensor is required to be symmetric or $\boldsymbol{D^t=D}$, $(\boldsymbol{D_{ij}=D_{ji}}$, i, j=1, 2, and 3). The symmetry results from a fundamental physical requirement of time-irreversibility and the universal third law of thermodynamics on entropy increase. Thus, the matrix has six unique elements (three diagonal and three off diagonal). Once computed for each voxel, the diffusion tensor can be diagonalized into three eigenvalues (λ_1, λ_2, and λ_3) and an orthonormal eigenvector set (e_1, e_2 and e_3: $e_k = \delta_{ijk}\ e_i\ x\ e_j$; $\boldsymbol{E} = [e_1\ e_2\ e_3]$). The characteristic equation can be represented as $DE = E\Lambda$ where $D = \sum_{i=1}^{3} \lambda_i \hat{e}_i{}^t \hat{e}_i$ or in matrix form (Figure 7):

$$\begin{bmatrix} D_{xx} & D_{xy} & D_{xz} \\ D_{xy} & D_{yy} & D_{yz} \\ D_{xx} & D_{yz} & D_{zz} \end{bmatrix} \begin{bmatrix} e_{1x} & e_{2x} & e_{3x} \\ e_{1y} & e_{2y} & e_{3y} \\ e_{1z} & e_{2z} & e_{3z} \end{bmatrix} = \begin{bmatrix} e_{1x} & e_{2x} & e_{3x} \\ e_{1y} & e_{2y} & e_{3y} \\ e_{1z} & e_{2z} & e_{3z} \end{bmatrix} \begin{bmatrix} \lambda_1 & 0 & 0 \\ 0 & \lambda_2 & 0 \\ 0 & 0 & \lambda_3 \end{bmatrix} \qquad [8]$$

Tensor diagonalization is an important procedure to enable representation of the tensor in the local coordinate tissue system and the quantification of tensor anisotropy in rotationally independent anisotropy indices.

Tensor Rotational Invariants and Anisotropy Indices

An n by n square matrix has n rotational scalar invariants subject to arbitrary rotations. Thus, a 3x3 second rank tensor has 3 invariants which are first, second, and third order polynomials in the eigenvalues or the corresponding tensor elements. Using the important matrix cyclic multiplication property $A{*}BC=C{*}AB$ and the fact that the rotated tensor transforms *as* $(\boldsymbol{D_R}=\boldsymbol{R}\ \boldsymbol{D}\ \boldsymbol{R^t})$ where ($R^t{*}R = U_{3x3}$ unity or identity matrix), the following tensor invariants can be defined. The Cartesian diffusion tensor $\boldsymbol{D}$ has three principal invariants $\{I_1, I_2, I_3\}$ which are related to the eigenvalues, $\{\lambda_1, \lambda_2, \lambda_3\}$ and defined by the characteristic equation (Basser 1995; Borisinko and Tarapov 1968; Hasan et al. 2001b):

$$\det(D - \Lambda U_{3x3}) = (\lambda - \lambda_1)(\lambda - \lambda_2)(\lambda - \lambda_3) = \lambda^3 - \lambda^2 I_1 + \lambda I_2 - I_3 = 0 \qquad [9]$$

where U_{3x3} is the 3x3 identity matrix. The first invariant is the square matrix trace (Tr) or

$$I_1 = Tr(D_R) = Tr(RDR^t) = Tr(RR_t D) = D_{xx} + D_{yy} + D_{zz} \qquad [10a]$$

In terms of the eigenvalues and eigenvectors, $D = E \Lambda E^{-1}$, thus

$$I_1 = Tr(D) = Tr(E\Lambda E^{-1}) = Tr(E^{-1}E\Lambda) = Tr(\Lambda) = \lambda_1 + \lambda_2 + \lambda_3 \qquad [10b]$$

The mean diffusivity is defined as $MD = D_{av} = \mu(D) = \frac{I_1}{3}$. The second and third tensor rotationally invariants can be related to the determinant and trace of the inverse of the tensor:

$$I_2 = (D_{xx}D_{yy} + D_{xx}D_{zz} + D_{yy}D_{zz}) - (D_{xy}{}^2 + D_{xz}{}^2 + D_{yz}{}^2) = \lambda_1\lambda_2 + \lambda_2\lambda_3 + \lambda_1\lambda_3$$

[11]

$$I_3 = \det(D_R) = \det(RDR') = \det(R'RD) = der(E\Lambda E^{-1}) = \det(E^{-1}E\Lambda) = \det(\Lambda) = \lambda_1\lambda_2\lambda_3$$

[12a]

which can also be written in terms of the diffusivities as:

$$I_3=\det(\mathbf{D})=(D_{xx}D_{yy}D_{zz}+D_{xy}D_{xz}D_{yz}) - (D_{zz}D_{xy}{}^2+D_{yy}D_{xz}{}^2+D_{xx}D_{yz}{}^2) = \lambda_1\lambda_2\lambda_3$$ [12b]

Note that the inverse of a matrix or $\boldsymbol{D}^{-1}$ has the same eigenvectors as the matrix $\boldsymbol{D}$ with inverted eigenvalues; this property can be demonstrated since $D = E\Lambda E^{-1}$ and its inverse is given by $D^{-1} = E^{-1}\Lambda^{-1}E$ which can be used to show that $I_2 = \det(D) * Tr(D^{-1})$. Other dependent invariants can be formed from the three principal invariants $\{I_1, I_2, I_3\}$; for example, the Frobenius norm or

$$I_4 = Tr(D^2) = I_1{}^2 - 2I_2 = \|D\|^2.$$ [12c]

Diffusion Tensor Anisotropy Measures in terms of the Principal Invariants

Anisotropy measures are normalized (minimum=0, isotropic to maximum=1 (anisotropic)) scale and order-independent functions of the eigenvalues, invariants or the diffusivities. The major normalized anisotropy indices (AI) (relative anisotropy, RA, fractional, FA, and volume fraction anisotropy, VF) are defined below (Hasan 2000).

$$RA(D) \propto \frac{\sigma(D)}{\mu(D)} = \sqrt{\frac{1}{2}}\frac{\sqrt{(\lambda_1-\lambda_2)^2+(\lambda_2-\lambda_3)^2+(\lambda_1-\lambda_3)^2}}{(\lambda_1+\lambda_2+\lambda_3)} = \sqrt{1-3\frac{I_2}{I_1^2}}$$

[13a]

$$FA \propto \frac{\sigma(D)}{\|D\|} = \sqrt{\frac{1}{2}}\frac{\sqrt{(\lambda_1-\lambda_2)^2+(\lambda_2-\lambda_3)^2+(\lambda_1-\lambda_3)^2}}{\sqrt{(\lambda_1{}^2+\lambda_2{}^2+\lambda_3{}^2)}} = \sqrt{1-3\frac{I_2}{I_4}}$$

[13b]

$$VF = 1 - \frac{\det(D)}{\mu(D)} = 1 - 27\frac{\lambda_1\lambda_2\lambda_3}{(\lambda_1 + \lambda_2 + \lambda_3)^3} = 1 - 27\frac{I_3}{I_1^{\ 3}}$$

[13c]

Note that these anisotropy indices are scale-independent with respect to scalar multiplication of the eigenvalues with an arbitrary constant (i.e. $AI(c\lambda_1, c\lambda_2, c\lambda_3) = AI(\lambda_1, \lambda_2, \lambda_3)$). Scale-independence is an important property to predict the anisotropy as physical variables such as temperature may vary. Since the diffusion distance increases with temperature as the probability of random collision increases with an increased thermal agitation, thus, in the steady state, if the medium diffusivities change with temperature at the same rate, it is expected that tensor anisotropy will be temperature independent. This important property of anisotropy indices may also hold when performing high resolution experiments on excised but fresh tissue (Lin et al. 2003; Schwartz et al. 2005). These anisotropy measures are the most commonly used in DTI literature and are defined here to be normalized. The indices attain a value of one for the extreme cylindrical anisotropic tensor case $(\lambda_1 >> \lambda_2 \cong \lambda_3)$ and zero for the spherical or isotropic tensor case $(\lambda_1 \cong \lambda_2 \cong \lambda_3)$. Simple arbitrary and normalized anisotropy measures such as eccentricity $e = \sqrt{1 - \frac{\lambda_3}{\lambda_1}}$ are discouraged, although scale-independent, due to extreme sensitivity to acquisition noise. Notice that due to acquisition thermal noise, the total axial (*FA=1*) and spherical tensor (*FA=0*) situations are never encountered but offer a framework for simulating the effect of measurement noise on both scalar and vector attributes of the tensor. As detailed in later sections, the working signal-to-noise ratio (SNR) should be selected so that measurement noise will not produce negative eigenvalues or extreme biases. In general, perturbation theory can be used to predict the bias introduced in the eigenvector-eigenvalue estimation due to noise. Noise will roughen the ideal spherical tensor case (*FA=0*) and will result in non-zero but finite residual anisotropy ($FA_{est} \geq 0$) due to "eigenvalue repulsion" even for pure water samples in large spherical containers acquired at high SNR. In the extreme anisotropy case (*FA=1*), measurement noise will increase the value of the estimated smallest eigenvalue which will reduce the estimated anisotropy ($FA_{est}<1$). These simple extreme cases indicate an interesting property of DTI which is commonly encountered in the science of inverse problems. Since the tensors and, hence, their anisotropy values are unknown, the estimation bias seemingly depends on the estimated tensor. This important topic will be explored in later sections of this chapter which will introduce the important topic of tensor estimation. Moreover, the normalized RA and FA anisotropy measures have been shown recently to be related by a closed form algebraic relationship (Hasan et al. 2004)

$$FA = \sqrt{\frac{3}{2 + RA^{-2}}} \Leftrightarrow RA = \frac{FA}{\sqrt{3 - 2FA^2}}$$

$$\sigma_{FA} = \frac{1}{3}(\frac{FA}{RA})^3 \sigma_{RA} \Leftrightarrow \frac{FA}{\sigma_{FA}} = (1 + 2RA^2)\frac{RA}{\sigma_{RA}} \quad [14]$$

These simple but important relations and their error propagation can be used to relate and unify a veritable plethora of published quantitative DTI reports that used RA or FA. Hasan et al. (2004) have also demonstrated that FA has better noise immunity properties than RA, confirming empirical observations by many groups (see Hasan et al. 2004).

Analytical Diagonalization of the Tensor Using the Invariants

There are at least three general methods for diffusion tensor diagonalization: Jacobi-QL, singular value decomposition and the analytical approach. Hasan et al. (2001) have validated an algebraic algorithm (dating back to the 14th century) to compute the eigenvectors, and eigenvalues directly from tensor elements without iteration. The method which is detailed elsewhere introduces invariant functions such as: $v = \left(\frac{I_1}{3}\right)^2 - \frac{I_2}{3}$, $s = \left(\frac{I_1}{3}\right) - \frac{I_1 I_2}{6} + \frac{I_3}{2}$, and $\phi = \arccos(\frac{s}{v^{3/2}})$. The tensor eigenvalues arc simply given by the equation (Hasan et al. 2001b):

$$\begin{bmatrix} \lambda_1 \\ \lambda_2 \\ \lambda_3 \end{bmatrix} = \frac{I_1}{3}\left[1 + 2.0 * RA \begin{bmatrix} \cos(\phi) \\ -\cos(\frac{\pi}{3} + \phi) \\ -\cos(\frac{\pi}{3} - \phi) \end{bmatrix}\right] \quad [15]$$

This simple relationship can be used to relate additional commonly used normalized, scale-independent and rotationally-invariant anisotropy measures such as cylindrical (A_{cyl}~1), linear (CL) and planar (CP) anisotropy indices (Westin et al. 2002; Hasan et al. 2001b).

$$\begin{bmatrix} A_{cyl} \\ CL \\ CP \end{bmatrix} = \frac{1}{I_1} * \begin{bmatrix} \lambda_1 - \dfrac{\lambda_2 + \lambda_3}{2} \\ \dfrac{\lambda_1 - \lambda_2}{2} \\ 2*(\lambda_2 - \lambda_3) \end{bmatrix} = RA * \begin{bmatrix} \cos(\phi) \\ \sin(\dfrac{\pi}{3} - \phi) \\ \dfrac{\sin(\phi)}{\sin(\dfrac{\pi}{3})} \end{bmatrix} \qquad [16]$$

A geometric and unified interpretation of anisotropy measures in terms of the trilinear coordinate system was presented in addition to a detailed analytical computation of the three orthonormal eigenvectors (Hasan et al. 2001b). As an illustration and summary of the different DTI-metrics presented in this section is provided in Figure 9.

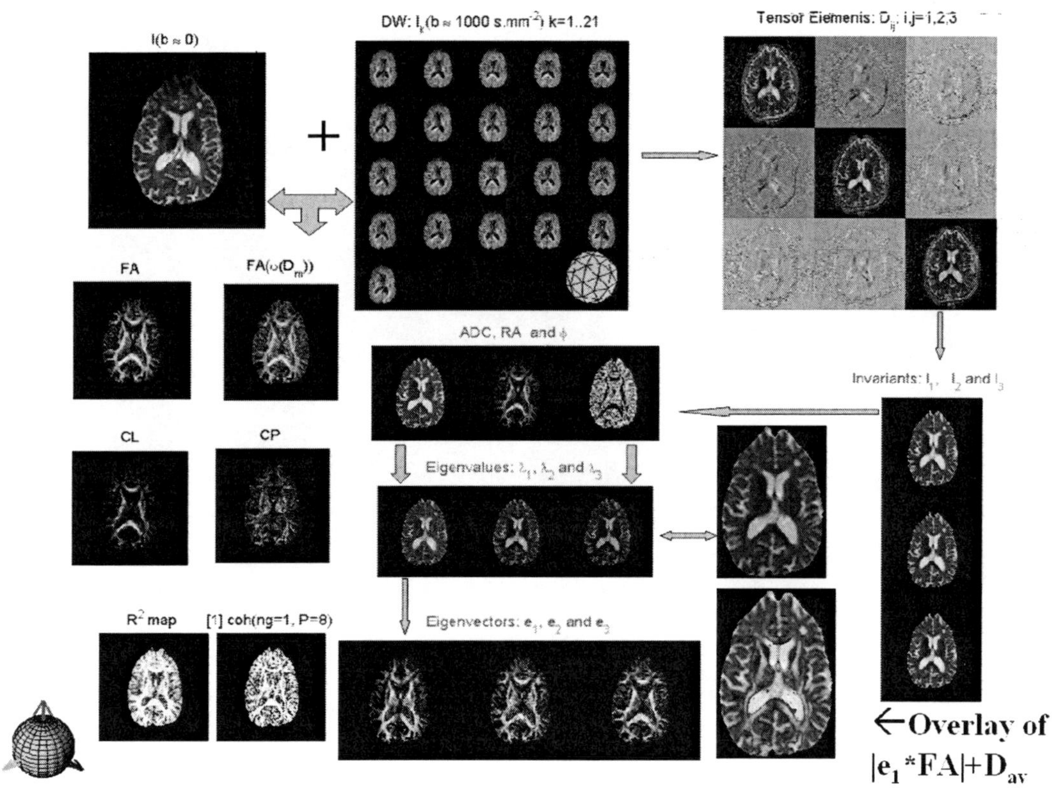

Figure 9. A schematic illustration of the different tissue contrast obtained from diffusion weighted, vector and scalar DTI maps. The major DTI processing steps using an encoding scheme with 21 uniformly distributed directions in 3D. The text (theory) details the construction and defines all variables used.

Special Cartesian Cylindrical Tensor Case

Due to its simplicity and relevance for modeling and simulations of water diffusion in simple lamellar structures such as the spinal cord, corpus callosum, skeletal muscle, celery and asparagus, the cylindrical tensor hypothetical case has been the focus of many studies (Conturo et al. 1996; Hsu and Mori 1995; Callaghan 1994; Gulani et al. 2001; Hasan and Narayana 2006). The cylindrical tensor has 4 independent degrees of freedom that can be represented by two eigenvalues $(\lambda_1, \lambda_2 \cong \lambda_3) or (\lambda_{\|}, \lambda_{\perp})$ and two rotational degrees of freedom (φ, θ). In this special case, all anisotropy measures can be inter-related and expressed as functions of a single variable which is the ratio of the major (parallel) to the minor (perpendicular) diffusivity ($x = \dfrac{\lambda_1}{\lambda_2}$). Thus, in the cylindrical case and using the previous equations with: $\phi = 0$, CP=0, RA=CL=A_{cyl}, FA and VF are given by:

$$\begin{bmatrix} RA \\ FA \\ VF \end{bmatrix} = \begin{bmatrix} \dfrac{\lambda_1 - \lambda_2}{\lambda_1 + 2\lambda_2} \\ \dfrac{\lambda_1 - \lambda_2}{\sqrt{\lambda_1^{\ 2} + 2\lambda_2^{\ 2}}} \\ 1 - 27\dfrac{\lambda_1 \lambda_2^{\ 2}}{(\lambda_1 + 2\lambda_2)^3} \end{bmatrix} = \begin{bmatrix} \dfrac{x-1}{x+2} \\ \dfrac{x-1}{\sqrt{x^2+2}} \\ 1 - 27\dfrac{x}{(x+2)^3} \end{bmatrix} \qquad [17a]$$

The fudge variable x, RA and mean diffusivity can also be related as:

$$\begin{bmatrix} RA \\ D_{av} \\ x \end{bmatrix} = \begin{bmatrix} 1 - \dfrac{3}{x+2} \\ \lambda_2 (x+2) \\ \dfrac{2 * RA + 1}{1 - RA} \end{bmatrix} \qquad [17b]$$

The two independent eigenvalues are given as a special case of the analytical mathematical forms above:

$$\begin{bmatrix} \lambda_1 \\ \lambda_2 \end{bmatrix} = D_{av} \begin{bmatrix} 1 + 2.0 * RA \\ 1 - RA \end{bmatrix} \qquad [18a]$$

Using standard error propagation, the standard error in the mean diffusivity ($D_{av} = \frac{\lambda_1 + 2\lambda_2}{3}$) and RA can also be expressed in terms of the variances in the eigenvalues:

$$\begin{bmatrix} \sigma(D_{av}) \\ \sigma(RA) \end{bmatrix} = \begin{bmatrix} \frac{1}{3}\sqrt{\sigma(\lambda_1)^2 + 4*\sigma(\lambda_2)^2} \\ \frac{1}{3D_{av}}\sqrt{(1-RA)^2*\sigma(\lambda_1)^2 + (2*RA-1)^2*\sigma(\lambda_2)^2} \end{bmatrix} \quad [18b]$$

For completeness and notational consistency with published diffusion weighted literature, the anisotropy index AI has been also defined as $AI = \frac{\lambda_1 - \lambda_2}{\lambda_1 + \lambda_2}$. Thus, it is seen that the cylindrical tensor case provides a simple and practical framework for DTI computation and analysis. Through simple algebraic relations, all anisotropy measures can be functionally related. Figure 10 provides a handy plot that can be used to relate and lookup all anisotropy indices from different publications. In a later section the tensor acquisition and encoding methodology of this case will be outlined.

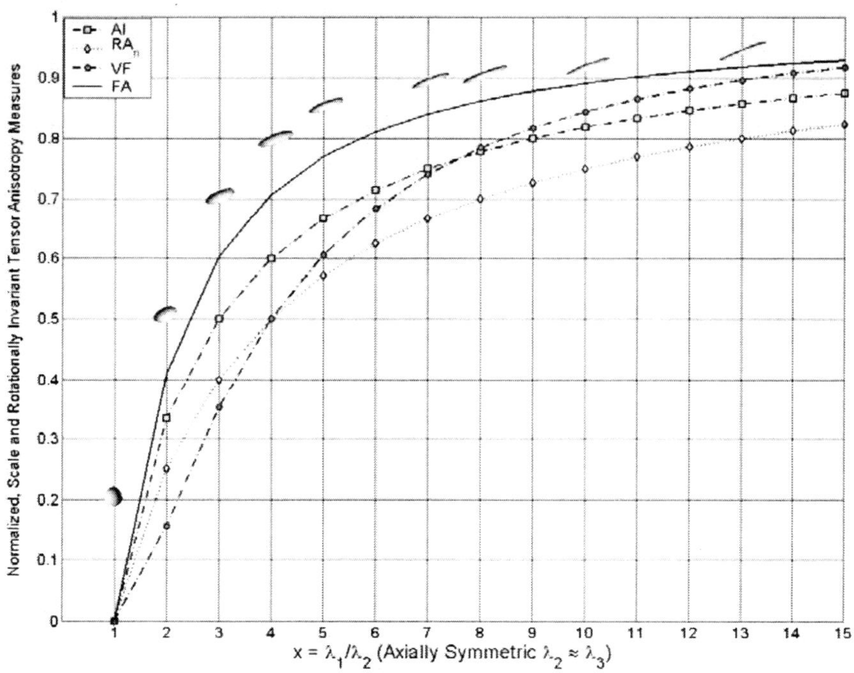

Figure 10. A plot of commonly used normalized, scale independent and rotationally invariant tensor anisotropy indices for axially symmetric tensors (AI, RA$_n$, VF, FA) (λ_1, $\lambda_2 \sim \lambda_3$) as function of the ratio x= λ_1/λ_2. The tensor ellipsoids for some selected eigenvalue ratio values are also shown.

Exact Diagonalization of the Two Dimensional Cartesian Tensor Case

The two-dimensional tensor is the simplest intuitive case which can be solved exactly and analytically for the eigenvalues and eigenvectors (Hasan 2002). Although apparently not encountered in mapping the 3 dimensional human brains, interest in this case motivates understanding the effect of small perturbations on the estimated eigenvalues and eigenvectors. In this case, diffusion is confined to the two -dimensional plane (x, y). The unknown tensor has three independent elements and two invariants:

$$D = \begin{bmatrix} D_{xx} & D_{xy} \\ D_{xy} & D_{yy} \end{bmatrix}$$
$$I_1 = D_{xx} + D_{yy}$$
$$I_2 = \det(D) = D_{xx}D_{yy} - D_{xy}^{\;2} \qquad [19]$$

Using the fact that the eigenvectors of this tensor can be determined by applying an orthogonal rotation matrix (R) and the requirement that the eigenvalue matrix is diagonal (with vanishing off-diagonal elements) lead to:

$$R(\varphi) = \begin{bmatrix} \cos(\varphi) & -\sin(\varphi) \\ \sin(\varphi) & \cos(\varphi) \end{bmatrix} = \begin{bmatrix} e_{1x} & e_{2x} \\ e_{1y} & e_{2y} \end{bmatrix} \Leftrightarrow D_R(\varphi) = \Lambda = R(\varphi)DR(\varphi)^t$$
$$\Lambda = \begin{bmatrix} \lambda_1 & 0 \\ 0 & \lambda_2 \end{bmatrix} = \frac{I_1}{2}\begin{bmatrix} 1+ec & 0 \\ 0 & 1-ec \end{bmatrix} \Leftrightarrow \vec{e}_1 = \begin{bmatrix} K \\ \sqrt{1+K^2}\,sign(D_{xx} - D_{yy}) - 1 \end{bmatrix} \qquad [20]$$

Where *K*, *ec*, and the normalized eigenvectors $\{e_1, e_2\}$ are given by:

$$ec = \sqrt{1 - 4\frac{I_2}{I_1^{\;2}}} = \frac{\lambda_1 - \lambda_2}{\lambda_1 + \lambda_2} = \frac{D_{xx} - D_{yy}}{D_{xx} + D_{yy}}\sqrt{1+K^2}$$
$$K = \tan(2\theta) = 2\frac{D_{xy}}{D_{xx} - D_{yy}}$$
$$\hat{e}_1 = \frac{\vec{e}_1}{\sqrt{\vec{e}_1^{\,t}\vec{e}_1}}$$
$$\hat{e}_2 = \begin{bmatrix} -e_{1y} \\ e_{1x} \end{bmatrix} \qquad [21]$$

Since K is linearly dependent on the off-diagonal element D_{xy}, and inversely proportional to the spacing contrast (or spectral width) between the diagonal elements (D_{xx}-D_{yy}), this will result in extreme sensitivity to measurement and computational errors (Noble and Daniel

1977). Anisotropy measures are functions of the invariant quantity *ec* and show more immunity to noise than eigenvectors. These simple considerations are clearly important in the design, processing and analysis of the information obtained from the DTI data (anisotropy, coherence, fiber tracks) as will be seen in later sections. For example, DTI-based fiber tracking based on the principal eigenvector (FACT-fiber assignment by continuous tracking) starts from a selected voxel in white matter (FA>0.2) and then connects this voxel with the neighboring most similar voxel based on the anisotropy and relative path curvature to form a connected track or streamline (Moorhead and Zhifan 1995; Mori and Van Zijl 2002).

$$\vec{r}_{k+1} = \vec{r}_k \pm s_k * \hat{e}_{1k} \qquad [22]$$

The procedure is continued by finding the next voxel and the step size following standard ray tracing procedures (Lori et al. 2002). For example, in a uniform tensor field (ellipsoids oriented along the x direction) and perturbed by a normally distributed noise distribution, the accumulated dispersion error due to measurement noise (low SNR) mimics a random walk and results in a net deviation that is roughly given by (Anderson 2001; Fukushima 1990; Lori et al. 2002; Lazar and Alexander 2005)

$$\delta y \approx \frac{voxel_{size}}{SNR} \frac{\sqrt{N}}{\lambda_1 - \lambda_2} \qquad [23]$$

Physical Considerations of DTI

DTI Parameter Space

The goal of DTI encoding is to obtain a bulk or apparent diffusion tensor from each volume element within the object or volume-of-interest. The diffusion weighted data are obtained by sensitizing the MRI active spins using a set of encoding pulses with known and controlled strength, spatial and temporal attributes (see Figure 7 and Figure 11). Figure 12 provides different conventional MRI and DTI images from the same subject acquired along 21 uniformly distributed directions (also see Figure 9). Figure 12 illustrates the dependence of the measured diffusion weighted signal on the diffusion pulse strength and orientation. For example, the corpus callosum (see Figures 1-2); (right-to-left) fibers are attenuated when the encoding is applied along the fibers, whereas it is bright when applied perpendicularly. The frontal (minor) and posterior (major) forceps which run anterior-posterior through the genu and splenium of the CC respectively are attenuated when the pulse is applied along the y. The posterior limb of the internal capsule which runs inferior-to-superior (foot-to-knee) is attenuated when the encoding pulse is applied along the z-direction (or $g_d = [0, 0, 1]$). The diffusion tensor is usually represented by an ellipsoid which is characterized by three orthonormal eigenvectors and three eigenvalues (Figure 7). The eigenvalues or tensor invariants are used to compute the tensor anisotropy and the eigenvectors are used to connect neighboring voxels with similar orientation coherence properties (Figures 1-2, 9) (Le Bihan

1995; 2003). The measurement thermal noise and system stability will reduce the accuracy and reproducibility of the estimated apparent tensors and hence DTI requirements for SNR are usually higher than conventional MRI methods (Conturo et al. 1995; Pierpaoli and Basser 1996; Bastin et al. 1998; Hasan 2000; Anderson 2001; Hasan and Narayana 2003; Hasan et al. 2004).

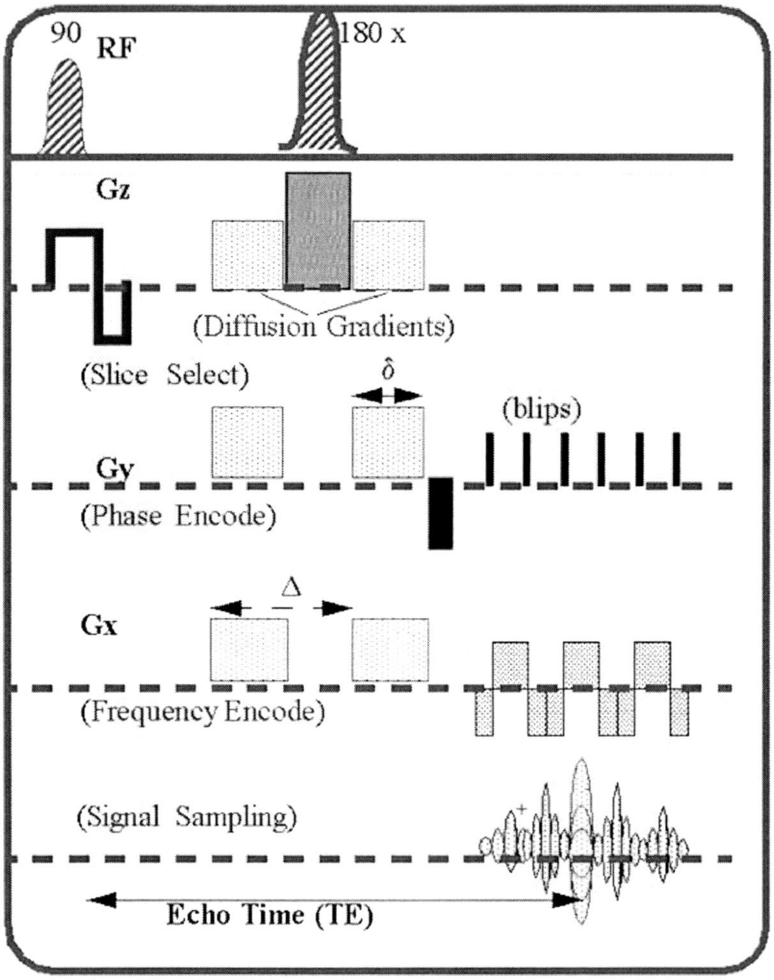

Figure 11. Schematic of the spin-echo prepared echo-planar sequence used for DTI and the parameters involved (see also Figure 8). The sequence uses a Stejskal-Tanner bipolar magnetic gradient diffusion pulses of equal area and known separation, order, number and orientation sandwiched around the 180° focusing pulse. The magnetic pulses have a linear spatial profile to facilitate encoding of water molecular translational diffusion during the dephasing (prior to the 180° pulse) and rephasing times (post 180° pulse).

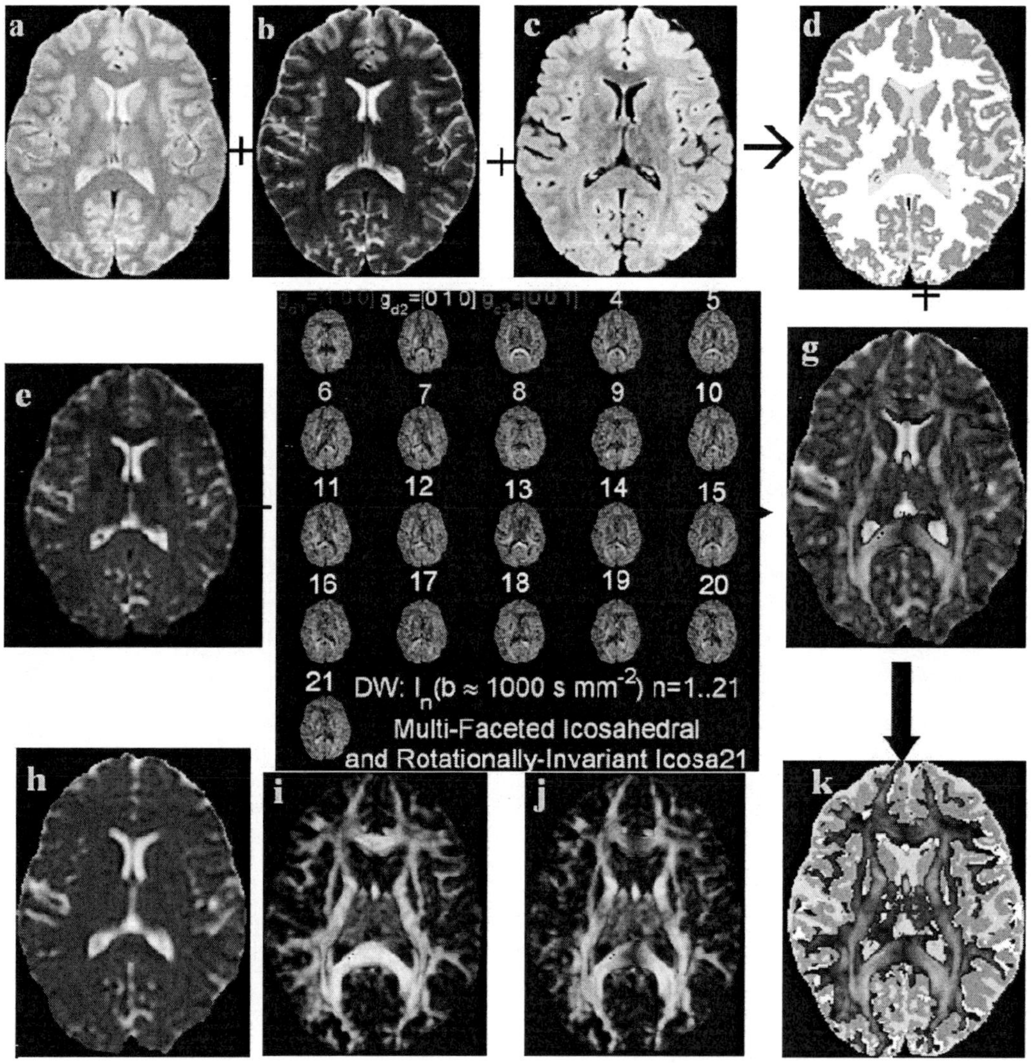

Figure 12. Illustration of combined conventional (turbo double spin echo and fluid attenuated inversion recovery) and optimized DTI data sets on a healthy subject at 3.0 T. A representative section from an entire brain data set. (a) a proton density map (b) T2w turbo spin echo map (c) FLAIR map(d) tissue segmentation map (white matter is white, gray matter is gray and CSF is cyan). The tensor decoding of the reference map (e) and the diffusion weighted images (central block-f) and fusion of the DTI data results in g which is formed by fusing the mean diffusivity map h with the fractional anisotropy map (FA) modulated by the principal vector e_1. Further Fusion of image g and d provides the map in k.

Due to the physical requirement that translational diffusion results in some predictable signal loss, the diffusion tensor is required to be symmetric with positive eigenvalues (Le Bihan 1995; Basser and Pierpaoli 1996). Therefore, a minimum of six non-collinear encoding magnetic pulses with calibrated strength, G_d, duration and directions ($\vec{G}_d = G_d \hat{g}$) are needed to obtain the six independent elements of the diffusion tensor (Le Bihan 1995). To facilitate using linear algebraic methods, the self-diffusion tensor, **D**, which was represented above as a 3x3 symmetric matrix with six unique tensor elements can be expressed by the column vector (Nye 1957):

$$\hat{\boldsymbol{d}} = \begin{bmatrix} D_{xx} & D_{yy} & D_{zz} & D_{xy} & D_{xz} & D_{yz} \end{bmatrix}^t \quad [24]$$

In the presence of local gradients ($\boldsymbol{G}_l$: imaging, inhomogeniety, or external), the single tensor model that relates the unknown tensor, ***D***, to the encoding diffusion unit vector, $\hat{\boldsymbol{g}}(\mathrm{n}) = \begin{bmatrix} g_x(n) & g_y(n) & g_z(n) \end{bmatrix}^t$, the diffusion weighting b-factor, b, the reference image pixel signal, *S(0)*, and the measured diffusion weighted signal, *S(n)*, can be expressed for $n=1...N_e$ as:

$$S(\hat{g}(n)) = S(0)\exp(-b\hat{g}(n)^t D\hat{g}(n) + c\vec{G}_d(n)^t D\vec{G}_l) \quad [25]$$

where N_e is the number of encoding directions, and c represents a complicated function of the diffusion pulse temporal parameters. The diffusion sensitized signal is generally dependent on the sign of the applied magnetic pulse, the coupling functional and the relative orientation of the pulse and the diffusion tensor. Notice that each diffusion signal measurement *(S(g(n))* is analogous to a sample or a projection of the tensor in this generalized diffusion space. By alternating the encoding polarity (Neeman et al. 1990; Le Bihan 1995; Madi et al. 2005) and combining the two measurements we can construct the element:

$$y(n) = \log(\frac{S(+\hat{g}(n))S(-\hat{g}(n))}{S(0)^2}) = -b\hat{g}(n)^t D\hat{g}(n) = -b * Trace(\hat{g}(n)\hat{g}(n)^t D) = -b\hat{h}(n)^t \hat{d} \quad [26a]$$

Since $D = \sum_{i=1}^{3} \lambda_i \hat{e}_i{}^t \hat{e}_i$, the measured signal can also be viewed as a projection on the tensor ellipsoid

$$y(n) = -b\hat{g}(n)^t D\hat{g}(n) = -b\hat{g}(n)^t \sum_{i=1}^{3} \lambda_i \hat{e}_i{}^t \hat{e}_i \hat{g}(n) = -b\sum_{i=1}^{3} \lambda_i \left\| \hat{e}_i \cdot \hat{g}(n) \right\|^2 = -b\sum_{i=1}^{3} \lambda_i \cos^2(\gamma_{ni}) \quad [26b]$$

Note that these equations involve a logarithmic operation which decouples any low frequency modulation of the measured signal by a space dependent bias field due to the RF coil sensitivity (Bammer et al. 2002; Ashburner and Friston 1998). The latter property would increase the confidence in the scale-independence and rotational invariance of the metrics provided by DTI, especially at high magnetic fields and using implanted surface coils (Madi et al. 2005). For accurate tensor encoding, estimation and decoupling, DTI usually involves the acquisition of many images with different encoding orientations, where $n=1...N_e$. The relationship between the vector of measurements, $\hat{Y}$, and the independent *unknown* diffusion tensor elements, $\hat{d}$ can be expressed in matrix notation as (Nye 1957; Basser et al. 1994; Le Bihan 1995; Papadakis 1999; Hasan et al. 2001a),

$$\hat{Y} = H\hat{d} + \hat{\eta}, \quad [27]$$

where $\boldsymbol{H}$ is the design encoding matrix, which is formed from the encoding row vectors $h(n)^t$ and $\hat{Y}$, is formed from the measured data. Hasan et al. (2003) demonstrated that the mean diffusivity and relative anisotropy indices can be estimated directly from the measured attenuated data directly if and only if the diffusion encoding set is icosahedral (see below). Thus, if the data is sampled uniformly the mean diffusivity is given by

$$D_{av} = \frac{\sum_{n=1}^{N_e} y(n)}{N_e} = \frac{\sum_{n=1}^{N_e}\left[\log(S(0)) - \log(S(n))\right]}{b * N_e} = \frac{1}{b}\left[\log(S(0)) - \frac{\sum_{n=1}^{Ne}\log(S(n))}{N_e}\right] \quad [28]$$

and the normalized relative anisotropy:

$$RA = \sqrt{\frac{5}{4}}\sqrt{\frac{\sum_{n=1}^{N_e}\left[\log(S(0)) - \log(S(n))\right]^2}{(bD_{av})^2 N_e} - 1} \quad [29]$$

The latter formulae and their error propagation provide a simple but important method for designing DTI protocols. Alternatively, the least-squares optimization and the singular value decomposition methods (Papdakis et al. 1999; Hasan et al. 2001a) can now be used to estimate the diffusivity vector, $\hat{d}$, where the superscript *-1* refers to matrix pseudo-inversion:

$$\breve{d} = (H^t H)^{-1} H^t \hat{Y} \quad [30]$$

The total scan time in single shot volume acquisitions depends directly on the total number of images. In general, the total number of DT-MRI images acquired, N_T, is composed of the sum $N_T = \sum_{s=1}^{N_s} N_e(s) N_d(s)$, where $N_e(s)$ is the number of encoding directions each averaged $N_d(s)$ times at some diffusion weighting step *(s)*. For symmetric trapezoidal, unipolar diffusion gradient pulses of strength g_d, rise time ε, duration δ, and separation Δ, the diffusion b-factor is given by (Le Bihan 1995; Mattiello et al. 1994),

$$b = (\gamma G_d)^2 (\delta^2 \left(\Delta - \frac{\delta}{3}\right) - \frac{\delta\varepsilon^2}{6} + \frac{\varepsilon^3}{30}), \quad [31]$$

where ε is the gyromagnetic ratio. The two-step DT-MRI experiment (N_s=2) is acquired by varying the direction, sign, order, strength *(G_d)*, number of reference ($N_{ref;}$ *b~0*) and diffusion weighted images (N_d), at fixed imaging parameters: repetition time (T_R), effective echo time (T_E), diffusion pulse duration (δ) and separation time (Δ), slice thickness, and sampling parameters. (see Figure 2). The total imaging time, T_t, for a two b-factor DT-MRI experiment

(N_s=2) can be expressed as $T_t = T_R{*}N_T$, where the total number of images acquired, $N_T = (N_{ref}+N_dN_e)$.

Signal-to-Noise Ratio in DTI

At a given main magnetic field (***B₀***), and in the absence of translational random diffusion, the signal-to-noise ratio (SNR_0) obtained using a spin echo prepared signal is proportional to the number of free and excited spins within the field-of-view (FOV_x by FOV_y) and the root of the total k-space sampling time (Hinshaw and lent 1983; Parker and Gullberg 1990). Additionally, it will be modulated by the spin-spin (T_2) and spin-lattice relaxation functions (T_1); hence, assuming that MRI noise is dominated by RF electric field dissipation in the sample (Callaghan 1994):

$$Conventional_{SNR_0} \sim B_0\left(1-\exp\left(-\frac{T_R}{T_1}\right)\right)*\exp\left(-\frac{TE}{T_2}\right)*\frac{FOV_x}{N_x}\frac{FOV_y}{N_y}*slice_{thickness}\sqrt{\frac{N_{ref}*N_x*N_y}{Sampling_{BW}}} \quad [32]$$

For parallel imaging with a coil characterized by a geometric noise factor ($Coil_g$) and using a k-space under-sampling or acceleration factor R, the same formula can be adjusted to provide (Jaermann et al. 2004; Sodickson et al. 2001; Pruessman et al. 1999):

$$SENSE_{SNR_0} \sim Conventional_{SNR_0}\frac{1}{Coil_{g-factor}\sqrt{R}} \quad [33]$$

Error Estimation of the Diffusivities and Encoding Quality Figures-of-Merit

The covariance matrix of the estimated diffusivities (Le Bihan 1995; Basser et al. 1994; Hasan 2001a) is given by:

$$\text{cov}(\hat{d}) = \left((H^tH)^{-1}H^t\right)\text{cov}(\hat{Y})\left((H^tH)^{-1}H^t\right)^{-1} \quad [34]$$

Equations (3-4) predict that $cov(\hat{Y})$ depends on the b-factor, the *I(0)* and *I(k)* SNR levels. The log-linear functional relationship also couples the $cov(\hat{d})$ to the estimated unknown values $\hat{d}$ (Basser et al. 1994; Papadakis et al. 1999; Hasan et al. 2001). In the case where the noise measurements are independent, we can write

$$\text{cov}(\hat{d}) = (H^tH)^{-1}\sigma(\hat{Y})^2 \quad [35]$$

The structure of the encoding matrix (***H***) is important in performing the inversion procedure as well as defining figures-of-merit, such as condition number, energy, and variance, to optimize the spatial distribution of the encoding vectors. Thus, the diffusion-to-noise ratio (*DNR*) defined as the coefficient of variation of the estimated apparent diffusion tensor element $DNR_{ij} = \frac{D_{ij}}{\sigma(D_{ij})}$ (*i,j=1,23*) or $d_k = \frac{d_k}{\sigma(d_k)}$ (*k=1,2,3,4,5,6*) is expected to be a complicated function of many parameters:

$DNR \sim SNR0\ f(b, H, \mathbf{D}, N_d, N_{ref}, N_e)$. For a non-tensor but two b-experiment acquired with $N_{ref} = n_1$ averages ($b \sim 0$) and n_2 diffusion weighted images (N_d) applied along one (N_e=1) specified encoding direction ($N_T = n_1 + n_2$), Xing et al. (1997) and Conturo et al. (1995) have shown that the projected apparent diffusion coefficient (*adc*) $DNR_{adc} = \frac{adc}{\sigma(adc)}$ ratio per unit SNR0 can be expressed as:

$$\kappa_{adc} = \frac{DNR}{SNR_0} = \frac{b * adc}{\sqrt{\frac{1}{N_{ref}} + \frac{\exp(2b * adc)}{N_d}}} \quad [36a]$$

For estimating the mean diffusivity estimation variance, this expression can be extended using error propagation of the expressions above and icosahedral encoding schemes:

$$\kappa_{D_{av}} = \frac{D_{av}}{\sigma(D_{av})SNR_0} = \frac{bD_{av}}{\sqrt{\frac{1}{N_{ref}} + \frac{\exp(2bD_{av})}{N_e N_d}}} \quad [36b]$$

Notice the dependence on the unknown diffusivity, b-factor and total diffusion time partition $N_d * N_e = N_T - N_{ref}$. This multi-dimensional function can be solved for the optimal b-factor and total diffusion time partition ratio $\frac{N_{ref}}{N_d * N_e}$ for some known adc or mean diffusivity range. Special cases and numerical solutions have been attempted (Jones et al. 1999; Armitage and Bastin 2001; Brihuega-Moreno et al. 2003; Poonawalla and Zhou 2004; Kingsley and Moohan 2004). In general, normal aging, pathology and tissue recovery alters the quantitative DTI-metrics and the b-factor, total time partition may need to be optimized to maximize abnormal-to-normal tissue diffusion contrast-to-noise ratio. For example, maximization of white-to-gray matter diffusion contrast by increasing the b-factor may enhance WM-GM visibility but would compromise the visualization of focal ischemic areas relative to white matter structures (Yoshiura et al. 2001). A complete analysis of the general optimization problem is beyond the scope of this chapter. Thus, it is clear that even for the simplest non-tensor case, the selection of the diffusion related parameters involve the solution of a complex multi-parameter optimization problem with some a priori knowledge and constraints imposed (Conturo 1995; Xing et al. 1997; Jones 1999; Hasan 2000).

The DTI Parameter Space Optimization Problem

The DTI full brain problem optimization seeks the most accurate estimation of the unknown tensors in a clinically tolerable and affordable time. Since we do not have *a priori* knowledge of the tensor distribution and to simplify the problem, we assume that the tensor ellipsoids are uniformly distributed in space (Hasan 2000). It is always desirable to reduce motion-related image distortion and partial volume averaging artifacts (Le Bihan 1995; Alexander et al. 2001) avoiding nerve stimulation and keeping the radio frequency power deposition below the FDA approved level (Basser 2002). Single-shot echo-planar imaging combined with coil sensitivity encoding (SENSE) and high magnetic fields seem to be the mainstay for clinical applications of DTI (Pruessmann et al. 1999; Jaermann et al. 2004). The SENSE reduction can be used to shorten the effective echo time and achieve the benefits of multi-shot imaging (Bammer et al. 2002). A reduction in effective echo time would also allow covering more slices per unit T_R which would allow thinner slices and reduce blurring, signal losses and susceptibility-related artifacts at larger magnetic fields (Hunsche et al. 2001). An intrinsic increase in SNR due to doubling the main magnetic field ($\boldsymbol{B_0}$) has the same theoretical advantage as multiplexing 4 repeated and temporally averaged and coherent data sets as indicated by the SNR Equation [32] above. Reduction in scan times would encourage the investigation and implementation of techniques such as eddy current self-compensated sequences (Wider 1994; Le Bihan 1995; Price 1997; 1998; Alexander et al. 1997; Reese et al. 2003), flow, CSF, gray or white matter suppressed preparation (Falconer and Narayana 1997; Zacharopoulos and Narayana 1998) or magnetization transfer preparation (Gupta et al. 2005) to increase the specificity of the signal sources and provide accurate interpretation of the contributors of anisotropy (Beaulieu 2002; Norris et al. 1995; Norris 2001; Le Bihan 1995). The reduced effective scan time and large gradients would also motivate the implementation of bipolar diffusion pulses, twice-focused eddy current compensation, single-shot spin echo or stimulated echo acquisition (Price 1997; 1998; Le Bihan 1995; Basser and Jones 2002).

An important advantage of reduced scan time at high magnetic fields is the ability to reduce the need for repeated acquisitions to improve SNR. Temporal averaging assumes extreme system hardware and exciter stability and minimal phase fluctuations (Weisskoff 1996). Notice that the same scan time can be invested in multiple b-factor acquisitions, or high angular resolution encoding sets. For single tensor estimation, it has been demonstrated that it is more efficient to use the entire time on the two b-factor partition (Le Bihan 1995); the problem is reduced further by solving for the optimal b-factor, number and orientation of the encoding set and the partition of the total scan time ($T_t=N_T*T_R$, $N_T=N_{ref}+N_dN_e$). A complete analysis of this problem is beyond the scope of this chapter, but general recommendations and guidelines will be stated (Hasan 2000). Our main focus will be on the selection of the tensor encoding set.

The b-factor can be estimated roughly by the diffusion matching filter property $b*Trace(D)\sim 1.1$ (see Equation [36] above). The b-factor, on the other hand, is determined by the gradient pulse duration, separation and strength (Equation [31]). To allow the most specific interpretation of the results on clinical scanners, the sequence should use the smallest possible pulse duration (δ) and the largest possible diffusion gradient with the largest gradient slew rates that are consistent with patient safety and comfort (Price 1997; 1998; Basser 2002). To reduce distortion and image artifacts, the echo spacing between k-space samples should be minimized (Le Bihan 1995; Bammer et al. 2002). The echo time should always be selected to maximize the SNR_0 based on the knowledge of the tissue relaxation parameters (T_2) of the compartment of interest (Jaermann et al. 2004). Due to practical considerations, a 10 minute upper limit for the DTI acquisition seems tolerable for many applications. An entire brain exam under four minutes is ideal for imaging non-sedated infants (Gilmore et al. 2004), uncooperative and unstable patients (acute stroke, traumatic, autistic, claustrophobic, schizophrenic, demented, etc). The reduction of the DTI scan time may also allow inclusion of other conventional MRI data acquisition schemes such as phase maps, phase sensitive fluid attenuated inversion recovery, metabolic, anatomical, functional and vascular imaging to be fused with DTI after proper registration.

Criteria and Figures-of-Merit for the Selection of the Tensor Encoding Matrix

The following figures-of-merit have been used to characterize and design the encoding matrix for DTI. The tensor total variance has been used by many groups even prior to DTI inception (Alderman et al. 1990; Papadakis et al. 1999; Hasan et al. 2001),

$$TV(D) = \sum_{i=1}^{3} \sum_{j=1}^{3} \sigma(D_{ij})^2 , \qquad [37]$$

Additionally, the encoding matrix condition number (Skare et al. 2000; Papdakis et al. 1999; Hasan et al. 2001; Batchelor et al. 2003) can be defined as:

$$\kappa = cond(H) = \frac{\max(eigvals(H))}{\min(eigvals(H))} \qquad [38]$$

The condition number of an acceptable encoding set is further required to be rotationally invariant (Hasan et al. 2003; Batchelor et al. 2003). It has been shown (Batchelor et al. 2003; Hasan and Narayana 2003) that the minimum condition is a weak criterion in the design of uniformly distributed encoding sets, and minimum condition sets are actually not uniformly distributed and rotationally variant. Borrowing from the analogy with the electrostatic repulsion problem of N_e identical unit charged pairs, we compute the interaction energy, E, of

N_e identical pair charges positioned at $\hat{g}$ on the surface of a unit sphere (Conturo et al. 1996; Jones et al. 1999; Hasan et al. 2001).

$$E = \sum_{k>r}^{2N_e} \sum_{r=1}^{2N_e} \frac{1}{\left\| \hat{g}(k) - \hat{g}(r) \right\|} \quad [39]$$

Note that since the unit charges are constrained to the surface of a unit sphere, $||\hat{g}(k)||=1$, we obtain the value for the relative distance matrix element, $R_{kr} = \left\|\hat{g}(k) - \hat{g}(r)\right\| = 2\sin(\frac{\alpha_{kr}}{2})$, where α_{kr} is the angle between the two unit vectors $\hat{g}(k)$ and $\hat{g}(r)$. To attain an equilibrium state or configuration with minimum energy, and uniform configuration, the angle (α) between any two encoding vertices of some encoding set has to be as large as possible (Papadakis et al. 2000; Hasan et al. 2001).

Analytical Example of the Relationship between Tensor Encoding Schemes

To study the relationship between different encoding schemes, the analytical encoding method was used (Hasan *et al.* 2001; Hasan and Narayana 2003). The method constructs the simplest encoding vector matrix for $N_e=6$ from cyclic permutations of the normalized vector $\hat{g}(x) = \frac{1}{\sqrt{1+x^2}}\left[\pm x \quad \pm 1 \quad 0\right]^t$, which can be constructed from the rows of the generating encoding set

$$\mathbf{E}_m(x) = \frac{1}{\sqrt{1+x^2}} \begin{bmatrix} x & x & 0 & 0 & 1 & 1 \\ 1 & -1 & x & x & 0 & 0 \\ 0 & 0 & 1 & -1 & x & -x \end{bmatrix}^t \quad [40a]$$

where x is a variable that allows analytical computation. The $\boldsymbol{H}$ matrix is formed as described above (Eq. 4) and is given by:

$$\mathbf{H}(x) = \frac{1}{1+x^2} \begin{bmatrix} x^2 & 1 & 0 & 2x & 0 & 0 \\ x^2 & 1 & 0 & -2x & 0 & 0 \\ 0 & x^2 & 1 & 0 & 0 & 2x \\ 0 & x^2 & 1 & 0 & 0 & -2x \\ 1 & 0 & x^2 & 0 & 2x & 0 \\ 1 & 0 & x^2 & 0 & -2x & 0 \end{bmatrix} \quad [40b]$$

This analytical and general encoding matrix gives three familiar cases after computing the energy, condition number and total variance as function of the variable x (see Figure 13). Figure 13 plots four scalar functions versus the fudge variable x for the minimum energy, variance, condition number and minimum angle between any two pairs constrained to the unit encoding sphere. For $x=1$ we obtain the cube edge bisectors (Basser and Pierpaoli 1998) with a condition number of 2.0; this commonly used encoding scheme is referred to here as the oblique double gradient scheme (ODG). The minimum condition set (Skare et al. 2000) is obtained with $x = x_{mc} = \sqrt{(5 \pm \sqrt{21})/2}$ with condition number $= \frac{\sqrt{7}}{2} \sim 1.3229$. The principal icosahedral encoding scheme (**Icosa6**) (Hasan et al. 2001; Hasan and Narayana 2003) is obtained at the golden ratio or $x = x_{icosa} = 2\cos(\pi/5) = \frac{\sqrt{5}+1}{2}$ and $x = \tau = 1/x_{icosa} = \frac{\sqrt{5}-1}{2}$, with condition number $= \frac{\sqrt{10}}{2} \sim 1.5811$. The icosahedral set is the only uniformly distributed and rotationally invariant scheme with $N_e=6$. The latter result has also been documented in the literature prior to DTI in another analogous area such as chemical shift tensor imaging (Alderman et al. 1990). The minimum energy spatial distribution algorithm will also provide uniformly distributed sets for arbitrary N_e including $N_e=6$. To summarize this section, notice that (1). The minimum energy and minimum variance scheme is provided by the icosahedral set (Icosa6), (2). The encoding sets at $x=1$ and $x=x_{mc}$ have the same tensor variance and are biased as illustrated by the minimum angle plot, (3). The minimum condition criterion does not yield uniformly distributed encoding directions, nor does the commonly used (ODG) encoding scheme for $x=1$ (Basser and Pierpaoli 1998), and (4) the icosahedral solution at $x = \tau$ is expected to be more stable to small perturbations or errors in the design of diffusion gradient directions (Figure 13).

Encoding Directions for Some Special Cases and N_e=6 General Case

The two dimensional and cylindrical tensor cases discussed earlier in the theory turn out to be intuitive and easily solvable. A uniformly distributed two-dimensional Cartesian tensor has three unique unknowns (D_{xx}, D_{yy}, D_{xy}; an ellipsoid with two eigenvalues and one orientation in the plane) and requires three unit encoding vectors that form an equilateral triangle in the unit circle (Table 3). The cylindrical case requires 4 vectors in the unit cube that form tetrahedral structure. The estimation of the mean diffusivity of the general tensor directly requires three independent measurements with orthogonal configuration. The general 3D Cartesian tensor case with $N_e=6$ unknowns can be encoded using the six vertices of the icosahedron. If the cross-terms are to be minimized, an alternating polarity icosahedral scheme can also be adopted (Neeman et al. 1991).

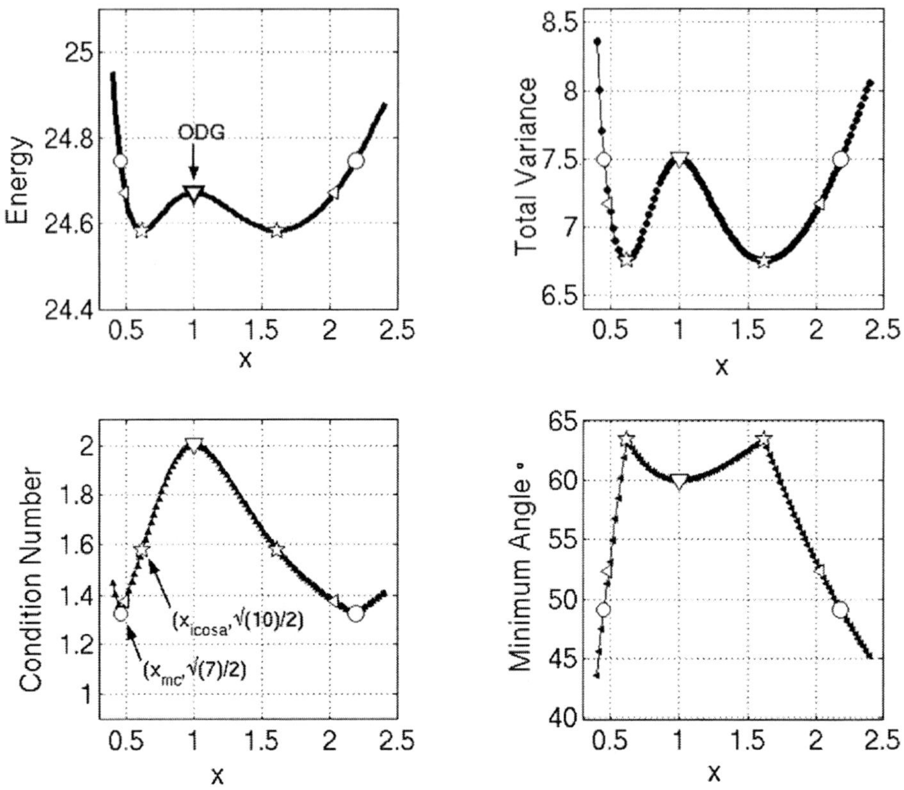

Figure 13. Plot of scalar functions obtained from the analytical encoding matrix approach. The Energy, Total Variance, Condition Number and Minimum Angle as function of the variable, x. Notice that the oblique double gradient, minimum condition and principal icosahedral schemes are special and related cases in this approach. The Icosahedral set is the most stable configuration (see theory).

Table 3. A listing of Encoding Directions for special tensor and the general case

Case	Encoding Vectors {(gx,gy,gz)}	Minimum Angle	Comments
Two dimensional planar tensor (x,y)	(1,0,0) , (-cos(π/3), sin(π /3),0) (-cos(π/3), sin(π/3),0)	120°	*Three* unit vectors separated by 120 ° over the unit circle forming equilateral triangle.
Efficient estimation of mean diffusivity D_{av}	(-1,1,-0.5), (1,0.5,-1), (0.5,1,1) (this set is more efficient than XYZ set={(1,0,0), (0,1,0), (0,0,1) }	90°	*Three* orthogonal vectors.
Three dimensional cylindrical tensor	(1,1,1), (-1,-1,1), (1,-1,-1), (-1,1,-1)	70.5°	*Four* tetrahedral vectors.
General three dimensional full tensor	(0, -1.0, -X), (-X, 0, -1.0), (-1.0, X, 0),(1.0, X, 0), (-X, 0, 1.0),(0, -1.0, X) (X = [√5-1]/2 or golden ratio)	63.4°	*Six* uniformly distributed vectors with icosahedral configuration.

Review of Encoding Optimization and Spatial Distribution Methods for $N_e \geq 6$

In general, the distribution of tensor shapes and orientations are not known *a priori* for a given tissue volume of interest. Consequently, it is normally assumed that the optimum encoding set will have uniformly distributed (UD) directions over a sphere. Several optimization methods have been reported to distribute the encoding N_e vertices on the diffusion gradient encoding sphere (see Hasan et al. 2001 for a more comprehensive review; also see Figure 14). These methods can be classified into three main approaches: heuristic, polyhedral, and numerical. The heuristic sets use combinations of the cubic vertices; these sets use the sides (orthogonal: x or y or z), corners (tetrahedral: x and y and z) (Conturu et al. 1996) and edge bisectors of the cube (x and y, x and z, y and z) (Basser and Pierpaoli 1998). Heuristic sets can provide N_e = 6, 7, 10, or 13 directions; these sets are not generally uniformly distributed in space (Hasan et al. 2001). The analytical solution for uniformly distributing unit vectors on the unit sphere is an unsolved problem in mathematics for an arbitrary number N_e required for tensor encoding (see references in Hasan et al. 2001; Papadakis 1999; 2000). The solution exists only for the icosahedron (Euler's Equation: V-E+F=2; 20 Faces, 12 Vertices, 30 Edges; see Hasan et al. 2001) and its dual, the dodecahedron (12-faces, 20-vertices) (Figure 15). The icosahedral vertex, face and edge centroids can thus provide 6, 10 and 15 directions (Figure 15, Tables 4-5). Face triangularization (Figure 16) with folding or frequency f can also provide more discrete sets with $N_e = 5f^2+1$, $f=1, 2, 3, ..$ ($V=10n^2+2$; $F=20n^2$; $E =3/2F$); the icosahedral set with f=2 is referred to has *Icosa21* (Tables 4-5 and Figure 15). For icosahedral schemes, the minimum angle in degrees between any adjacent pair of vertices can be expressed as

$$\alpha = \frac{180}{\pi}\arctan(2.0)\sqrt{\frac{5}{N_e-1}} \cong 63.4349^o\sqrt{\frac{5}{N_e-1}} \qquad [41]$$

This formula can be used to diagnose any proposed set against the icosahedral set. For an arbitrary number of encoding directions $N_e > 6$, the spatial distribution problem can be solved by numerically optimizing and ordering tiles of equal solid angles on a unit sphere (Hasan et al. 2001). The optimization cost function can be minimized using the constrained least-squares method subject to the scalar figure-of-merits discussed above. A comparison of numerical optimization criteria, including minimum condition number (MC), minimum tensor variance (MV), minimum force (MF) and minimum energy (ME), has been investigated previously (Hasan et al. 2001; Hasan 2000). The minimum force and energy approaches establish an analogy with the electrostatic interaction problem of N_e identically charged pair dipoles constrained on the surface of a sphere. Notice that the minimum energy approach provided the natural icosahedral set for $N_e = 6$. The numerical sets generated have to be further balanced to minimize the effect of linear cross term couplings. The balancing adjusts the sign of each encoding diffusion gradient vector and seeks to minimize the magnitude of the net sum:

$$\left\| \sum_{k=1}^{N_e} \hat{g}(k) \right\| \qquad [42]$$

The balanced numerical sets can then be called uniformly distributed tensor encoding sets.

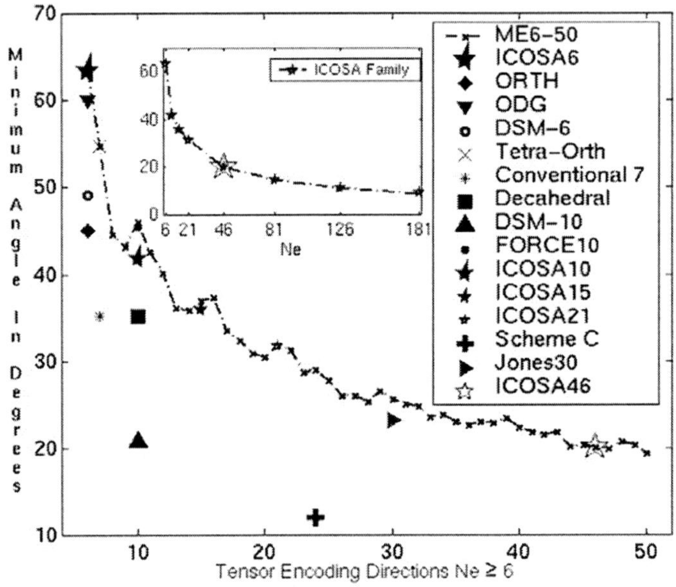

Figure 14. A summary of the minimum angle subtended between any two pairs of different heuristic, minimum energy and icosahedral tensor encoding schemes. The minimum angle should be as large as possible to warrant uniform distribution. The Icosahedral sets ($N_e = 5f^2+1$) provide an asymptotic theoretical value of the minimum angle subtended to test any arbitrary encoding set

Multi-Faceted Icosahedral Tensor Encoding Schemes

The vertices of icosahedral schemes are uniformly distributed over the unit encoding hemisphere. Thus, they are infinitely rotationally invariant subject to arbitrary orthogonal rotations (Figure 15). The Icosa21b (Table 4) and Icosa16b (Table 5) sets, by design, contain two independent icosahedral subsets (i.e. Icosa21b=Icosa6+Icosa15; Icosa16=Icosa6+ Dodecahedron (or Icosa10) (Hasan and Narayana 2003; Akkerman 2003; Batchelor et al. 2003). Notice that a rotation applied to a uniformly distributed scheme always results in a uniformly distributed set and preserves its geometrical, physical and topological properties. The schemes enjoy some unique and novel properties that are useful in the clinical setup. The data acquired with these encoding schemes can be used to estimate the diffusion tensor using the same acquired N_{ref} images but with different combinations of N_e and hence total number of images, N_T; thus providing a method for self-calibration, data navigation and quality control (Hasan and Narayana 2003; Hasan et al. 2004; Madi et al. 2005).

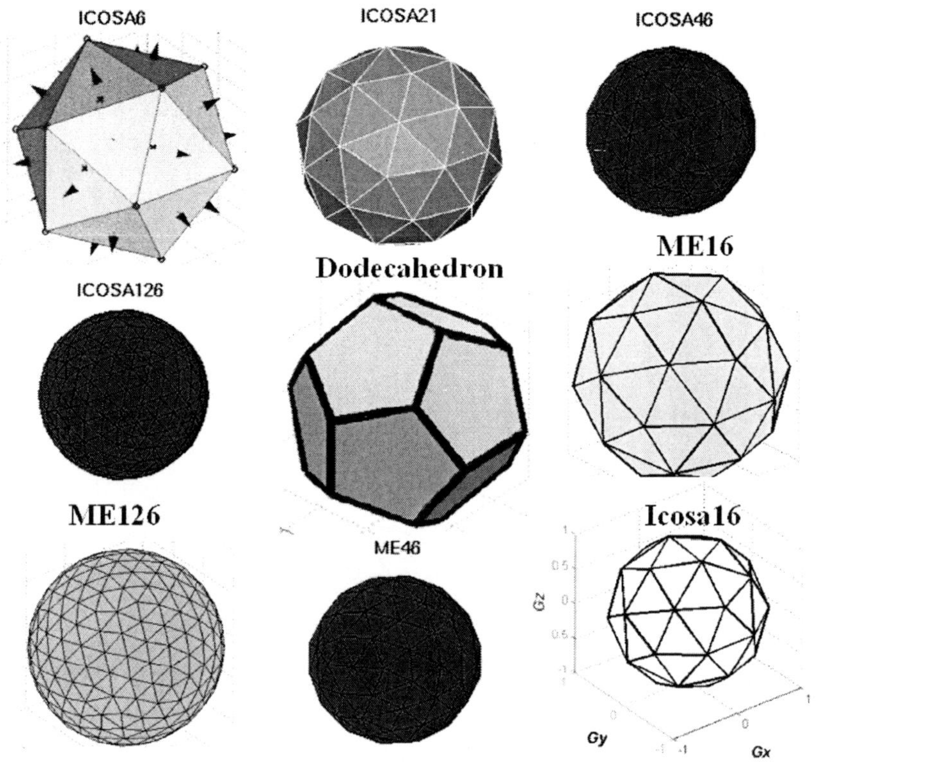

Figure 15. Triangularization of several isotropically distributed tensor encoding sets; mainly icosahedral (with discrete N_e values of 6, 10, 16, 21, 46, and 126) and minimum energy (numerical) sets with N_e =6, 16, 46, 126. Notice that the ME and Icosahedral sets for the same N_e are functionally equivalent (e.g. ME16 vs. Icosa16, Icosa46 vs. ME46, Icosa126 vs. ME126). The Icosahedral sets and their duals with $N_e > 6$ are rotationally invariant and multi-faceted which can be used to provide tensor estimates from the same data at different SNR. The vertices of Icosa21 and Icosa16 and their subsets (Icosa6, Icosa10 (or Dodecahedron), Icosa15), are listed in Tables 4 and Table 5 respectively.

Table 4. Listing of the Balanced and Normalized and Multi-Faceted Icosa21 Tensor Encoding Scheme (N_e=21)

	1	2	3	4	5	6	7	8	9	10
g_x	1	0	0	0	0	A	A	-B	-B	C
g_y	0	1	0	A	-A	-B	B	0	0	-D
g_z	0	0	1	-B	-B	0	0	A	-A	-.5

	11	12	13	14	15	16	17	18	19	20	21
g_x	C	-C	C	-.5	.5	.5	.5	-D	D	D	-D
g_y	D	-D	-D	C	-C	C	C	.5	-.5	.5	-.5
g_z	-.5	-.5	.5	D	D	-D	D	C	C	-C	-C

Define τ=2cos(π/5); A= $1/\sqrt{(1+\tau^2)}$; B= $\tau/\sqrt{(1+\tau^2)}$; C=$(\tau-1)/2$; D= $\tau/2$
The orthogonal **xyz** set is # [1,2,3]; **Icosa6** = # [4,5,6,7,8,9]; **Icosa15** = [**Icosa21-Icosa6**];
Condition number κ(**Icosa6,15,21**) ~ 1.58. To attain a 42 direction encoding scheme (uniform over the unit sphere) or Icosa21bpn follow each orientation by an opposite orientation

Table 5 Listing of the Balanced and Normalized and Multi-Faceted Icosa16 Tensor Encoding Scheme (N_e=16)

#	g_x	g_y	g_z
1	1.0000	0	0
2	-0.4472	0.8944	0
3	-0.4472	-0.7236	-0.5257
4	-0.4472	-0.7236	0.5257
5	-0.4472	0.2764	-0.8507
6	-0.4472	0.2764	0.8507
7	0.7947	0.6071	0
8	-0.1876	-0.9822	0
9	0.1876	0.3035	0.9342
10	0.1876	0.3035	-0.9342
11	-0.7947	0.4911	-0.3568
12	-0.7947	0.4911	0.3568
13	0.7947	0.1876	0.5774
14	0.1876	-0.7947	-0.5774
15	0.1876	-0.7947	0.5774
16	0.7947	0.1876	-0.5774

Icosa6 = # [1,2,3,4,5,6]; Icosa10 = [Icosa16-Icosa6];
Condition number κ(Icosa6,10,16) ~ 1.58. To attain a 32 direction encoding scheme (uniform over the unit sphere) or Icosa16bpn follow each orientation by an opposite orientation (alternating polarity).

Combining these multi-faceted schemes with an alternating polarity approach has been utilized at high fields (7.0 T) in imaging the spinal cord of living rats using implanted coils (Madi et al. 2005). Additionally, it has been demonstrated that icosahedral schemes can provide the fractional anisotropy from the raw diffusion weighted data without diagonalization or tensor decoding and hence offering a real time method for the computation of the mean diffusivity and tensor anisotropy (Hasan and Narayana 2003; Akkerman 2003).

DTI Extensions and Acquisition Flavors

A typical DT-MRI experiment is commonly performed using a spin-echo prepared single-shot echo-planar imaging (SS-EPI) sequence with bipolar diffusion encoding gradient pulses applied along the three physical gradient channels (Stejskal and Tanner 1965; Taylor and Bushell 1985; Callaghan 1994; Le Bihan 1995) (Figure 8, Figure 11). The measured diffusion sensitized signal is a superposition of spatially dependent incoherent phases, acquired due to random translational Brownian motion during the application of spatially dependent diffusion encoding magnetic field (Torrey 1956; Stejskal and Tanner 1965; Price 1997; 1998). Although there are different acquisition methodologies (Table 1), processing strategies (Le Bihan 1995; Hasan and Narayana 2003) and interpretation flavors (Cohen and Assaf 2002; Assaf et al. 2002) such as q-space (Q-ball, high angular resolution diffusion (HARDI), diffusion spectrum imaging or DSI (Lin et al. 2003), spherical harmonic decomposition, non-Gaussian and higher order tensor imaging) (Frank 2002; Tuch 2004), and multiple tensors (Le Bihan 1995; Mulkern et al. 1999; Clark et al. 2002), the "conventional" single tensor model approach was adopted in this chapter (Le Bihan 1995; Basser 1995;1996; Hasan et al. 2001; 2002; 2003; 2004; 2005). Direct data driven methods such as principal components, independent components (Arfanakis et al. 2002c) and real time computation of anisotropy using icosahedral schemes have also been reported (see Hasan and Narayana 2003). It has been shown by P. J. Basser (2002) that the single tensor model is a practical option in a clinical setup if the acquisition parameters are carefully selected. Current clinical scanners enable the acquisition of the single tensor (conventional cDTI) for the entire brain in about five minutes. The main goal of the extension of cDTI is to increase the specificity of the estimated information, and overcome the limitations encountered due to partial volume averaging as a result of multiple crossing fibers or compartmental exchange in the voxel (Shimony et al. 1999; Wiegell et al. 2000; Alexander et al. 2001; Frank 2002; Lin et al. 2003; Tuch 2004). In simple excised tissue, geometric diffusion restrictions and barriers have also been shown to be resolved with q-space imaging and in providing clues to a more specific interpretation of the signal sources without the assumption of Gaussian or free diffusion (Assaf et al. 2002; Cohen and Assaf 2002). In the slow exchange regime (compartment size is smaller than the diffusion distance), the signal obtained upon applying a gradient pulse over the diffusion time and sampled at some echo time T_E and replication time T_R can be modeled as a superposition from different compartments which have multiple fiber tensor orientations (Le Bihan 1995; Karger 1988; Callaghan 1994).

$$S(n)=\sum_{c=1}^{N_c}\sum_{f=1}^{N_f}S_0(f,c)\exp(-\frac{T_E}{T_2(c,f))})(1-\exp(-\frac{T_R}{T_1(c,f)})\exp(-(\gamma Gd\delta)^2(\Delta-\frac{\delta}{3})\hat{g}_d(n)^t D(c,f)\hat{g}_d(n)) \qquad [43]$$

The separation of all fiber tensor orientations and compartments may be intractable and clearly requires higher spatial resolution, strong and short diffusion magnetic gradient pulses, and more scanning time for multiple b-factors, temporal averaging and high angular encoding vector distribution, which is clinically prohibitive. In general, these variant methods may be model or data dependent, require a specialized sampling grid (e.g. concentric icosahedral shells) and involve operations such as Laplace, Fourier or specialized transform methods, spherical harmonic deconvolution and non-linear least-squares. Simplifications, phantom models and special cases have been validated and used on excised animal spinal cords, single neurons and optic nerves (Lin et al. 2003; Schwartz et al. 2005; Grant et al. 2001). The utility of q-space for understanding multiple sclerosis pathology has also been demonstrated by Assaf et al. (2002). Notice that to attain the largest possible b-factor with the shortest echo time, some encoding schemes (tetra-orth, ODG, icosahedral) need not be normalized on the unit sphere and a multi-b tensorial approach can be sought on a cube to maximize the time efficiency of the DTI experiment (Hasan et al. 2002; Conturo et al. 1996; Hasan et al. 2001). In summary, this section was intended as an overview of these nascent, time-consuming variants; the interested readers should consult Cohen and Assaf (2002) and Tuch (2004 and Thesis) for more recent reviews.

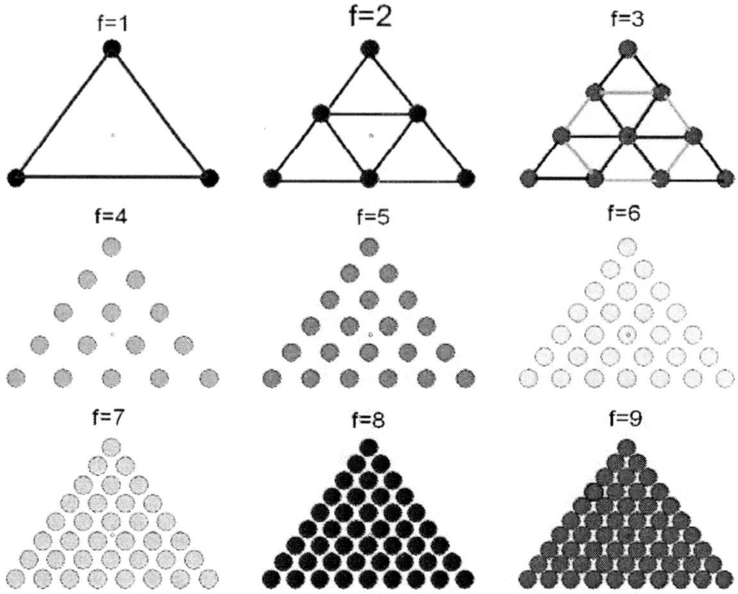

Figure 16. Illustration of the triangularization procedure applied on all faces of the principla icosahedraon to generate discrete uniform sets with with frequency f (N_e =5f^2+1). The figure shows the procedure for f=1,2,..,9. The case when f=2 corresponds to Icosa21 which is further mapped onto the unit sphere

Materials and Methods

Subjects

A total of 91 entire brain DTI sets were obtained from 10 healthy children (9-16.5 years), 32 healthy adults (21-64 years; 16 males and 16 females), and 49 clinically diagnosed multiple sclerosis patients aged (19-69 years). The MS group included twenty six clinically-definite relapsing-remitting (RRMS) patients (22 females, 4 males; mean age ± SD = 37.9±11.7) while the 32 age-matched healthy adult controls (16 females, 16 males; age = 38.1±12.1 years) were included in these studies. The median extended disability status score (EDSS) for the 26 RRMS patients was 1.25 (range 0.0, 6.0) and the median disease duration (DD) to imaging was 7.6 yrs (range 0.3, 17.6). All RRMS patients were on medication for a variable period at the time of MRI data acquisition. The four pediatric traumatic brain injured (TBI) cases that have been investigated in these studies had a mean age at injury of 8.1 years; the mean age at DT-MRI was 12.9 years. The ten normal controls, NDC1-NDC10, (nine males and one female, average age at scan ± SD: 13.9±2.1 years; range 9-16.5 yrs), included fraternal (NDC6) and identical twins (NDC7) to TBI3 and TBI4 respectively. The age difference between the two groups was not significant (two-tailed t-test, p=0.4). Our studies were approved by the Committee for the Protection of Human Subjects, University of Texas Health Science Center at Houston, and written consent was obtained from all subjects or their guardians.

Diffusion Tensor Image Acquisition Experiments: 1.5T and 3.0 T

Full human brain conventional MRI (FLAIR, turbo spin echo, Gadolinium enhanced on MS patients) and same graphically prescribed DTI measurements were acquired on both General Electric 1.5 T (neurovascular optimized MR scanner, LX echo speed, version 8.4-9.1) using a quadrature (transmit/receive) head coil and a gradient system with a slew rate of 150 T/m/s and a maximum gradient amplitude of 40 mT/m. Further details of the data acquisition are provided in Hasan et al. (2005). Data were also collected on a Philips 3.0 Tesla Intera scanner with a Quasar gradient system. An optimum tensor encoding scheme with $N_e=21$ directions (Hasan et al. 2001) (*Icosa21b_ord,* Table 4 and Figure 15) was incorporated into the spin-echo prepared EPI (see Figures 7, 11) that utilized a ramp and under k_y sampling using a parallel imaging multi-channel receiver head coil with a SENSE acceleration or k-space undersampling factor of R=2. The image matrix = 256x256, $FOV=240$ mm, # axial sections/slice thickness/space between slices = 44/3 mm/0 mm. The gradient strength was tuned to achieve a b-factor of $b=1000\ s\ mm^{-2}$. The number of b ~ 0 images, $I(0)$, used was N_{ref} = 8 and the N_d=2; another set was acquired by alternating the polarity (N_d=1), keeping the imaging time constant.

Data Processing and Analysis

The diffusion-weighted (DW) data were transferred to a work station via ftp. The data were then spatially filtered using a median 3x3 filter. Novel image spatial denoising methods have also been reported by Hahn et al. (2004). While acquisition of the DTI data at 1.5 T with the dual echo EPI sequence (Reese et al. 2003) and ramp sampling considerably reduce, but do not eliminate, the geometric distortions. The residual distortions were corrected by registering the diffusion-weighted images with the reference image using the 2-D module of the automated image registration (AIR) package (8 parameter with perspective; Wood et al. 1998). Another efficient approach uses the b=0 volumes and mutual information maximization (Netsch et al. 2004). Furthermore, since the corpus callosum is located close to the center of the image, the susceptibility-induced distortions in this region are expected to be fairly minimal. Based on our observations, the distortion was minimal along the frequency encoding or x-direction and largest along the phase encoding or y-direction. The DWI data processing pipeline is illustrated in Figure 9 on a normal brain data set acquired with the *Icosa21b* scheme. Diffusion tensor decoding, cubic voxel interpolation, diagonalization and D_{av} and *FA* computation were performed using the in-house developed DTI design and analysis toolbox that is based on the generalized decoding (Hasan et al. 2001) and the analytical diagonalization methods (Hasan et al. 2001b) written under IDL (Research Systems: Boulder, Co). Figures 17-18 describe the DTI design, processing and modules in the DTI toolbox.

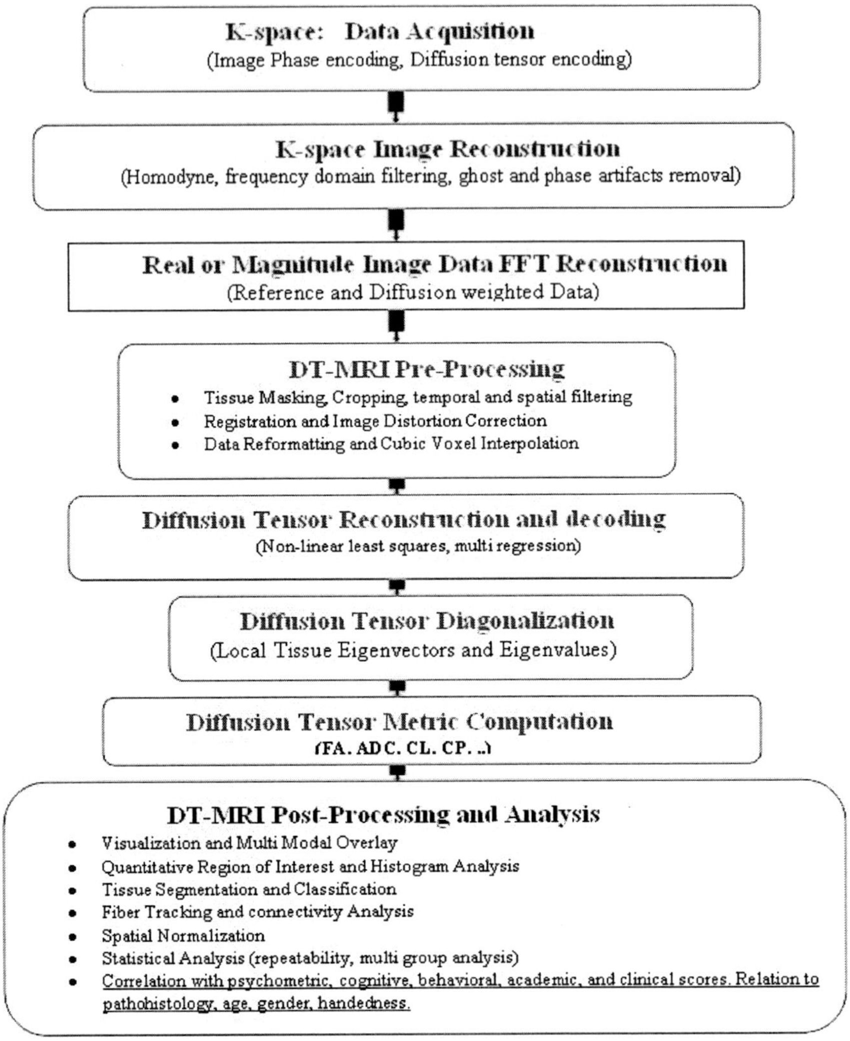

Figure 17. A schematic illustration of the major preprocessing, processing, and postprocessing steps involved in DTI (see also Figure 9).

Region-of-Interest Selection and DTI Data Overlay Method

In general, there are three approaches to present the DTI information. The first method uses entire brain histograms and has limited utility and lacks spatial specificity (Bammer and Fazekas 2002; Henry et al. 2003; Nusbaum et al. 2001). The second method invokes anatomical landmarks and trained rater skills for region-of-interest placement (Chepuri et al. 2002; Hasan et al. 2005; Moeller et al. 2005). The ROI method is the most common method in published DTI reports. The third method is hypothesis-generating and analyzes the data voxel-wise after spatial normalization to a standardized template (Jones et al. 2002; Xu et al. 2003; Ashtari et al. 2005; Ardekani et al. 2003; Agartz et al. 2001). A detailed analysis of the merits, pitfalls and limitations of these methods and their challenging application to pathology and DTI is beyond the scope of this chapter (Bookstein 2001; Ashburner and Friston 2001; Davatzikos 2004). To increase the utility of DTI in neurological disorders, we have implemented ROI procedures that allow the visualization of three-dimensional maps of fiber orientation along any direction and have fused the DTI maps with any other data set including conventional FLAIR and dual spin echo images. Since the DTI maps are self-registered, we have found the FA modulated principal vector (e_1) map fused with D_{av}, T2w, FLAIR, exp($-b*D_{av}$) maps or any co-registered map to be useful in the ROI placement and visualization of compact fiber bundles in the vicinity of MS lesions. An example of this image fusion is shown in Figures 1-2, 4-6). This method considerably helped identify and avoid partial averaging from adjacent gray matter or CSF in the ROI placement.

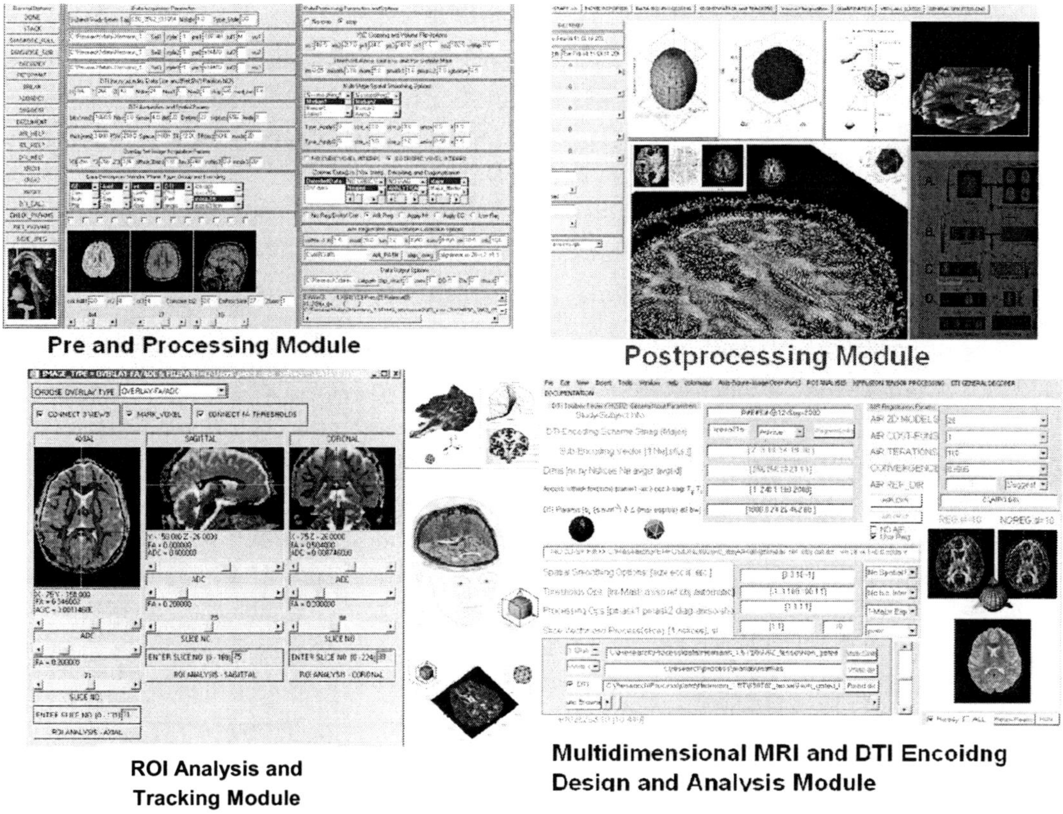

Figure 18. Illustration of the different DTI design, processing and analysis modules that are used to obtain quantitative ROI and qualitative connectivity information.

Witelson Subdivision of the Corpus Callosum and ROI Placements

A semi-automated sub-regional division of the corpus callosum as described by Witelson (1985) and used in other non-DTI studies (Highley et al. 1999; Aboitiz et al. 1992; Levin et al. 2000; Hardan et al. 2000; Giedd et al. 1994), was implemented (Hasan et al. 2004; Hasan et al. 2005) in which the CC was divided into seven segments. The DTI-guided Witelson subdivisions described above was identified on the midsagittal section from the reformatted axial DTI data after isotropic voxel interpolation and used the column of the fornix and inter-thalamic mass as anatomical landmarks (see Figure 2 and Hasan et al. 2005 for more details).

Compact Fiber Bundle Tracking

To demonstrate the feasibility of connecting adjacent and directionally similar voxels in the normal appearing white matter (NAWM) of the CC, we used the fiber assignment by continuous tracking (FACT) approach (Mori and Van Zijl 2002; Xu et al. 2002). The initial seeds for fiber tracking were placed in the seven segments of the CC (Figure 2) with a tracking threshold of $FA \geq 0.2$. Additional seeds were also placed in the corticospinal tract and in the posterior limb of the internal capsule (Figure 2).

DTI Data Collection and Processing Quality Control

Since the data were collected over a period of one year and involved region-of-interest (ROI) placement by trained raters, the results of the ROI analysis on the same subjects from two independent sessions were compared. For b-factor calibration and residual eddy current distortion correction, we have also collected the DTI data on a spherical water phantom. The large diffusion encoding gradients induce mechanical motion that could compromise the estimated DTI measures. In order to ascertain that mechanical vibrations have minimal effect on the DTI measures, we performed temporal and spatial stability and bootstrap analyses on water phantoms and human brains as described elsewhere (Hasan et al. 2004; Madi et al. 2005; Pejevic and Basser 2003; Hasan 2002).

Statistical Analysis

For group age and gender differences, a student t-test and a Chi square test were used respectively. The confidence level was set at 95% unless otherwise stated. Statistical significance for the intracallosal comparisons of the seven segments of the CC was evaluated using analysis of variance (ANOVA). To investigate the effect of gender on the intracallosal heterogeneity of the CC segments on the FA, a two-way ANOVA followed by post-hoc multiple paired t-tests were performed. For comparison between two populations in the same ROI $(N_{1,2}{}^{k}, \mu_{1,2}{}^{k}, \sigma_{1,2}{}^{k})$ with known number of samples, group means and standard errors, the effect size and t-test ($F=t^2$) are given by (Glantz 2002):

$$es^k = \frac{\mu_1{}^k - \mu_2{}^k}{\sqrt{\dfrac{(N^k{}_1 - 1)(\sigma_1{}^k)^2 + (N^k{}_2 - 1)(\sigma_2{}^k)^2}{(N^k{}_1 + N^k{}_2 - 2)}}}$$

$$t_{1,2}{}^k = \frac{es^k}{\sqrt{\dfrac{1}{N_1} + \dfrac{1}{N_2}}} \qquad [44]$$

For paired comparisons of mean differences of two different regions (1, 2) on the same subjects with correlation coefficient r, the t-statistic is given by:

$$t_{1,2(paired)}^{\ \ k} = \frac{\mu_1^{\ k} - \mu_2^{\ k}}{\sqrt{\frac{\left(\sigma_1^{\ k}\right)^2 + \left(\sigma_2^{\ k}\right)^2 - 2r^k \sigma_1^{\ k} \sigma_2^{\ k}}{N^k}}} \quad [45]$$

The Bonferroni procedure was adopted to adjust the significant alpha whenever multiple comparisons were done (Glantz 2002). For intracallosal comparisons, spatial covariances between adjacent CC segments were also incorporated and the smallest p value provided by the four methods Tukey-Kramer, Bonferroni, Scheffe and Dunn-Sidak was used for significance. In general, the Bonferroni method is the most conservative and the significance p for the 21 (7*6/2) comparisons was set ≤ 0.002 (alpha $< 0.05/21$). Statistical significance of FA and D_{av} values for comparisons between different regions of the CC was determined by using a one-way ANOVA. The differences between group means were computed by a two-tailed t-test for unpaired comparisons. Notice that the t-test in this case is equivalent to ANOVA for two groups. For intercallosal comparisons between groups, the Bonferroni adjustment of the significant alpha was accounted for by setting the significance level $\leq 0.05/7 \sim 0.007$ (7 group comparisons or subdivisions of the corpus callosum used in this work). The DTI measures (FA, D_{av}) were also correlated with EDSS, and disease duration using Spearman's rank correlation coefficient. For repeatability analysis, we have used the Bland-Altman analysis.

Results

Encoding Schemes Comparison and Minimum Angle Test

Figure 14 compares the minimum angle computed from the vector dot product of all pairs in a family of isotropic icosahedral encoding sets constrained to the unit encoding sphere, as well as other heuristic approaches. The icosahedral family is used to provide the theoretical asymptotic values for all encoding sets. Note that the observations made in the previous section are still valid. Figures 15-16 shows a triangularization of some minimum energy (ME) and icosahedral encoding sets. Notice that the ME procedure can generate isotropically distributed encoding sets with *arbitrary* N_e; whereas, the icosahedral based sets are limited to the *discrete* values of $N_e=5f^2+1$, $f=1, 2, 3, 4$...(Hasan 2000; Hasan 2001). In addition, the minimum energy encoding sets (ME) are indistinguishable from the icosahedral for $N_e = 6$, 15, 16, 21, and 46 (Figure 15). The conventional-7 (x, y, z, xy, xz, yz, xyz), Jones30, and Force10 encoding schemes are described in (Jones et al. 1999). The decahedral, DSM-6 and DSM-10 are minimum condition sets (Skare et al. 2000). The ORTH scheme uses x, y, z, xy, xz, and yz cubic vertices. The scaled tetra-orth scheme (Hasan et al. 2001) is used in Nye (1957) and Shimony et al. (1999). The minimum angle is a sensitive, simple and practical test to characterize the bias and sensitivity of tensor encoding sets. The angle has to be as large as possible when an optimal UD configuration is attained (Papadakis et al. 2000) (Figure 14-16).

Application of Entire Brain DTI at 1.5 T and 3.0 T to Mapping the Human Brain

Figure 19 provides preliminary examples of the utility of DTI at 1.5 T and 3.0 T (Hasan and Narayana 2005). The figures demonstrate using and fusing optimized DTI and conventional MRI protocols in mapping the human brain in less than six minutes at 3.0 T. The entire brain DTI data set was further used to perform compact fiber tracking.

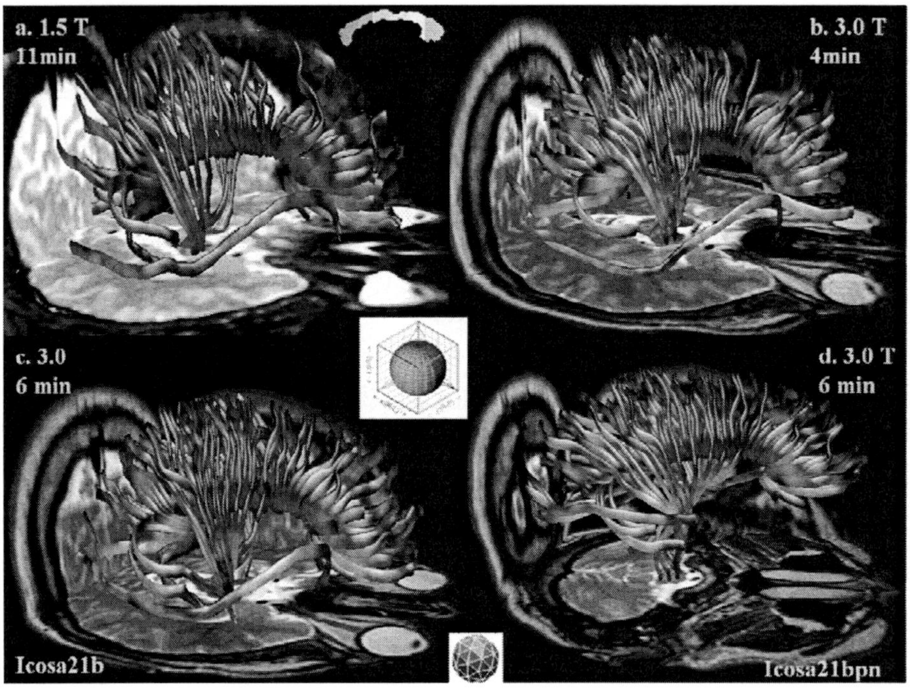

Figure 19. Illustration of the feasibility of entire brain DTI fiber tracking on the same subject at 3.0 T in 4.0 minutes (a) data acquired in 11 minutes @ 1.5 T (b) 4 minutes @ 3.0 T © 6 minutes at 3.0 T and 6 minutes without diffusion weighted averaging and at equal time to c but with alternating the Icosa21b polarity. Notice the high quality of compact fiber tracks (projection, commissural and association) at 3.0 T in the short time of 4 minutes. Notice that each data set two additional data subsets that were used for quality control (data not shown).

Figure 20 shows the excellent quality of compact fiber tracks acquired at 3.0 T on another healthy subject imaged using the same b-factor, encoding scheme (Icosa21b) T_E, T_R, slice thickness and other image parameters. The total imaging time was varied via altering N_{ref} and N_d and using the alternating polarity option instead of multiple repeated averaging. The scan time can further be reduced by shortening T_R, keeping the slice coverage largest and the echo time shortest. The latter option appeals to a future upgrade in system gradient hardware which will attain acceptable DTI scan using single-shot EPI in approximately three minutes.

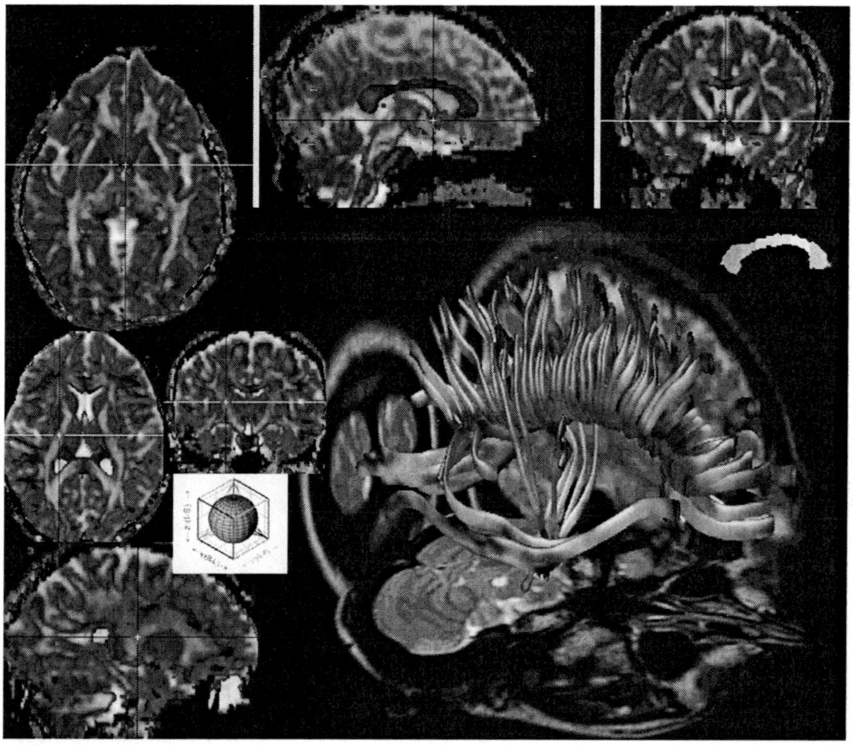

Figure 20. Illustration of the utility of optimized DTI at 3.0 T in 6 minutes in building the digital fiber atlas of the normal human brain. The data set is the same as in Figure 12. The connected multi plane views are used in seed placement for fiber tracking. Notice the connections of the callosal fibers (red-commissural fibers RL) and the cortico-spinal track (blue-projection fibers-SI) and association pathways (green-AP)

Quantitative and Qualitative Results

DTI anisotropy maps have good contrast between white and gray matter, and magnitude images have good contrast between cerebrospinal fluid and gray or white matter. The DTI maps are also co-registered and are free from coil related biases. Thus, multiparametric volumetry MRI methods can be used with DTI maps. The feature vector in this case can be anisotropy, eigenvalues or the local coherence (Carano et al. 2000; Sajja et al. 2004). In addition, semiautomated regional segmentation or specific structures such as the corpus callosum and combined with subdivision paradigms such as that of Witelson. Figure 21 provides a preliminary example of a promising application of DTI in tissue classification, regional and global tissue morphometry (Hasan et al. 2005).

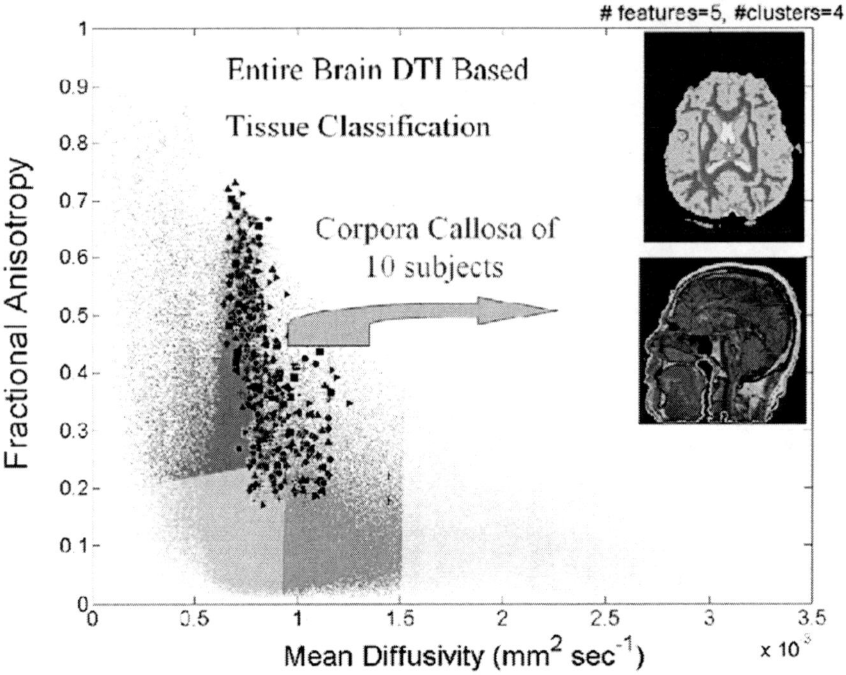

Figure 21. Illustration of the feasibility of using DTI co-registered information (eigenvalues, FA) to perform tissue global classification and regional segmentation. The segmentation done here uses a k-means approach

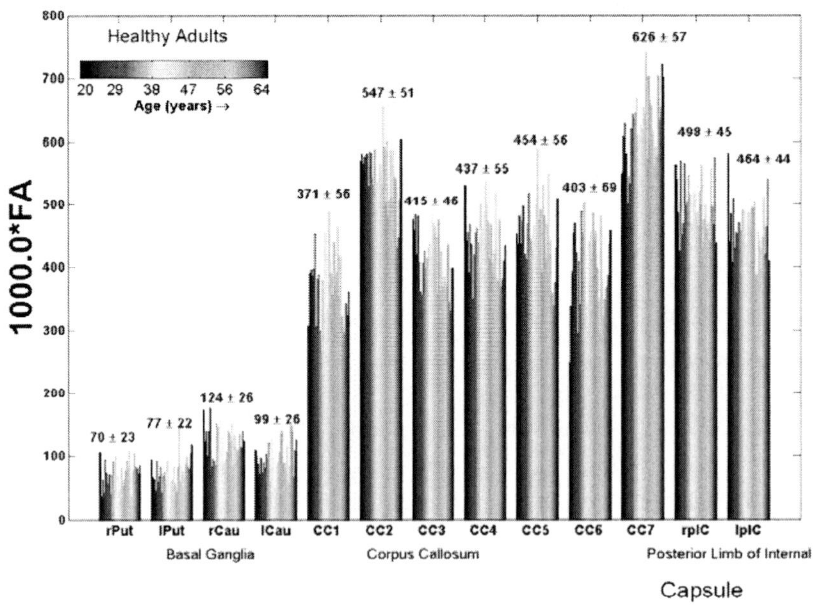

Figure 22. A bar plot of regional FA values (13 structures in Figure 2) obtained from the 32 healthy adults grouped by age. Notice the FA heterogeneity of the corpus callosum. The splenium of the CC attains the highest anisotropy of any other structure

Inter and Intracallosal Comparisons on Age-Matched Male and Female Healthy Adults

Figure 22 shows the pooled regional FA results of the post-hoc analysis of the values of FA of different segments of the CC and other tissue structures (see Figure 2) for both the healthy age-matched male and female controls. The stratification by gender (Figure 23) was conducted to assure that the results are not due to the bias in the gender distribution in our adult MS patients. The spatial heterogeneity of FA tensor anisotropy in the CC is observed to be gender-independent in the healthy controls as evaluated by the two-way ANOVA analysis (Figure 23).

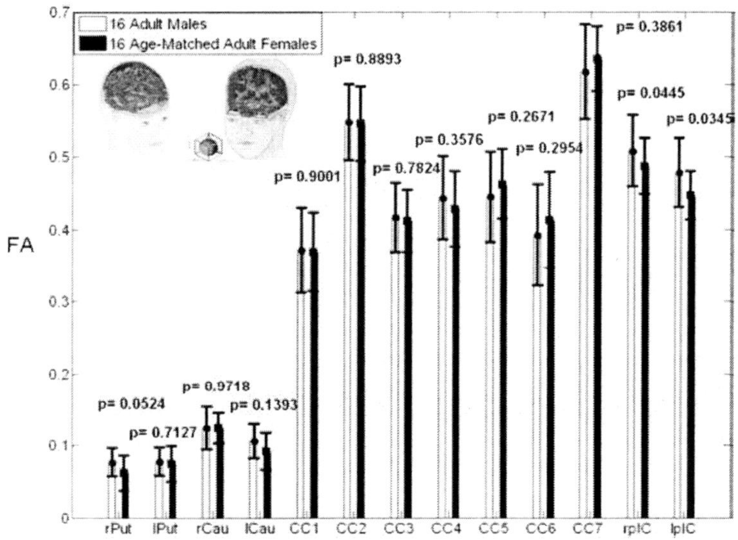

Figure 23. A bar plot showing the comparison of FA group means and SD (□ ± □) of the 13 gray and white matter structures (Figure 2) including the seven subdivisions of the corpus callosum between the age-matched healthy males and females. Notice the lack of statistical significance between the age-matched male and female adults in these brain regions

The corresponding follow-up paired t-test comparisons are shown in Figure 23. For intracallosal comparisons, the FA values of the anterior, middle and posterior CC subdivisions were significantly different ($p<0.002$) and FA (splenium) > FA (genu) > FA (body) in normal adults, children and patients (see below). This trend was observed for both genders. Thus, both male and female data were pooled to reduce redundant comparisons and possible loss of statistical power due to small populations.

Normative vs. Pathological FA and D_{av} CC Spatial Distribution and Inter-Group Comparisons

Figure 24 graphically summarizes the results of the comparison of FA between the 32 healthy adults and the 26 RRMS patients. The figure shows group means, standard error of the mean and the corresponding p values of the group differences. The FA values of posterior, anterior, and midbody were significantly different ($p<0.002$) in normal controls. This regional heterogeneity was also observed in MS patients, FA(posterior CC) > FA(anterior CC) > FA(middlle CC) for both controls and patients. The FA values were significantly *decreased* in the MS patients compared to the controls in the CC4 (anterior; $p=0.0039$) and CC5 (posterior; $p=0.0018$) midbody segments, and that did not reach statistical significance in the CC1, CC6 and CC7 segments.

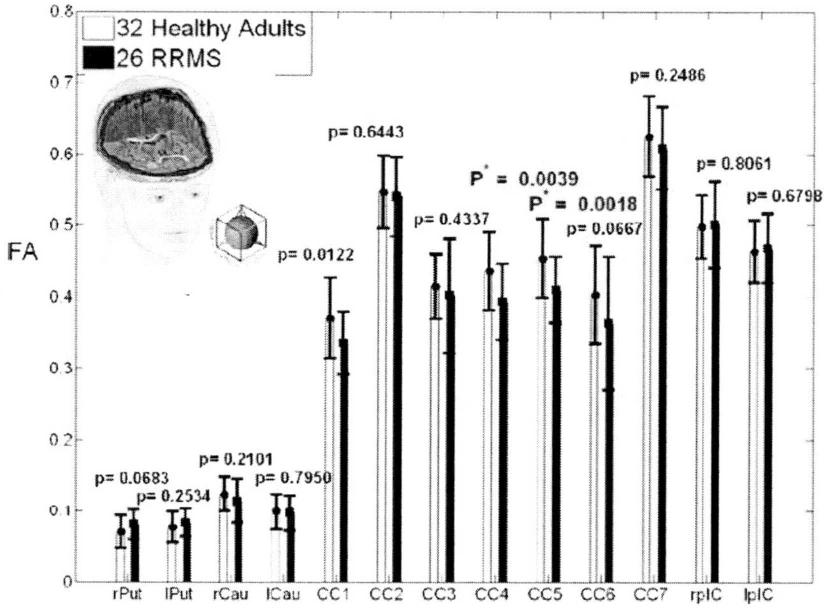

Figure 24. A bar-plot of the mean and SD fractional anisotropy values of the 13 structures (Figure 2) including the seven segments of the CC in the 26 RRMS group and the 32 age-matched healthy adult controls. The p values are computed using the two-tailed t-test for unequal samples. The significance level is taken as 0.007. FA(MS) < FA(Controls): FA(splenium) > FA(genu) > FA(body of CC) and CC4-CC5 are significantly different between the two groups

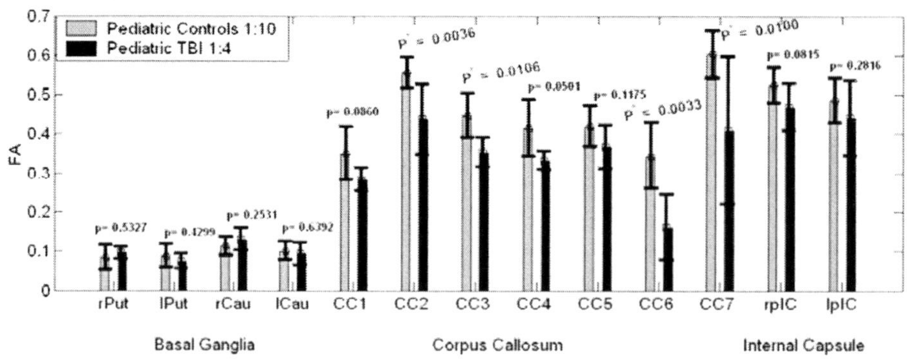

Figure 25. A bar-plot of the mean and SD fractional anisotropy values of the 13 structures (Figure 2) including the seven segments of the CC in the 4 pediatric TBI and the 10 age-matched healthy children controls. The p values are computed using the two-tailed t-test for unequal samples. The significance level is taken as 0.007. FA(TBI) < FA(Controls): The frontal and posterior segments of the corpus callosum have reduced anisotropy reflecting.

Healthy Children vs. Pediatric Trauma

Figure 25 shows the FA ROI values of the 13 structures obtained from the healthy age-matched and TBI children. Notice the reduction in anisotropy in the splenium and genu of the CC and the relative similarity of anisotropy in other white and gray matter structures.

Longitudinal Fiber Tracking of MS and Traumatic Brain Injury

Figure 26 provides an illustration of the potential of conventional MRI and DTI in multiple sclerosis and pediatric brain trauma research conducted on the same patients longitudinally on both 1.5 T and 3.0 T. The ability to fuse and use conventional MRI data, and segmented cMRI with DTI along with longitudinal DTI fiber tracking provided important longitudinal information about the effect of lesion proximity and fiber connectivity (Charil et al. 2003; Oh et al. 2004) that can be useful for diagnosis, treatment and patient management. Notice the effect of reduced anisotropy in the body of CC (MS) and splenium-genu in the TBI child on the tracking. The correlation of these preliminary observations with disease duration, clinical and behavioral dysfunction is being examined (Hasan et al. 2004; Hasan et al. 2005). Figure 27-28 illustrates another novel application of DTI and cMRI in the study of the pathogenesis and longitudinal evolution of MS lesions, callosal and brain atrophy.

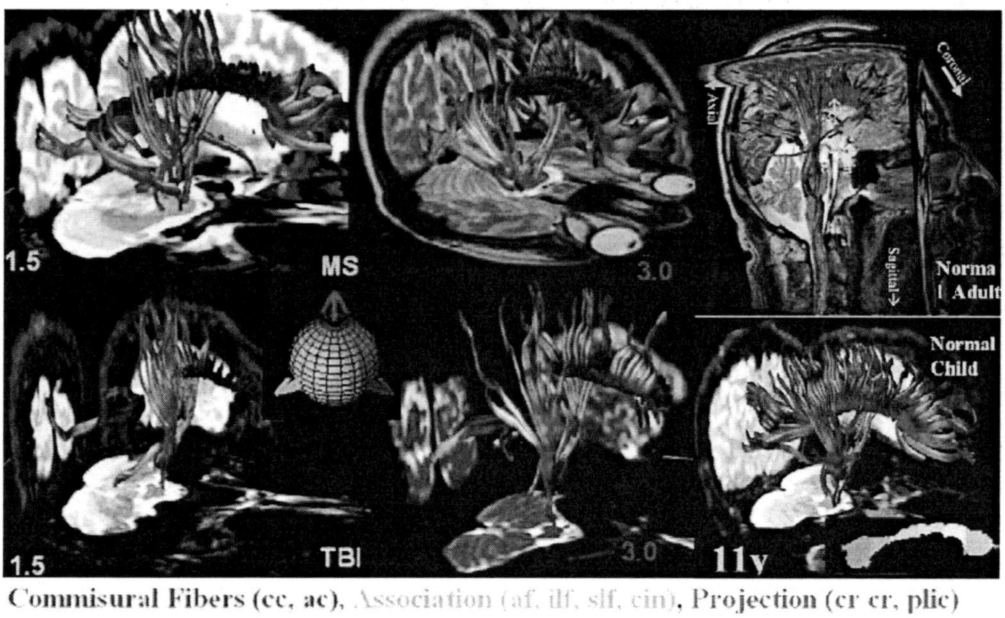

Figure 26. Illustration of the feasibility of compact fiber tracking using entire brain high angular resolution icosahedral DTI data acquisition on both relapsing and remitting adult patients and TBI children. The figure also shows the complementary role of fused DTI and conventional MRI in localizing lesions and providing clues on the pathogenesis and evolution of MS lesions (adult) and diffuse axonal injury in TBI (child) on the same subjects at both 1.5 T and 3.0 T. The figure has also the corresponding age-matched control data sets (se also Figures 19, 20).

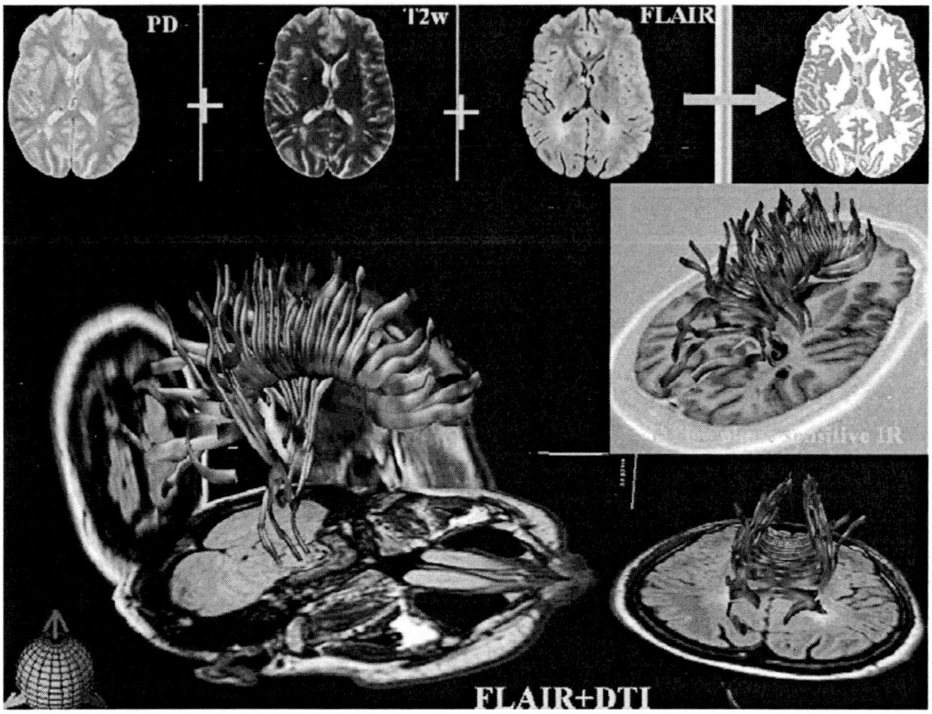

Figure 27. Illustration of the potential of compact fiber tracking and the utility of conventional MRI in lesion localization and segmentation at 3.0 T. DTI provides structural connectivity of the affected lesion and can quantify the effect of lesion proximity on the tensor anisotropy and eigenvalues

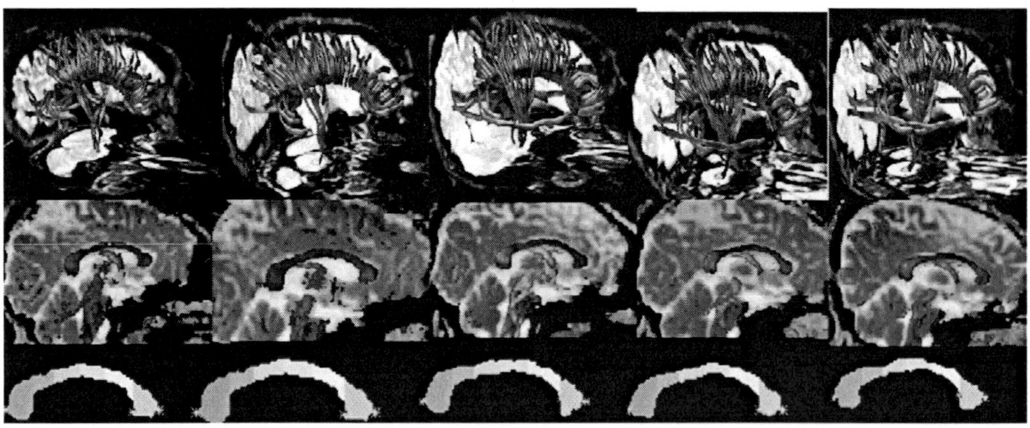

Figure 28. An illustration of the ability and future of DTI in longitudinal mentoring of entire brain or regional atrophy. The Figure shows the same RRMS scanned over 5 times separated by three months using the same protocol and 1.5 T MRI scanner

Age Dependence of the Splenium and Genu FA

The genu and splenium corpus callosum regional FA anisotropy values are plotted as function of age for the 91 subjects in Figure 29. Notice the relative uniformity of the splenium FA across the 9-69 years life span. The genu curve indicates a decreasing trend with age. Figure 30 provides a qualitative medio-lateral view of the human CC of the ages 4 days to 60 years. Notice the adult-like appearance of the frontal and posterior portion of the human brains during the first year. The body of the CC anisotropy seemingly requires more time to mature possibly due to axonal elimination and active myelination and migration of Oligodedrocytes.

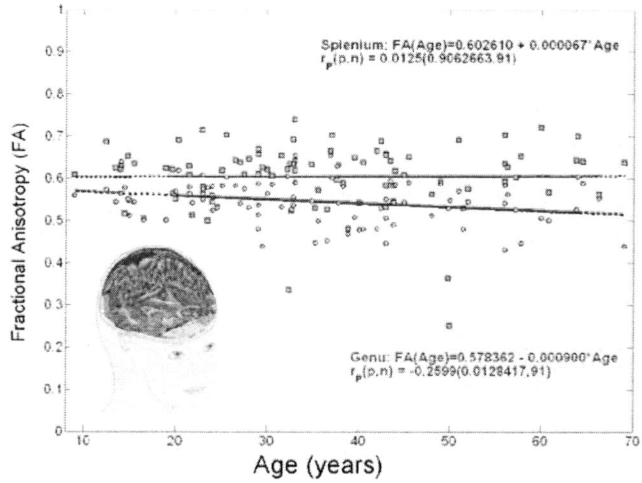

Figure 29. A plot of the regional FA values in the normally appearing genu and splenium of the corpus callosum of the 91 subjects spanning the age 9-69 years. Notice the significant decrease in the genu anisotropy compared to the relative constancy of the splenium

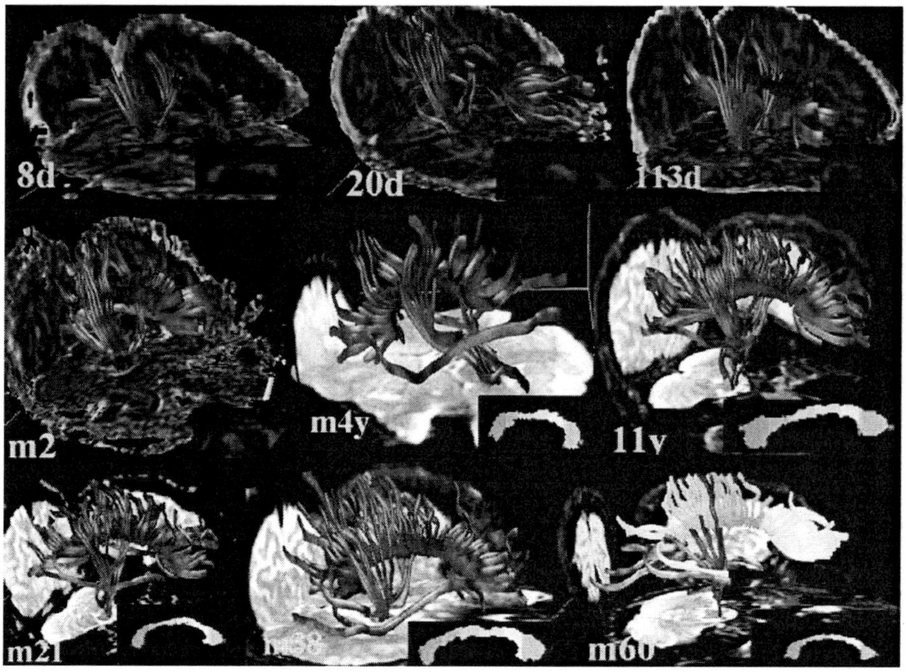

Figure 30. An illustration of the potential of DTI in mapping the healthy developing and aging human brain from birth (~ 4 days) till the 6th decade (~ 64 years). Notice the evolution and appearance of the body of the corpus callosum and the relative maturation of the genu, splenium and corticospinal tracts

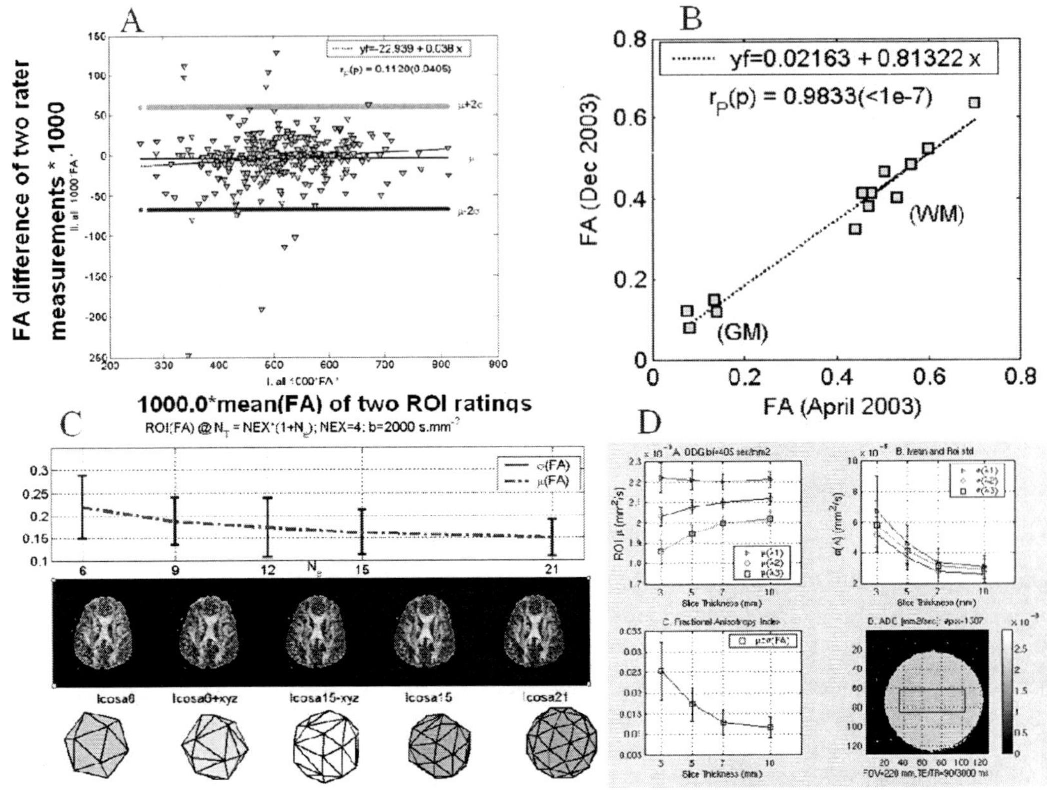

Figure 31. An illustration of the different quality control tests and protocols used to assure the consistency and accuracy of the DTI data. (A) A Bland-Altman bias analysis of the FA results (x 1000.0) obtained from all regions and all subjects studied upon repeating the analysis. The horizontal axis shows the mean of two rating sessions, the vertical axis shows the difference of the two sessions. The linear regression least squares fit curve shows no significant trend between the two rating sessions. (B) Same subject, same rater and same regions FA repeatability analysis which shows excellent reproducibility and scanner stability over an 8 month span. (C) an analysis showing the dependence of the estimated FA anisotropy on the signal-to-noise ratio (total imaging time); notice the reduction in FA as SNR increases and the effect of rotational variance on the estimated SD. (D) The effect of SNR through variation of the slice thickness on the estimated DTI metrics (eigenvalues, anisotropy). These empirical results on the water phantom confirm simulation studies and the brain measurements.

Quality Control and Repeatability of FA

A Bland-Altman bias analysis of the FA results obtained from 13 ROIs of 69 subjects is performed to assess the reproducibility; in addition, same subject measurements were also conducted periodically to test the stability of the hardware. Figure 31 shows the reproducibility of our results and the dependence of anisotropy on predictable DTI parameters (slice thickness, encoding scheme, total time, etc.) as explained by the theory. Figure 32 illustrates the effect of measurement noise (small voxel size) on the fidelity of fiber tracking results confirming the theoretical predictions mad in the theory (Anderson 2001). Other empirical methods such as the Bootstrap analysis and the water phantom anisotropy plot as function of total number of images show reproducible results (Hasan et al. 2004; Madi et al. 2005; Hasan 2000).

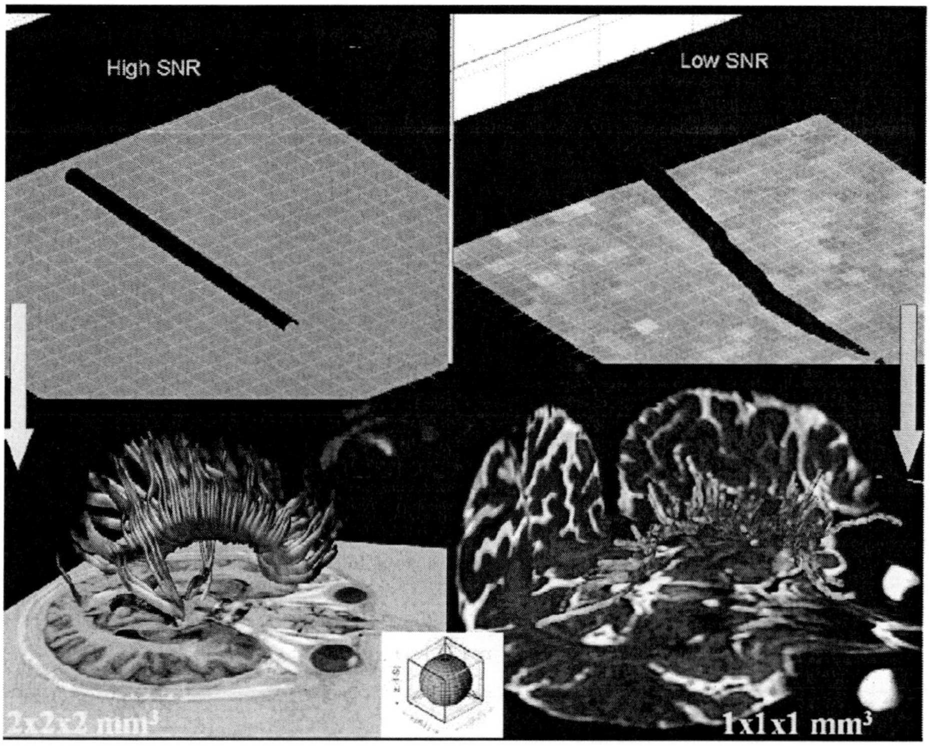

Figure 32. An illustration of the effect of measurement noise and low SNR through slice thickness on the fiber tracking fidelity shown on both simulated and human brain data acquired at 3.0 T with isotropic voxel volumes of 8 mm^3 (High SNR) and 1 mm^3 (low SNR) Notice the track deviation (or dispersion) at low SNR of the compact corpus callosum tracts which is also predicted by the theory section (see also Anderson 2001).

Discussion

Normal CC Anisotropy Heterogeneity and Age Dependence

Using optimized DTI acquisition and combined with accurate and reproducible CC subdivision and ROI placement methodologies we have shown that FA shows regional heterogeneity with location (splenium FA > genu FA > body) for the children and adult age groups. Since our subjects are mostly right-handed we could not measure regional differences between age-matched males and females. These results are consistent with known and published trends in regards to myelination of inferior, posterior and sensory regions which precede that of superior, anterior and motor areas (Filley 2001; Neil JJ et al. 2002 and refs therein; Chepuri et al. 2002; Hasan et al. 2005). Notice that our results on the heterogeneity of CC confirm those of Chepuri et al. (2002), Pfefferbaum et al. (2003). Also, note that the age pattern seen here was not detected by Chepuri et al (2002), and the age trend is consistent with Abe et al. (2002) for the adult group. The gender brain regional anisotropy similarity between adult males and females are consistent with those published by Peled et al. (1998) and Abe (2002). The FA (CC) relationship with age (9-69 years) seems to be region specific and may reflect fundamentally a trend related to axonal structure, and programmed function. Prefrontal cortical connections seem to be reflected by the genu are more involved and affected by aging. The Splenium FA is relatively independent (9-69 years) after some projected maturation phase (<9 years) which is not reported here. The genu FA maturation curve from 0-69 can be extrapolated using our data and published trends. Our results show that age of subjects must be incorporated in DT-MRI metric comparisons and studies. Our data can also be projected and extrapolated with those published separately by other groups on the infant and child age group (birth to 9 years) (Mukherjee et al. 2001; Gilmore et al. 2004; Schneider et al. 2003; Partridge et al. 2004). A detailed explanation of the regional anisotropy heterogeneity may require further modeling, simulations and histopathological studies (Hasan et al. 2005). The explanation of the preservation of anisotropy may have to do with continued preservation and remyelination of the posterior and occipito-parietal portion of the brain. The loss in anisotropy of the genu may reflect a trend towards already reduced myelination and possibly accelerated loss or elimination of small myelinated axons due to normal aging as genu evolves and ages faster (Miller et al. 2003; Miller et al. 2002). The validation of these preliminary observations with postmortem histology would provide a definite answer. Our results on the age dependence of the CC genu and splenium are also consistent with those of Abe et al. (2002) on adults who reported gender independence. The age trends contradict the observations of Chepuri et al. (2002) who did not report age-related changes (on eight subjects per age group). We attribute differences to sample size, SNR and methodological accuracy of ROI placement (Peled et al. 1998; Moseley 2002; Hasan et al. 2004; 2005).

Findings in Relapsing and Remitting MS and TBI Children

In our studies we have also observed reduced anisotropy in the NAWM of the CC of the adult RRMS group compared to the age-matched adults, possibly reflecting loss of axons directly or indirectly due to slow Wallerian dgeneration (Pierpaoli et al. 2001; Ge et al. 2003; Henry et al. 2003; Cicarelli et al. 2003). Axonal degeneration may be attributed to distal cortical lesion activity or to proximal lesion load that may --through inflammatory mechanisms-- have intoxicated the ability of the Oligodedrocytes to remyelinate the denuded axons. Our preliminary results are consistent with published reports and known histological findings on MS (Evangelou et al. 2000). A detailed account of these studies can be found elsewhere (Hasan et al. 2005). Our results in regards to the pediatric TBI corpora callosa confirm known trends in closed-head injuries which affect the splenium of the CC (Levin et al. 2000). The loss of anisotropy may be due to a diffuse axonal loss or a disconnection of axons with their corresponding axonal bodies. In summary, our observations on the heterogeneity of the CC, and age dependence combined with basic histology, clinical-psychometric battery and modeling should eventually provide clues toward understanding the relation between the measured anisotropy and local axonal myelin and morphology (Figure 33; Figure 7).

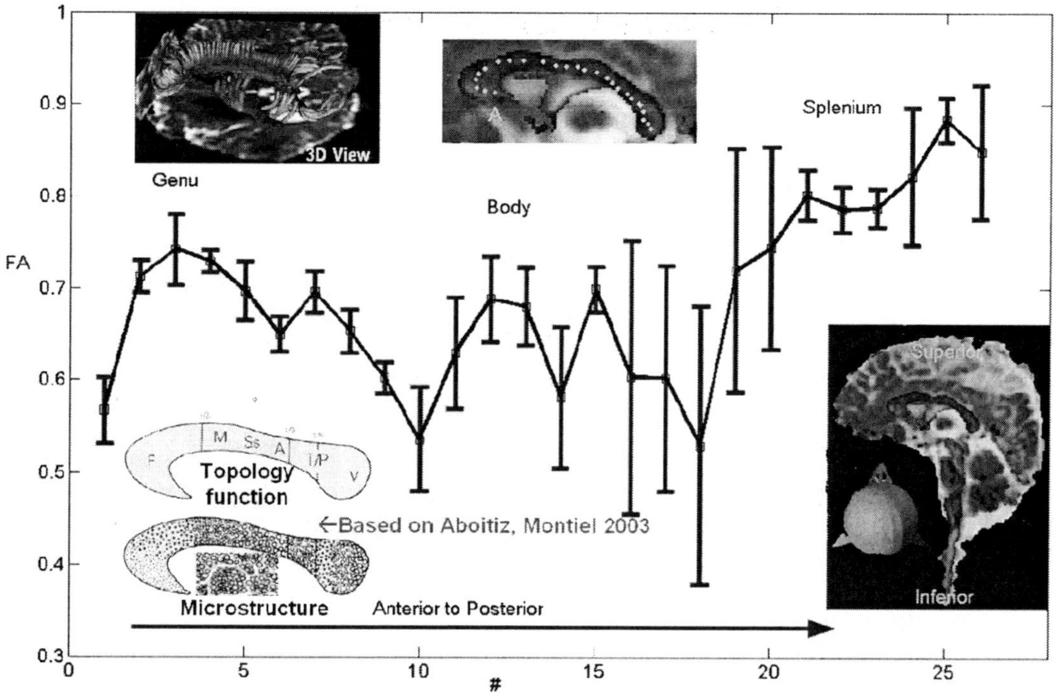

Figure 33. An illustration of the future potential of DTI metrics (eigenvalues, anisotropy) in providing axonal morphological information (diameter, myelination, density). The figure shows the mean and SD anisotropy along a traced line from the genu to the splenium of the corpus callosum and the corresponding histology expected fiber density (Aboitiz and Montiel 2003).

Conclusion

Diffusion tensor imaging is a sensitive modality that is very promising in radiological and psychiatric applications (Tables 1-2). A full brain DT-MRI exam can be obtained in less than six minutes using the single shot echo-planar method (see Figure 11). An efficient, accurate and specific DTI experiment seeks to partition the total imaging time into the different parameter space variables to obtain high quality images with minimal artifacts. The data sufficiency condition for tensor decoding requires at least seven independent measurements. Without *a priori* knowledge about the full brain fiber distribution, the encoding directions are required to be uniformly distributed over the encoding unit sphere in order to reduce the encoding directional bias. This work has presented the fundamental aspects of the MRI based single diffusion tensor encoding and estimation theory and applied to imaging both healthy and sick children and adults. This work discussed some criteria (figures-of-merit) for the evaluation and optimization of single tensor encoding directions assuming a two-diffusion weighting scheme. The icosahedral and minimum energy sets have been found to be optimal (uniformly distributed, least biased and rotationally invariant) for single tensor encoding when the tensor distribution is uniformly distributed. This work also related the minimum condition set with $N_e=6$ to a commonly used tensor encoding scheme (ODG) (Figure 13). The minimum condition criterion does not lead to uniformly distributed tensor encoding sets. We have shown, implemented and used multi-faceted icosahedral schemes with alternating polarity and demonstrated that useful entire brain DTI on both healthy volunteers and MS patients can be acquired in 4-6 minutes, hence making DTI as affordable as any conventional MRI exam. The application of DTI fiber tracking in multiple sclerosis research, and traumatic brain injury may provide important objective and quantitative data on the pathogenesis, fiber type and lesion proximity relations (Barkhoff et al. 2002) and will help build the digital atlas of MS plaques (Charil et al. 2003) in relation to normal-appearing white matter (Evangelou et al. 2005; Ciccarelli et al. 2003; Ge et al. 2003; Henry et al. 2003; Hasan et al. 2005), spinal cord (Evangelou et al. 2005), cortex (De Stefano et al. 2004) and vasculature (Law et al. 2004). Time efficient entire brain DTI at 3.0 T is also promising in the understanding and management of challenging conditions such as brain development, genetic disorders, aging, Alzheimer's disease schizophrenia, autism, learning disabilities, infant and child traumatic brain injury and neurotoxins research (Tables 1-2; Barker RA and Dunnett SB 1999; Compston 2004).

Acknowledgments

I wish to thank Marci A. Harris for carefully editing the manuscript. I am also thankful to my colleagues and mentors Ponnada A. Narayana, Ph. D.; Jerry S. Wolinsky, MD; Linda Ewing-Cobbs, Ph. D.; Gerry F. Moeller, MD; Joel S Steinberg, MD; Jack Fletcher, Ph. D.; Rafael M. Santos, MD, FRCS; Larry Kramer, MD and Rakesh K. Gupta, Ph. D. for the chance to learn from their experience and for providing access and feedback on the human data used in this chapter. The author also acknowledges the assistance of Bhavik P. Kanabar, Meghna Mehta, Wimla Ahobila, Vipul Kumar Patel and Drs. Ping Hou, Sajja Rao, Sushmita Datta and Renjie He. This work is funded in part by the department of diagnostic and interventional imaging through a grant from the Dunn Research Foundation awarded to the Chair Dr Susan John. The main funding of this work is from the National Institute of Health Grants R01 EB02095, 1RO1-NS046308-01, P01-HD35946 and P50DA 009262. This Chapter is dedicated to the memory of my teacher Dr Jack H Petajan, PhD, MD.

References

Abe O, Aoki S, Hayashi N, Yamada H, Kunimatsu A, Mori H, Yoshikawa T, Okubo T, Ohtomo K (2002). Normal aging in the central nervous system: quantitative MR diffusion-tensor analysis. *Neurobiol Aging* 23:433-441.

Aboitiz F, Scheibel AB, Fisher RS, Zaidel E (1992). Fiber composition of the human corpus callosum. *Brain Res* 598:143-153.

Aboitiz F, Montiel J (2003). One hundred million years of interhemispheric communication: the history of the corpus callosum. *Braz J Med Biol Res* 36(4):409-420.

Agartz I, Andersson JL, Skare S (2001). Abnormal brain white matter in schizophrenia: a diffusion tensor imaging study. *Neuroreport* 12:2251-2254.

Ahn CB, Cho ZH (1989). A generalized formulation of diffusion effects in micron resolution nuclear magnetic resonance imaging. *Med Phys* 16(1):22-28.

Akkerman EM. Efficient measurement and calculation of MR diffusion anisotropy images using the Platonic variance method. *Magn Reson Med.* 2003;49(3):599-604.

Alderman DW, Sherwood M, Grant D (1990). Two-dimensional chemical-shift tensor correlation spectroscopy: analysis of sensitivity and optimal measurement directions. *J Magn Reson* 86:60-69.

Alexander AL, Tsuruda JS, Parker DL (1997). Elimination of eddy current artifacts in diffusion-weighted echo-planar images: the use of bipolar gradients. *Magn Reson Med.* 1997;38(6):1016-1021.

Alexander AL, Hasan KM, Lazar M, Tsuruda JS, Parker DL (2001). Analysis of partial volume effects in diffusion-tensor MRI. *Magn Reson Med* 45(5):770-780.

Alexopoulos GS, Kiosses DN, Choi SJ, Murphy CF, Lim KO (2002). Frontal white matter microstructure and treatment response of late-life depression: a preliminary study. *Am J Psychiatry* 159(11):1929-1932.

Alfano B, Brunetti A, Larobina M, Quarantelli M, Tedeschi E, Ciarmiello A, Covelli EM, Salvatore M (2000). Automated segmentation and measurement of global white matter lesion volume in patients with multiple sclerosis. *J Magn Reson Imaging* 12(6):799-807.

Anderson AW (2001). Theoretical analysis of the effects of noise on diffusion tensor imaging. *Magn Reson Med* 46:1174-1188.

Ardekani BA, Nierenberg J, Hoptman MJ, Javitt DC, Lim KO (2003). MRI study of white matter diffusion anisotropy in schizophrenia. *Neuroreport* 14: 2025-2029.

Arfanakis K, Haughton VM, Carew JD, Rogers BP, Dempsey RJ, Meyerand ME (2002a). Diffusion tensor MR imaging in diffuse axonal injury. *AJNR Am J Neuroradiol* 23:794-802.

Arfanakis K, Hermann BP, Rogers BP, Carew JD, Seidenberg M, Meyerand ME (2002b). Diffusion tensor MRI in temporal lobe epilepsy. *Magn Reson Im*aging 20:511-519.

Arfanakis K, Cordes D, Haughton VM, Carew JD, Meyerand ME (2002c). Independent component analysis applied to diffusion tensor MRI. *Magn Reson Med* 47(2):354-363.

Armitage PA, Bastin ME (2001). Utilizing the diffusion-to-noise ratio to optimize magnetic resonance diffusion tensor acquisition strategies for improving measurements of diffusion anisotropy. *Magn Reson Me*d 45(6):1056-65.

Ashburner J, Friston K (1998). MRI sensitivity correction and tissue classification. *NeuroImage* 7:S706.

Ashburner J, Friston KJ (2001). Why voxel-based morphometry should be used. *Neuroimage* 14(6):1238-1243.

Ashtari M, Kumra S, Bhaskar SL, Clarke T, Thaden E, Cervellione KL, Rhinewine J, Kane JM, Adesman A, Milanaik R, Maytal J, Diamond A, Szeszko P, Ardekani BA (2005). Attention-deficit/hyperactivity disorder: A preliminary diffusion tensor imaging study. *Biol Psychiatry* 57(5):448-455.

Assaf Y, Ben-Bashat D, Chapman J, Peled S, Biton IE, Kafri M, Segev Y, Hendler T, Korczyn AD, Graif M, Cohen Y (2002). High b-value q-space analyzed diffusion-weighted MRI: application to multiple sclerosis. *Magn Reson Med* 47(1):115-126.

Axer H, Keyserlingk DG (2000). Mapping of fiber orientation in human internal capsule by means of polarized light and confocal scanning laser microscopy. *J Neurosci Methods* 94: 165-175.

Bammer R, Fazekas F (2002). Diffusion imaging in multiple sclerosis. *Neuroimaging Clin N Am* 12: 71-106 (*entire volume is on clinical applications of DTI*)

Bammer R, Auer M, Keeling SL, Augustin M, Stables LA, Prokesch RW, Stollberger R, Moseley ME, Fazekas F (2002). Diffusion tensor imaging using single-shot SENSE-EPI. *Magn Reson Med* 48(1):128-136.

Barker GJ (2001). Diffusion-weighted imaging of the spinal cord and optic nerve. *J Neurol Sci* 186 Suppl 1:S45-49.

Barker RA, Dunnett SB (1999). Neural repair, transplantation and rehabilitation. *Psychology Press* Ltd, East Sussex, UK.

Barkhof F (2002). The clinico-radiological paradox in multiple sclerosis revisited. *Curr Opin Neurol* 15: 239-245.

Barkhof FJ, Elton M, Lindeboom J, Tas MW, Schmidt WF, Hommes OR, Polman CH, Kok A, Valk J (1998). Functional correlates of callosal atrophy in relapsing-remitting multiple sclerosis patients. *J Neurol* 245:153-158.

Barkovich AJ, Norman D (1988). Anomalies of the corpus callosum: correlation with further anomalies of the brain. *AJR Am J Roentgenol* 151(1):171-179.

Barnard RO, Triggs M (1974). Corpus callosum in multiple sclerosis. *J Neurol Neurosurg* Psychiatry 37: 1259-1264.

Barnea-Goraly N, Kwon H, Menon V, Eliez S, Lotspeich L, Reiss AL (2004). White matter structure in autism: preliminary evidence from diffusion tensor imaging. *Biol Psychiatry* 55(3):323-326.

Basser PJ, Mattiello J, Le Bihan D (1994). Estimation of the effective self-diffusion tensor from the NMR spin echo. *J Magn Reson B* 103(3):247-254.

Basser PJ, Pierpaoli C (1998). A simplified method to measure the diffusion tensor from seven MR images. *Magn Reson Med* 39:928-934.

Basser PJ (2002). Relationships between diffusion tensor and q-space MRI. *Magn Reson Med* 47(2):392-397.

Basser PJ, Pierpaoli C (1996). Microstructural and physiological features of tissues elucidated by quantitative-diffusion-tensor MRI. *J Magn Reson* B 1996; 111(3):209-219.

Basser PJ, Jones DK (2002). Diffusion-tensor MRI: theory, experimental design and data analysis - a technical review. *NMR Biomed.* 15: 456-467.

Basser PJ (1995). Inferring microstructural features and the physiological state of tissues from diffusion-weighted images. *NMR Biomed* 8: 333-344.

Basser PJ (2004). Scaling laws for myelinated axons derived from an electrotonic core-conductor model. *J Integr Neurosci* 3(2):227-244.

Bastin ME, Armitage PA, Marshall I (1998). A theoretical study of the effect of experimental noise on the measurement of anisotropy in diffusion imaging. *Magn Reson Imaging* 16(7):773-785.

Batchelor PG, Atkinson D, Hill DL, Calamante F, Connelly A (2003). Anisotropic noise propagation in diffusion tensor MRI sampling schemes. *Magn Reson Med* 49(6):1143-1151.

Beaulieu C, Does MD, Snyder RE, Allen PS (1996). Changes in water diffusion due to Wallerian degeneration in peripheral nerve. *Magn Reson Med* 36(4):627-631.

Beaulieu C (2002). The basis of anisotropic water diffusion in the nervous system - a technical review. *NMR Biomed* 15(7-8):435-455.

Behrens TE, Johansen-Berg H, Woolrich MW, Smith SM, Wheeler-Kingshott CA, Boulby PA, Barker GJ, Sillery EL, Sheehan K, Ciccarelli O, Thompson AJ, Brady JM, Matthews PM (2003). Non-invasive mapping of connections between human thalamus and cortex using diffusion imaging. *Nat Neurosci* 6(7):750-757.

Beppu T, Inoue T, Shibata Y, Kurose A, Arai H, Ogasawara K, Ogawa A, Nakamura S, Kabasawa H (2003). Measurement of fractional anisotropy using diffusion tensor MRI in supratentorial astrocytic tumors. *J Neurooncol* 63(2):109-116

Berg HC (1993). *Random Walks in Biology*. Princton University Press, New Jersey

Bermudez P, Zatorre RJ (2001). Sexual dimorphism in the corpus callosum: methodological considerations in MRI morphometry. *Neuroimage* 13(6 Pt 1):1121-1130.

Bishop KM, Wahlsten D (1997). Sex differences in the human corpus callosum: myth or reality? *Neurosci Biobehav Rev* 21: 581- 601.

Bjartmar C, Trapp BD (2001). Axonal and neuronal degeneration in multiple sclerosis: mechanisms and functional consequences. *Curr Opin Neurol* 14: 271-278.

Bland JM, Altman DG. Statistical methods for assessing agreement between two methods of clinical measurement. *Lancet* 1(8476):307-310.

Bookstein FL (2001). "Voxel-based morphometry" should not be used with imperfectly registered images. *Neuroimage* 14(6):1454-1462.

Borisenko AI and Tarapov IE (1968). Vector and Tensor Analysis with Applications. *Dover Publications* Inc, New York.

Bozzali M, Falini A, Franceschi M, Cercignani M, Zuffi M, Scotti G, Comi G, Filippi M (2002). White matter damage in Alzheimer's disease assessed in vivo using diffusion tensor magnetic resonance imaging. *J Neurol Neurosurg Psychiatry* 72(6):742-746.

Brihuega-Moreno O, Heese FP, Hall LD. Optimization of diffusion measurements using Cramer-Rao lower bound theory and its application to articular cartilage (2003). *Magn Reson Med* 50(5):1069-1076.

Buchsbaum MS, Tang CY, Peled S, Gudbjartsson H, Lu D, Hazlett EA, Downhill J, Haznedar M, Fallon JH, Atlas SW (1998). MRI white matter diffusion anisotropy and PET metabolic rate in schizophrenia. *Neuroreport* 9(3):425-430.

Callaghan PT (1994). *Principles of Nuclear Magnetic Resonance Microscopy*. 492 pp. Oxford University Press.

Callaghan PT (1996). NMR imaging, NMR diffraction and applications of pulsed gradient spin echoes in porous media. *Magn Reson Imaging* 14(7-8):701-709.

Carano RA, Li F, Irie K, Helmer KG, Silva MD, Fisher M, Sotak CH (2000). Multispectral analysis of the temporal evolution of cerebral ischemia in the rat brain *J Magn Reson Imaging* 12(6):842-858.

Carr H, Purcell EM (1954). Effects of Diffusion on Free Precession in Nuclear Magnetic Resonance Experiments. *Phys Rev* 94:630-638.

Catani M, Jones DK, Ffytche DH (2005). Perisylvian language networks of the human brain. *Ann Neurol* 57(1):8-16.

Catani M, Jones DK, Donato R, Ffytche DH (2003). Occipito-temporal connections in the human brain. *Brain* 126(Pt 9):2093-2107.

Charil A, Zijdenbos AP, Taylor J, Boelman C, Worsley KJ, Evans AC, Dagher A (2003). Statistical mapping analysis of lesion location and neurological disability in multiple sclerosis: application to 452 patient data sets. *Neuroimage* 19:532-544.

Chepuri NB, Yen YF, Burdette JH, Li H, Moody DM, Maldjian JA (2002). Diffusion anisotropy in the corpus callosum. *AJNR Am J Neuroradiol* 23: 803-808.

Choi SJ, Lim KO, Monteiro I, Reisberg B (2005). Diffusion tensor imaging of frontal white matter microstructure in early Alzheimer's disease: a preliminary study. *J Geriatr Psychiatry Neurol* 18(1):12-9.

Chudler EH (2005). http://faculty.washington.edu/chudler/ehceduc.html. An excellent Neuroscience education web page (ehc.html, facts.html, quotes.html, etc)

Ciccarelli O, Werring DJ, Barker GJ, Griffin CM, Wheeler-Kingshott CA, Miller DH, Thompson AJ (2003). A study of the mechanisms of normal-appearing white matter damage in multiple sclerosis using diffusion tensor imaging--evidence of Wallerian degeneration. *J Neurol* 250: 287-292.

Clark CA, Hedehus M, Moseley ME (2002). In vivo mapping of the fast and slow diffusion tensors in human brain. *Magn Reson Med* 47(4):623-628.

Cohen Y, Assaf Y (2002). High b-value q-space analyzed diffusion-weighted MRS and MRI in neuronal tissues - a technical review. *NMR Biomed* 15(7-8):516-542.

Compston A (2004). The pathogenesis and basis for treatment in multiple sclerosis. *Clin Neurol Neurosurg.* 2004;106(3):246-248.

Concha L, Beaulieu C, Gross DW (2005). Bilateral limbic diffusion abnormalities in unilateral temporal lobe epilepsy. *Ann Neurol* 57(2):188-196.

Conturo TE, McKinstry RC, Aronovitz JA, Neil JJ (1995). Diffusion MRI: precision, accuracy and flow effects.*NMR Biomed* 8: 307-332.

Conturo TE, McKinstry RC, Akbudak E, Robinson BH (1996). Encoding of anisotropic diffusion with tetrahedral gradients:a general mathematical diffusion formalism and experimental results. *Magn Reson Med* 35(3):399-412.

Cook ND (1986). The Brain Code: mechanisms of information transfer and the role of the corpus callosum. *Cook ND*, London.

Crank J (2002). *The Mathematics of Diffusion.* Oxford Science Publications. Oxford.

Crick F, Jones F (1993). Backwardness of Human Fiber Anatomy: *Nature* 14:361 p109.

Davatzikos C (2004). Why voxel-based morphometric analysis should be used with great caution when characterizing group differences. *Neuroimage* 23(1):17-20.

de L'acoste MC, Kirkpatrick JB, Ross ED (1985). Topography of the human corpus callosum. *J Neuropathol Exp Neurol* 44(6):578-591.

De Stefano N, Matthews PM, Filippi M, et al (2003). Evidence of early cortical atrophy in MS: relevance to white matter changes and disability. *Neurology* 60(7):1157-1162.

Dietemann JL, Beigelman C, Rumbach L, Vouge M, Tajahmady T, Faubert C, Jeung MY, Wackenheim A (1988). Multiple sclerosis and corpus callosum atrophy: relationship of MRI findings to clinical data. *Neuroradiology* 30(6):478-480.

Dong Q, Welsh RC, Chenevert TL, Carlos RC, Maly-Sundgren P, Gomez-Hassan DM, Mukherji SK (2004). Clinical applications of diffusion tensor imaging. *J Magn Reson Imaging* 19: 6-18.

Einstein A (1956). Investigations on the theory of Brownian movement. *Dover Publications*, New York.

Evangelou N, Konz D, Esiri MM, Smith S, Palace J, Matthews PM (2000a). Regional axonal loss in the corpus callosum correlates with cerebral white matter lesion volume and distribution in multiple sclerosis. *Brain* 123: 1845-1849.

Evangelou N, Esiri MM, Smith S, Palace J, Matthews PM (2000b). Quantitative pathological evidence for axonal loss in normal appearing white matter in multiple sclerosis. *Ann Neurol* 47: 391-395.

Evangelou N, DeLuca GC, Owens T, Esiri MM (2005). Pathological study of spinal cord atrophy in multiple sclerosis suggests limited role of local lesions. *Brain*128(1):29-34.

Falconer JC, Narayana PA (1997). Cerebrospinal fluid-suppressed high-resolution diffusion imaging of human brain. *Magn Reson Med* 37:119-123.

Field AS, Alexander AL (2004). Diffusion tensor imaging in cerebral tumor diagnosis and therapy. *Top Magn Reson Imaging* 15(5):315-324.

Filippi M, Cercignani M, Inglese M, Horsfield MA, Comi G (2001). Diffusion tensor magnetic resonance imaging in multiple sclerosis. *Neurology* 56: 304-311.

Filley CM (2001). *The Behavioral Neurology of White Matter*. Oxford.

Foong J, Maier M, Clark CA, Barker GJ, Miller DH, Ron MA (2000). Neuropathological abnormalities of the corpus callosum in schizophrenia: a diffusion tensor imaging study. *J Neurol Neurosurg Psychiatry* 68: 242-244.

Frank LR (2002). Characterization of anisotropy in high angular resolution diffusion-weighted MRI. *Magn Reson Med* 47(6):1083-1099.

Fukushima K (1990). *Introduction to statistical pattern Recognition*. Academic Press, San Diego.

Ge Y, Law M, Johnson G, Herbert J, Babb JS, Mannon LJ, Grossman RI (2004). Preferential occult injury of corpus callosum in multiple sclerosis measured by diffusion tensor imaging. *J Magn Reson Imaging*. 20(1):1-7.

Giedd JN, Castellanos FX, Casey BJ, Kozuch P, King AC, Hamburger SD, Rapoport JL (1994). Quantitative morphology of the corpus callosum in attention deficit hyperactivity disorder. *Am J Psychiatry* 151(5):665-669.

Gilmore JH, Zhai G, Wilber K, Smith JK, Lin W, Gerig G (2004). 3 Tesla magnetic resonance imaging of the brain in newborns. *Psychiatry Res* 132(1):81-85.

Georgy BA, Hesselink JR, Jernigan TL (1993). MR imaging of the corpus callosum. *AJR Am J Roentgenol.* 160(5):949-955.

Glantz SA (2002). *Primer of Biostatistics*. New York McGraw-Hill Med Pub 5th ed.

Grant SC, Buckley DL, Gibbs S, Webb AG, Blackband SJ (2001). MR microscopy of multicomponent diffusion in single neurons. *Magn Reson Med* 46(6):1107-1112.

Gulani V, Webb AG, Duncan ID, Lauterbur PC (2001). Apparent diffusion tensor measurements in myelin-deficient rat spinal cords. *Magn Reson Med* 45: 191-195

Guo AC, Petrella JR, Kurtzberg J, Provenzale JM (2001). Evaluation of white matter anisotropy in Krabbe disease with diffusion tensor MR imaging: initial experience. *Radiology* 218(3):809-815.

Gupta RK, Rao AM, Mishra AM, Chawla S, Sekar DR, Venkatesan R. (2005). Diffusion-weighted EPI with magnetization transfer contrast. *Magn Reson Imag* 23(1):35-39.

Gupta RK, Hasan KM, Trivedi R, Pradhan M, Das V, Parikh NA, Narayana PA (2005). Diffusion tensor imaging of the developing human cerebrum. J Neurosci Res. 15;81(2):172-178

Hahn E (1950). Spin Echoes. *Physics Review* 80(4) 580-594.

Hahn KR, Prigarin S and Hasan KM (2004). *A novel Denoising Technique for very noisy diffusion tensor MRI data. Proc.* 12th International Society of Magnetic Resonance in Medicine Meeting in Kyoto, Japan, p1208.

Hampel H, Teipel SJ, Alexander GE, Horwitz B, Teichberg D, Schapiro MB, Rapoport SI (1998) Corpus callosum atrophy is a possible indicator of region- and cell type-specific neuronal degeneration in Alzheimer disease: a magnetic resonance imaging analysis. *Arch Neurol* 55(2):193-198.

Hanyu H, Asano T, Sakurai H, Imon Y, Iwamoto T, Takasaki M, Shindo H, Abe K (1999). Diffusion-weighted and magnetization transfer imaging of the corpus callosum in Alzheimer's disease. *J Neurol Sci* 167(1):37-44.

Hardan AY, Minshew NJ, Keshavan MS (2000). Corpus callosum size in autism. *Neurology* 55(7):1033-1036.

Hasan K. Analysis, optimization and evaluation of water spin self-diffusion tensor imaging encoding and acquisition schemes. Dissertation, University of Utah, Salt Lake City, Utah, 2000. 216 p. (University of Utah Marriott Library Catalog: R117.5; 2000.H38).

Hasan KM, Parker DL, Alexander AL (2001a). Comparison of Optimization Procedures for Diffusion-Tensor Encoding Directions. *J Magn Reson Imaging* 13: 769-780.

Hasan KM, Basser PJ, Parker DL, Alexander AL (2001a). Analytical Computation of the Eigenvalues and Eigenvectors in DTI. *J Magn Reson* 152: 41-47.

Hasan KM, Arfanakis K, Alexander AL. A referenceless, balanced and efficient encoding scheme for diffusion tensor imaging. *In: Proceedings of the 10th Annual Meeting of ISMRM,* Honolulu, 2002. p 1107.

Hasan KM, Narayana PA (2003). Computation of the Mean Diffusivity and Fractional Anisotropy Maps Without Tensor Decoding and Diagonalization: Theoretical Analysis and Experimental Validation. *Magn Reson Med* 50: 589-598.

Hasan KM, Alexander AL, Narayana PA (2004). Does Fractional Anisotropy Have Better Noise Immunity Characteristics than the Relative Anisotropy in Diffusion Tensor MRI: An Analytical Approach? *Magn Reson Med* 51(2):413-417.

Hasan KM, Bhavik P. Kanabar, Rafeal M. Santos RM, Ewing-Cobbs L, Narayana PA (2004a). *Age Dependence of the Fractional Anisotropy of Genu and Splenium of Human Corpus Callosum Using Optimized DT-MRI. Proc.* 12th International Society of Magnetic Resonnance (ISMRM talk) in Kyoto, Japan: p338.

Hasan KM, Kanabar BP, Rafael M. Santos RM, Kramer L, Mary Prasad, Ewing-Cobbs L, Narayana PA (2004b). *Diffusion Tensor MRI after Pediatric Brain Injury. Proc.* 12th International Society of Magnetic Resonance in Medicine Meeting in Kyoto, Japan: p1350.

Hasan KM, Gupta RK, Santos RM, Wolinsky JS, Narayana PA (2005). Diffusion Tensor Fractional Anisotropy of the Seven Segments of the Normal-Appearing White Matter of the Corpus Callosum in Healthy Adults and Relapsing Remitting Multiple Sclerosis J Magn Reson Imaging 21(6):735-743.

Hasan KM, Narayana PA (2005). DTI parameter optimization at 3.0 T: potential application in entire normal human brain mapping and multiple sclerosis research. MedicaMundi 49(1):30-45.

Hasan KM, Narayana PA (2006). Retrospective Measurement of the Diffusion Tensor Eigenvalues from Diffusion Anisotropy and Mean Diffusivity in DTI. Magn Reson Med (*in press*).

Haueisen J, Tuch DS, Ramon C, et al (2002). The influence of brain tissue anisotropy on human EEG and MEG. *Neuroimage* 5(1):159-66.

Heimer L, Robards MJ (1981). *Neuroanatomical tract-tracing methods.* New York : Plenum Press.

Helenius J, Soinne L, Perkio J, Salonen O, Kangasmaki A, Kaste M, Carano RA, Aronen HJ, Tatlisumak T (2002). Diffusion-weighted MR imaging in normal human brains in various age groups. *AJNR Am J Neuroradiol* 23:194-199.

Helpern JA, Huang N. Diffusion-weighted imaging in epilepsy. *Magn Reson Imaging* 1995; 13 :1227–1231.

Henry RG, Oh J, Nelson SJ, Pelletier D (2003). Directional diffusion in relapsing-remitting multiple sclerosis: a possible in vivo signature of Wallerian degeneration. *J Magn Reson Imaging* 18: 420-426.

Highley JR, Esiri MM, McDonald B, Cortina-Borja M, Herron BM, Crow TJ (1999). The size and fibre composition of the corpus callosum with respect to gender and schizophrenia: a post-mortem study. *Brain* 122: 99-110.

Hinshaw W, Lent A (1983). An Introduction to NMR Imaging: From the Bloch Equation to the Imaging Equation. *Proceedings of the IEEE* 71(3): 338-350.

Hoehn-Berlage M (1995). Diffusion-weighted NMR imaging: Application to experimental focal Ischemia. *NMR in Biomed*; 8:345-58. http://www.ujf-grenoble.fr/ismrm/Diffusion/diffusion_outline.htm.

Holodny AI, Diffusion imaging in brain tumors. Ollenschlager M (2002). *Neuroimaging Clin N Am* 12(1):107-124.

Holodny AI, Ollenschleger MD, Liu WC, Schulder M, Kalnin AJ (2001). Identification of the corticospinal tracts achieved using blood-oxygen-level-dependent and diffusion functional MR imaging in patients with brain tumors. *AJNR Am J Neuroradiol* 22(1):83-8.

Holodny AI, Gor DM, Watts R, Gutin PH, Ulug AM (2005). Diffusion-Tensor MR Tractography of Somatotopic Organization of Corticospinal Tracts in the Internal Capsule: Initial Anatomic Results in Contradistinction to Prior Reports. *Radiology* 234(3):649-653.

Hoptman MJ, Volavka J, Johnson G, Weiss E, Bilder RM, Lim KO (2002). Frontal white matter microstructure, aggression, and impulsivity in men with schizophrenia: a preliminary study. *Biol Psychiatry* 52(1):9-14

Horsfield MA, Jones DK (2002). Applications of diffusion-weighted and diffusion tensor MRI to white matter diseases - a review. *NMR Biomed* 15: 570-577.

Hsu EW, Muzikant AL, Matulevicius SA, Penland RC, Henriquez CS (1998). Magnetic resonance myocardial fiber-orientation mapping with direct histological correlation. *Am J Physiol* 274(5 Pt 2):H1627-1634.

Hsu EW, Mori S (1995). Analytical expressions for the NMR apparent diffusion coefficients in an anisotropic system and a simplified method for determining fiber orientation. *Magn Reson Med* 34(2):194-200.

Huisman TA, Schwamm LH, Schaefer PW, Koroshetz WJ, Shetty-Alva N, Ozsunar Y, Wu O, Sorensen AG (2004). Diffusion tensor imaging as potential biomarker of white matter injury in diffuse axonal injury. *AJNR Am J Neuroradiol* 25(3):370-376.

Hunsche S, Moseley ME, Stoeter P, Hedehus M (2001). Diffusion-tensor MR imaging at 1.5 and 3.0 T: initial observations. *Radiology* 221(2):550-556.

Huppi PS, Maier SE, Peled S, Zientara GP, Barnes PD, Jolesz FA, Volpe JJ (1998). Microstructural development of human newborn cerebral white matter assessed in vivo by diffusion tensor magnetic resonance imaging. *Pediatr Res* 44(4):584-590.

Jaermann T, Crelier G, Pruessmann KP, Golay X, Netsch T, van Muiswinkel AM, Mori S, van Zijl PC, Valavanis A, Kollias S, Boesiger P (2004). SENSE-DTI at 3 T. *Magn Reson Med* 51(2):230-236.

Jancke L, Staiger JF, Schlaug G, Huang Y, Steinmetz H (1997). The relationship between corpus callosum size and forebrain volume. *Cereb Cortex* 7(1):48-56.

Jellison BJ, Field AS, Medow J, Lazar M, Salamat MS, Alexander AL (2004). Diffusion tensor imaging of cerebral white matter: a pictorial review of physics, fiber tract anatomy, and tumor imaging patterns. *AJNR Am J Neuroradiol* 25(3):356-369.

Jones DK, Horsfield MA, Simmons A (1999). Optimal strategies for measuring diffusion in anisotropic systems by magnetic resonance imaging. *Magn Reson Med* 42:515-525.

Jones DK, Griffin LD, Alexander DC, Catani M, Horsfield MA, Howard R. Williams SC (2002). *Spatial normalization and averaging of diffusion tensor MRI data sets Neuroimage* 17(2):592-617.

Kandel ER, Schwartz JH, Jessel TM (1991). *Principles of Neural Science*. Elsevier, New York.

Karger J, Pfeifer H, Heink W (1988). Principles and application of self-diffusion measurements by nuclear magnetic resonance. *Adv Magn Reson* 12: 1-89.

Kikinis R, Guttmann CR, Metcalf D, Wells WM 3rd, Ettinger GJ, Weiner HL, Jolesz FA (1999). Quantitative follow-up of patients with multiple sclerosis using MRI: technical aspects. *J Magn Reson Imaging*. 9(4):519-530.

Kingsley PB, Monahan WG (2004). Selection of the optimum b factor for diffusion-weighted magnetic resonance imaging assessment of ischemic stroke. *Magn Reson Med* 51(5):996-1001.

Klingberg T, Vaidya CJ, Gabrieli JD, Moseley ME, Hedehus M (1999). Myelination and organization of the frontal white matter in children: a diffusion tensor MRI study. *Neuroreport* 10: 2817-2821.

Koenig SH, Brown RD, III, Spiller M, Lundbom N (1990). Relaxometry of brain: why white matter appears bright in MRI. *Magn Reson Med* 14:482-495.

Lamantia AS, Rakic P (1990). Cytological and quantitative characteristics of four cerebral commissures in the rhesus monkey. *J Comp Neurol* 291(4):520-53.

Laule C, Vavasour IM, Moore GR, Oger J, Li DK, Paty DW, MacKay AL (2004). Water content and myelin water fraction in multiple sclerosis. A T2 relaxation study. *J Neurol* 251(3):284-293.

Law M, Saindane AM, Ge Y, Babb JS, Johnson G, Mannon LJ, Herbert J, Grossman RI (2004). Microvascular abnormality in relapsing-remitting multiple sclerosis: perfusion MR imaging findings in normal-appearing white matter. *Radiology* 231(3):645-652.

Lazar M, Alexander AL (2005). Bootstrap white matter tractography (BOOT-TRAC). *Neuroimage* 24(2):524-532.

Le Bihan D, Turner R, Douek P (1993). Is water diffusion restricted in human brain WM? *Neuroreport* 4:887-890.

Le Bihan D (2003). Looking into the functional architecture of the brain with diffusion MRI. *Nat Rev Neurosci* 4(6):469-480

Le Bihan D (ed 1995). Diffusion and Perfusion Magnetic Resonance Imaging: *Applications to Functional MRI*. New York: Raven Press 374p.

Le Bihan D, Van Zijl P (2002). From the diffusion coefficient to the diffusion tensor. *NMR Biomed* 15(7-8):431-434 (*entire issue is dedicated to DTI methods and applications*).

Lee L, Harrison LM, Mechelli A (2003). A report of the functional connectivity workshop, Dusseldorf 2002. *Neuroimage* 19(2 Pt 1):457-465.

Lehericy S, Ducros M, Van de Moortele PF, Francois C, Thivard L, Poupon C, Swindale N, Ugurbil K, Kim DS (2004). Diffusion tensor fiber tracking shows distinct corticostriatal circuits in humans. *Ann Neurol* 55(4):522-529.

Lemke G (1992). In Hall ZW. *Introduction to Molecular Neurobiology* 1992. Sinauer Asociates Inc, Sunderland, Mass. Sinauer Associates.

Levin HS, Benavidez D, Verger-Maestre K, Perachio N, Song J, Mendelsohn D, Fletcher JM (2000). Reduction of corpus callosum growth after severe traumatic brain injury in children. *Neurology* 54: 647-653.

Lim KO, Helpern JA (2002). Neuropsychiatric applications of DTI - a review. *NMR Biomed* 15(7-8):587-593.

Lin CP, Wedeen VJ, Chen JH, Yao C, Tseng WY (2003). Validation of diffusion spectrum magnetic resonance imaging with manganese-enhanced rat optic tracts and ex vivo phantoms. *Neuroimage* 19(3):482-495.

Lori NF, Akbudak E, Shimony JS, Cull TS, Snyder AZ, Guillory RK, Conturo TE (2002). Diffusion tensor fiber tracking of human brain connectivity: aquisition methods, reliability analysis and biological results. *NMR Biomed* 15(7-8):494-515.

Lovet DR (1989). *Tensor Properties of Crystals*. IOP Publishing, Bristol.

Luypaert R, Boujraf S, Sourbron S, Osteaux M (2001). Diffusion and perfusion MRI: basic physics. *Eur J Radiol* 38(1):19-27.

Maas LC, Mukherjee P, Carballido-Gamio J, Veeraraghavan S, Miller SP, Partridge SC, Henry RG, Barkovich AJ, Vigneron DB (2004). Early laminar organization of the human cerebrum demonstrated with diffusion tensor imaging in extremely premature infants. *Neuroimage* 22(3):1134-1140.

Maas LC (2003). Diffusion tensor imaging: Basic principles and emerging clinical applications. *Applied Radiology Online* 32(6):S49-S57.

Madi S, Hasan KM, Narayana PA. Diffusion tensor imaging of in vivo and excised rat spinal cord at 7 T with an icosahedral encoding scheme. *Magn Reson Med.* 2005;53(1):118-125.

Makris N, Worth AJ, Sorensen AG, Papadimitriou GM, Wu O, Reese TG, Wedeen VJ, Davis TL, Stakes JW, Caviness VS, Kaplan E, Rosen BR, Pandya DN, Kennedy DN (1997). Morphometry of in vivo human white matter association pathways with diffusion-weighted magnetic resonance imaging. *Ann Neurol* 42(6):951-692.

Marner L, Nyengaard JR, Tang Y, Pakkenberg B (2003). Marked loss of myelinated nerve fibers in the human brain with age. *J Comp Neurol* 462(2):144-152.

Mattiello J, Basser PJ, Lebihan D (1994). Analytical expressions for the b-matrix in NMR diffusion imaging and spectroscopy. *J Magn Reson Ser A* 108:131-141.

McKinstry RC, Mathur A, Miller JH, Ozcan A, Snyder AZ, Schefft GL, Almli CR, Shiran SI, Conturo TE, Neil JJ (2002). Radial organization of developing preterm human cerebral cortex revealed by non-invasive water diffusion anisotropy MRI. *Cereb Cortex* 12(12):1237-1243.

Melhem ER, Mori S, Mukundan G, Kraut MA, Pomper MG, van Zijl PC (2002). Diffusion tensor MR imaging of the brain and white matter tractography. *Am J Roentgenol* 178: 3-16.

Miller JH, McKinstry RC, Philip JV, Mukherjee P, Neil JJ (2003). Diffusion-tensor MR imaging of normal brain maturation: a guide to structural development and myelination. *AJR Am J Roentgenol* 180: 851-859.

Miller SP, Vigneron DB, Henry RG, Bohland MA, Ceppi-Cozzio C, Hoffman C, Newton N, Partridge JC, Ferriero DM, Barkovich AJ (2002). Serial quantitative diffusion tensor MRI of the premature brain: development in newborns with and without injury. *J Magn Reson Imaging* 16(6):621-32

Moeller GF, Hasan KM, Steinberg JL, et al (2005). Reduced Anterior Corpus Callosum White Matter Integrity as Measured by Diffusion Tensor Imaging is Related to Impulsivity in Cocaine-Dependent Subjects. *Neuropsychopharmacology* 30(3):610-617.

Moorhead RJ, Zhifan Z (1995). Signal Processing Aspects of Scientific Visualization. *IEEE Signal Proc* 12(5):20-41.

Mori S, Kaufmann WE, Davatzikos C, Stieltjes B, Amodei L, Fredericksen K, Pearlson GD, Melhem ER, Solaiyappan M, Raymond GV, Moser HW, van Zijl PC (2002). Imaging cortical association tracts in the human brain using diffusion-tensor based axonal tracking. *Magn Reson Med* 47(2):215-223.

Mori S, van Zijl PC (2002). Fiber tracking: principles and strategies - a technical review. *NMR Biomed* 15(7-8):468-480.

Moseley M (2002). Diffusion tensor imaging and aging - a review. *NMR Biomed* 15: 553-560.

Moseley M, Bammer R, Illes J (2002). Diffusion-tensor imaging of cognitive performance. *Brain Cogn* 50(3):396-413.

Mukherjee P, Miller JH, Shimony JS, Conturo TE, Lee BC, Almli CR, McKinstry RC (2001). Normal brain maturation during childhood: developmental trends characterized with diffusion-tensor MR imaging. *Radiology* 221: 349-358.

Mulkern RV, Gudbjartsson H, Westin C-F, Zengingonul HP, Gartner W, Guttmann CR, Robertson RL, Kyriakos W, Schwartz R, Holtzmann D, Jolesz FA, Maier SE (1999). Multi-component apparent diffusion coefficients in human brain. *NMR Biomed* 12:51-62.

Munoz Maniega S, Bastin ME, Armitage PA, Farrall AJ, Carpenter TK, Hand PJ, Cvoro V, Rivers CS, Wardlaw JM (2004). Temporal evolution of water diffusion parameters is different in grey and white matter in human ischaemic stroke. *J Neurol Neurosurg Psychiatry* 75(12):1714-1718.

Nagy Z, Westerberg H, Skare S, Andersson JL, Lilja A, Flodmark O, Fernell E, Holmberg K, Bohm B, Forssberg H, Lagercrantz H, Klingberg T (2003). Preterm children have disturbances of white matter at 11 years of age as shown by diffusion tensor imaging. *Pediatr Res* 54(5):672-679.

Neeman M, Freyer JP, Sillerud LO (1991). A simple method for obtaining cross-term-free images for diffusion anisotropy studies in NMR microimaging. *Magn Reson Med* 21: 138-143.

Neil JJ, Shiran SI, McKinstry RC, Schefft GL, Snyder AZ, Almli CR, Akbudak E, Aronovitz JA, Miller JP, Lee BCP, Conturo TE (1998). Normal brain in human newborns: apparent diffusion coefficient and diffusion anisotropy measured by using diffusion tensor MR imaging. *Radiology* 209: 57-66.

Neil JJ, Miller J, Mukherjee P, Huppi PS (2002). Diffusion tensor imaging of normal and injured developing human brain -a technical review. *NMR Biomed* 15: 543-52.

Netsch T, van Muiswinkel A (2004). Quantitative evaluation of image-based distortion correction in diffusion tensor imaging. *IEEE Trans Med Imaging* 23(7):789-798.

Neumann-Haefelin T, Moseley ME, Albers GW (2000). New magnetic resonance imaging methods for cerebrovascular disease. *Ann Neuro*l 47:559-570.

Nevo U, Hauben E, Yoles E, Agranov E, Akselrod S, Schwartz M, Neeman M (2001). Diffusion anisotropy MRI for quantitative assessment of recovery in injured rat spinal cord. *Magn Reson Med* 45:1-9.

Nimsky C, Ganslandt O, Hastreiter P, Wang R, Benner T, Sorensen AG, Fahlbusch R (2005). Intraoperative diffusion-tensor MR imaging:shifting of white matter tracts during neurosurgical procedures--initial experience. *Radiology* 234(1):218-225.

Noble B, Daniel W (1977). *Applied Linear Algebra.* New Jersey, Prentice Hall.

Norris DG, Niendorf T (1995). Interpretation of DW data: dependence on experimental conditions. *NMR Biomed* 8: 280-288.

Norris DG (2001). The effects of microscopic tissue parameters on the diffusion weighted magnetic resonance imaging experiment. *NMR Biomed* 14:77-93.

Nusbaum AO, Tang CY, Buchsbaum MS, Wei TC, Atlas SW (2001). Regional and global changes in cerebral diffusion with normal aging. *AJNR Am J Neuroradiol* 22(1):136-142.

Nye JF (1957). *Physical properties of crystals*. Oxford: Clarendon Press, 176p.

Oh J, Henry RG, Genain C, Nelson SJ, Pelletier D (2004). Mechanisms of normal appearing corpus callosum injury related to pericallosal T1 lesions in multiple sclerosis using directional diffusion tensor and 1H MRS imaging. *J Neurol Neurosurg Psychiatry* 75(9):1281-1286.

Ono J, Harada K, Mano T, Sakurai K, Okada S (1997). Differentiation of dys- and demyelination using diffusional anisotropy *Pediatr Neurol* 16: 63-66.

Ojima K, Abiru H, Matsumoto H, Fukui Y (1996). Effects of postnatal exposure to cocaine on the development of the rat corpus callosum. *Reprod Toxicol* 10(3):221-225.

Pajevic S, Basser PJ (2003). Parametric and non-parametric statistical analysis of DT-MRI data. *J Magn Reson* 161: 1-14.

Pandya D, Seltzer B (1986). *The topography of commissural fibers*. In Lepore F, Petito M, Jasper H (eds): Two hemispheres - one brain: Functions of the corpus callosum. New York, Alan R. Liss, Inc. pp. 47-73.

Papadakis NG, Murrills CD, Hall LD, Huang CL, Adrian Carpenter T (2000). Minimal gradient encoding for robust estimation of diffusion anisotropy. *Magn Reson Imaging* 18(6):671-679.

Papadakis NG, Xing D, Huang CL, Hall LD, Carpenter TA (1999). A comparative study of acquisition schemes for diffusion tensor imaging using MRI. *J Magn Reson* 137:67-82.

Parker DL, Gullberg GT (1990). Signal-to-noise efficiency in magnetic resonance imaging. *Med Phys* 17(2):250-257.

Parker GJ (2004). Analysis of MR diffusion weighted images. *Br J Radiol* 77 (Special Issue) No 2:S176-185.

Partridge SC, Mukherjee P, Henry RG, Miller SP, Berman JI, Jin H, Lu Y, Glenn OA, Ferriero DM, Barkovich AJ, Vigneron DB (2004). Diffusion tensor imaging: serial quantitation of white matter tract maturity in premature newborns. *Neuroimage* 22(3):1302-1314.

Peled S, Gudbjartsson H, Westin CF, Kikinis R, Jolesz FA (1998). Magnetic resonance imaging shows orientation and asymmetry of white matter fiber tracts. *Brain Res* 780:27-33.

Peters A, Rosene DL (2003). In aging, is it gray or white? *J Comp Neurol* 462(2):139-143 (comment on Marner et al. 2003).

Pierpaoli C, Basser PJ (1996). Toward a quantitative assessment of diffusion anisotropy. *Magn Reson Med* 36(6):893-906 (Erratum in: *Magn Reson Med* 1997;37(6):972)

Pierpaoli C, Jezzard P, Basser PJ, Barnett A, Di Chiro G (1996) Diffusion tensor MR imaging of the human brain. *Radiology* 201(3):637-648.

Pierpaoli C, Barnett A, Pajevic S, Chen R, Penix LR, Virta A, Basser P (2001). Water diffusion changes in Wallerian degeneration and their dependence on white matter architecture. *Neuroimage* 13(6 Pt 1):1174-1185.

Pfefferbaum A, Sullivan EV, Hedehus M, Lim KO, Adalsteinsson E, Moseley M (2000). Age-related decline in brain white matter anisotropy measured with spatially corrected echo-planar diffusion tensor imaging. *Magn Reson Med* 44:259-268.

Pfefferbaum A, Rosenbloom M, Sullivan EV (2002). Alcoholism and AIDS: magnetic resonance imaging approaches for detecting interactive neuropathology. *Alcohol Clin Exp Res* 26(7):1031-46.

Pomara N, Crandall DT, Choi SJ, Johnson G, Lim KO (2001). White matter abnormalities in HIV-1 infection: a diffusion tensor imaging study. *Psychiatry Res* 106(1):15-24.

Poonawalla AH, Zhou XJ (2004). Analytical error propagation in diffusion anisotropy calculations. *J Magn Reson Imaging* 19(4):489-98.

Price WS (1997). Pulsed-Field Gradient Nuclear Magnetic Resonance as a Tool for Studying Translational Diffusion: Part 1. *Basic Theory. Concepts in Magnetic Resonance*, v. 9:5.

Price WS (1998). Pulsed-Field Gradient Nuclear Magnetic Resonance as a Tool for Studying Translational Diffusion: Experimental Aspects. *Concepts in Magnetic Resonance* 10, 4: 197-237.

Pruessmann KP, Weiger M, Scheidegger MB, Boesiger P (1999). SENSE: sensitivity encoding for fast MRI.*Magn Reson Med* 42(5):952-962.

Reese TG, Heid O, Weisskoff RM, Wedeen VJ (2003). Reduction of eddy-current-induced distortion in diffusion MRI using a twice-refocused spin echo. *Magn Reson Med* 49: 177-182.

Rose SE, Chen F, Chalk JB, Zelaya FO, Strugnell WE, Benson M, Semple J, Doddrell DM (2000). Loss of connectivity in Alzheimer's disease: an evaluation of white matter tract integrity with colour coded MR diffusion tensor imaging. *J Neurol Neurosurg Psychiatry* 69: 528-530.

Rudick RA (1999). Disease-modifying drugs for relapsing-remitting multiple sclerosis and future directions for multiple sclerosis therapeutics. *Arch Neurol* 56: 1079.

Rugg-Gunn FJ, Symms MR, Barker GJ, Greenwood R, Duncan JS. Diffusion imaging shows abnormalities after blunt head trauma when conventional magnetic resonance imaging is normal. *J Neurol Neurosurg Psychiatry* 70(4):530-533.

Rugg-Gunn FJ, Eriksson SH, Symms MR, Barker GJ, Thom M, Harkness W, Duncan JS (2002). Diffusion tensor imaging in refractory epilepsy. *Lancet* 359(9319):1748-1751.

Sajja BR. Datta S, He R, Narayana PA (2004). A Unified Approach for Lesion Segmentation on MRI of Multiple Sclerosis. *Proceedings of the 26th Annual International Conference of the IEEE EMBS*, San Francisco, CA, USA. 1778-1781.

Scamvougeras A, Kigar DL, Jones D, Weinberger DR, Witelson SF (2003). Size of the human corpus callosum is genetically determined: an MRI study in mono and dizygotic twins. *Neurosci Lett* 338: 91-94.

Schmierer K, Niehaus L, Roricht S, Meyer BU (2000). Conduction deficits of callosal fibres in early multiple sclerosis. *J Neurol Neurosurg Psychiatry* 68: 633-638.

Schneider JF, Il'yasov KA, Hennig J, Martin E (2004). Fast quantitative diffusion-tensor imaging of cerebral white matter from the neonatal period to adolescence. *Neuroradiology* 46(4):258-266

Schwartz ED, Chin CL, Shumsky JS, Jawad AF, Brown BK, Wehrli S, Tessler A, Murray M, Hackney DB (2005). Apparent diffusion coefficients in spinal cord transplants and surrounding white matter correlate with degree of axonal dieback after injury in rats. AJNR *Am J Neuroradiol* 26(1):7-18

Schwartz ED, Cooper ET, Fan Y, Jawad AF, Chin CL, Nissanov J, Hackney DB (2005). MRI diffusion coefficients in spinal cord correlate with axon morphometry. *Neuroreport* 16(1):73-76.

Shimony JS, McKinstry RC, Akbudak E, Aronovitz JA, Snyder AZ, Lori NF, Cull TS, Conturo TE (1999). Quantitative diffusion-tensor anisotropy brain MR imaging: normative human data and anatomic analysis. *Radiology* 212(3):770-84

Skare S, Hedehus M, Mosley ME, Li TQ (2000). Condition number as a measure of noise performance of diffusion tensor data acquisition schemes with MRI. *J Magn Reson* 147(2):340-352.

Sodickson DK, McKenzie CA (2001). A generalized approach to parallel magnetic resonance imaging. *Med Phys* 28(8):1629-1643.

Song SK, Sun SW, Ramsbottom MJ, Chang C, Russell J and Cross AH (2002). Dysmyelination Revealed through MRI as Increased Radial (but Unchanged Axial) Diffusion of Water, *NeuroImage* 17:1429-1436.

Song SK, Sun SW, Ju WK, Lin SJ, Cross AH, Neufeld AH (2003). Diffusion tensor imaging detects and differentiates axon and myelin degeneration in mouse optic nerve after retinal ischemia. *Neuroimage.* 20(3):1714-1722.

Sotak CH (2002). The role of diffusion tensor imaging in the evaluation of ischemic brain injury - a review. *NMR Biomed* 15(7-8):561-569.

Sowell ER, Peterson BS, Thompson PM, Welcome SE, Henkenius AL, Toga AW (2003). Mapping cortical change across the human life span. *Nat Neurosci* 6(3):309-315.

Steinman L, Martin R, Bernard C, Conlon P, Oksenberg JR (2002). Multiple sclerosis: deeper understanding of its pathogenesis reveals new targets for therapy. *Annu Rev Neurosci* 25: 491-505.

Stejskal EO, Tanner JE (1965). Spin diffusion measurements: spin echoes in the presence of a time-dependent field gradient. *Journal of Chemical Physics* 42:288-92.

Sullivan EV, Adalsteinsson E, Hedehus M, Ju C, Moseley M, Lim KO, Pfefferbaum A (2001). Equivalent disruption of regional white matter microstructure in ageing healthy men and women. *Neuroreport* 12: 99-104.

Sullivan EV, Pfefferbaum A (2003). Diffusion tensor imaging in normal aging and neuropsychiatric disorders. *Eur J Radiol* 45(3):244-55

Sundgren PC, Dong Q, Gomez-Hassan D, Mukherji SK, Maly P, Welsh R (2004). Diffusion tensor imaging of the brain: review of clinical applications. *Neuroradiology* 46(5):339-350.

Suzuki Y, Matsuzawa H, Kwee IL, Nakada T (2003). Absolute eigenvalue diffusion tensor analysis for human brain maturation. *NMR Biomed* 16(5):257-260.

Takahashi M, Ono J, Harada K, Maeda M, Hackney DB (2000). Diffusional anisotropy in cranial nerves with maturation: quantitative evaluation with diffusion MR imaging in rats. *Radiology* 216(3):881-885.

Takahashi M, Hackney DB, Zhang G, Wehrli SL, Wright AC, O'Brien WT, Uematsu H, Wehrli FW, Selzer ME (2002). Magnetic resonance microimaging of intraaxonal water diffusion in live excised lamprey spinal cord. *Proc Natl Acad Sci USA* 10;99(25):16192-16196.

Takahashi S, Yonezawa H, Takahashi J, Kudo M, Inoue T, Tohgi H (2002). Selective reduction of diffusion anisotropy in white matter of Alzheimer disease brains measured by 3.0 Tesla magnetic resonance imaging. *Neurosci Lett* 332(1):45-48.

Taylor DG, Bushell MC (1985). The spatial mapping of translational diffusion coefficients by the NMR imaging technique. *Phys Med Biol* 30(4):345-349.

Teipel SJ, Hampel H, Pietrini P, Alexander GE, Horwitz B, Daley E, Moller HJ, Schapiro MB, Rapoport SI (1999). Region-specific corpus callosum atrophy correlates with the regional pattern of cortical glucose metabolism in Alzheimer disease. *Arch Neurol* 56(4):467-473.

Thomalla G, Glauche V, Weiller C, Rother J (2005). Time course of wallerian degeneration after ischaemic stroke revealed by diffusion tensor imaging. *J Neurol Neurosurg Psychiatry* 76(2):266-268.

Torrey HC (1956). Bloch equations with diffusion terms. *J. Chem. Phys* 104 (3):563–565.

Trapp BD, Peterson J, Ransohoff RM, Rudick R, Mork S, Bo L (1998). Axonal transection in the lesions of multiple sclerosis. *N Engl J Med* 338: 278-285.

Tuch DS (2004). Q-ball imaging. *Magn Reson Med* 52(6):1358-1372.

Wakana S, Jiang H, Nagae-Poetscher LM, van Zijl PC, Mori S (2003). Fiber tract-based atlas of human white matter anatomy. *Radiology* 230: 77-87.

Waxman SG (1998). Demyelinating diseases--new pathological insights, new therapeutic targets. *N Engl J Med.* 338(5):323-325.

Waxman SG, Kocsis JD, Stys PK (1995). *Axon: structure, function, and pathophysiology.* Oxford University Press, New York.

Weisskoff RM (1996). Simple measurement of scanner stability for functional NMR imaging of activation in the brain. *Magn Reson Med* 36: 643-645.

Werring DJ, Clark CA, Barker GJ, Miller DH, Parker GJ, Brammer MJ, Bullmore ET, Giampietro VP, Thompson AJ (1998). The structural and functional mechanisms of motor recovery: complementary use of diffusion tensor and functional magnetic resonance imaging in a traumatic injury of the internal capsule. *J Neurol Neurosurg Psychiatry* 65: 863-869.

Werring DJ, Clark CA, Barker GJ, Thompson AJ, Miller DH (1999). Diffusion tensor imaging of lesions and normal-appearing white matter in multiple sclerosis. *Neurology* 52(8):1626-1632.

Westin CF, Maier SE, Mamata H, Nabavi A, Jolesz FA, Kikinis R (2002). Processing and visualization for diffusion tensor MRI. *Med Image Anal* 6(2):93-108.

Westerhausen R, Walter C, Kreuder F, Wittling RA, Schweiger E, Wittling W (2003). The influence of handedness and gender on the microstructure of the human corpus callosum: A DT-MRI study. *Neurosci Lett* 351: 99-102.

Wider G, Dotsch V, Wuthrich K (1994). Self-Compensating Pulsed Magnetic-Field. Gradients for Short Recovery Times. *J. Magn. Reson* A 108: 255-258.

Wiegell MR, Larsson HB, Wedeen VJ (2000). Fiber crossing in human brain depicted with diffusion tensor MR imaging. *Radiology* 217(3):897-903.

Wiegell MR, Tuch DS, Larsson HB, Wedeen VJ (2003). Automatic segmentation of thalamic nuclei from diffusion tensor magnetic resonance imaging. *Neuroimage* 19(2 Pt 1):391-401.

Wieshmann UC, Symms MR, Parker GJ, Clark CA, Lemieux L, Barker GJ, Shorvon SD (2000). Diffusion tensor imaging demonstrates deviation of fibres in normal appearing white matter adjacent to a brain tumour. *J Neurol Neurosurg Psychiatry* 68(4):501-503

Wimberger DM, Roberts TP, Barkovich AJ, Prayer LM, Moseley ME, Kucharczyk J (1995). Identification of "premyelination" by diffusion-weighted MRI. *J Comput Assist Tomogr* 19(1):28-33.

Witelson SF (1985). The brain connection: the corpus callosum is larger in left-handers. *Science* 229: 665-668.

Witelson SF (1989). Hand and sex differences in the isthmus and genu of the human corpus callosum. A postmortem morphological study. *Brain* 112: 799-835.

Wolinsky JS, Narayana PA (2002). Magnetic resonance spectroscopy in multiple sclerosis: window into the diseased brain. *Curr Opin Neurol* 15: 247-251.

Woods RP, Grafton ST, Holmes CJ, Cherry SR, Mazziotta JC (1998). Automated image Registration: I General methods and intrasubject, intramodality validation. *J Comp Assist Tomog* 22: 141-154

Xing D, Papadakis NG, Huang CL, Lee VM, Carpenter TA, Hall LD (1997). Optimised diffusion-weighting for measurement of apparent diffusion coefficient (ADC) in human brain. *Magn Reson Imaging* 15:771-784.

Xu D, Mori S, Solaiyappan M, van Zijl PC, Davatzikos C (2002). A framework for callosal fiber distribution analysis. *Neuroimage* 17: 1131-1143.

Yang X (1996). Contrast in NMR Imaging and Microscopy. *Concepts in Magnetic Resonance* 8(3):205-225.

Yoshiura T, Wu O, Zaheer A, Reese TG, Sorensen AG (2001). Highly diffusion-sensitized MRI of brain: dissociation of gray and white matter. *Magn Reson Med* 45(5):734-40.

Zacharopoulos NG, Narayana PA (1998). Selective measurement of white matter and gray matter diffusion trace values in normal human brain. *Med Phys* 25:2237-2241.

Zaidel E, Iacoboni M (2003). The parallel brain: The Cognitive Neuroscience of the Corpus Callosum. *MIT press*, Cambridge.

In: Progress in Brain Mapping Research
Editor: F. J. Chen, pp. 81-121 ISBN 1-59454-580-4

Chapter 2

Mapping the Functional Organization of the Human Auditory Cortex

Selene Cansino[1]
Laboratory of NeuroCognition, Faculty of Psychology
National Autonomous University of Mexico, Mexico City, Mexico

Abstract

The knowledge on how the auditory system is functionally organized to respond to different acoustic parameters has mainly been derived from animal studies. Electrophysiological, cytoarchitectonic and histochemical experiments in animals have provided functional evidence of how the peripheral and central auditory systems process acoustic information. However, extrapolation to humans of findings obtained in animal studies remains to be confirmed. Although the anatomy of the auditory system shows strong similarities among primates, high order cognitive functions such as speech indicate that direct human experimentation is required to understand how the human auditory system processes simple and complex auditory stimulation. The development of techniques that allow to record human brain activity while subjects are subjected to auditory stimulation, such as event-related potentials (ERP), magnetoencephalography (MEG), positron emission tomography (PET) and functional magnetic resonance imaging (fMRI), have provided new insights on how the human auditory system processes auditory information. The present chapter reviews and updates the functional mappings of the human auditory cortex derived from these techniques. It focuses on human studies; however, results in animal subjects are also described when similarities were found. This chapter inspects auditory cortex mappings, since the mentioned techniques have provided their major findings in cortical regions, whereas activity from subcortical areas has been more difficult to survey. Functional auditory cortex mappings are revised for acoustic parameters such as frequency, amplitude, spectrum and temporality. The growing knowledge on high order auditory functions such as speech

[1] Corresponding author: Selene Cansino, Ph.D. Laboratory of NeuroCognition, Faculty of Psychology, National Autonomous University of Mexico, Avenida Universidad 3004, Colonia Copilco Universidad, Mexico D. F., 04510, Mexico, Phone: (52 55) 56 22 23 39; Fax: (52 55) 56 16 07 78; E-mail: selene@servidor.unam.mx

and music are beyond the scope of this chapter, for it would be impossible to provide an outright description of these extensive research areas. The chapter starts with an anatomical description of the auditory cortices derived from recent cytoarchitectonic and histochemical experiments. Next, a definition and description of each of the acoustic parameters to be reviewed are provided. The research intended to establish auditory cortical maps for each of these parameters is then analyzed. An integration of the current knowledge in this field of research is presented at the end.

Keywords: *Auditory cortex, frequency, spectrum, intensity, temporality, tonotopic maps, amplitopic maps.*

Introduction

For decades, invasive techniques such as cortical lesions, *in vivo* tracers and microelectrode recordings have been extensively employed in numerous non-human species to explore the correlates between structure and function in the auditory cortex, especially from a micro-anatomic and micro-physiologic perspective. Most of this research has been done in cats and recently in non-human primates. Although the subcortical auditory system is similar among various species [62] and the primary auditory cortex has been identified in bats, rodents, carnivores, non-human primates and humans [42], the organization of the cortical auditory system shows remarkable differences among species [62], which complicate comparative extrapolations. Non-human and human primates might be the exception to this rule since some cortical cythoarchitecture similarities have recently been identified in both species [119]. However, as pointed out by Griffiths et al. [42], the existence of generic auditory processing mechanisms across species should be tested before human auditory function is interpreted using non-human primate models. The important framework provided by the extensive research field on non-human species has been reviewed elsewhere [e.g. 24, 22, 119].

In contrast, the knowledge on human auditory cortex has derived mostly from non-invasive techniques, which provide a better understanding of the auditory system from the macro-anatomical and macro-physiological points of view; except for the studies with post-mortem subjects and the experiments with intracortical recordings. However, the results of these two kinds of studies should be considered with caution. The first because findings have mainly been derived from donors aged 70 years old or more and there is evidence that brain volume diminishes with age due to nervous cells lost [55]. The second, because intracortical recordings are usually performed under surgical conditions with the brain exposed to air, and there is evidence that physiological responses under these conditions are delayed [1]. The understanding of the organization of the human auditory cortex has improved in recent times because of the development of high-resolution non-invasive techniques. Event-related potentials (ERP) and magnetoencephaolography (MEG) offer high temporal resolution, of the order of one millisecond, of brain responses from neural populations. In addition, these techniques, especially MEG, provide spatial information on the sources that give rise to the brain activity recorded outside the head by means of inverse equation calculations. Positron emission tomography (PET) and particularly, functional magnetic resonance imaging (fMRI) provide high spatial resolution, of the order of a centimeter or less, of blood oxygenation responses associated to neural brain activity. Although numerous findings have emerged from studies which have employed these techniques to explore the human auditory cortex, few authors have reviewed this research field recently [47]; others, have reviewed not only studies with human subjects but also with non-human primates [119, 63]; and others have based their reviews on specific acoustic parameters such us periodicity [67] or spatial and temporal sound features [39].

The present chapter focuses on human studies, with the techniques cited above, intending to investigate functional maps of the auditory cortex specialized on the processes of the acoustic parameters: frequency, amplitude, spectrum and temporality. This review attempts to integrate the growing, and scarcely examined, knowledge on this topic. Although it is impossible to cite all publications relevant to this review, a careful selection has been made of those that deal with the different topics under discussion.

Anatomy of the Human Auditory Cortex

The advent of new methods and techniques to study the anatomy of the human auditory cortex from the micro-structural and macro-structural perspectives has enlarged our knowledge on this region. The classical architectonic studies based on visual inspection have been replaced for quantitative analysis performed by automated microscopes independent of observers. High-resolution structural magnetic resonance imaging (MRI) has been employed to explore this area in living [e.g. 95] and in post-mortem subjects [e.g. 86]. At present, various histological markers have contributed with a more precise definition of the architecture of this area: the parvalbumin inmunoreactivity stains of thalamocortical projection zones thus provide information about connectivity; cytochrome oxidase stains metabolic activity; Nissl staining offers cytoarchitectonic information; acetylcholinesterase (AChE) staining supplies information on pyramidal cells containing AChE.

Primary Auditory Cortex

The human primary auditory cortex was described by Brodman [13] as one koniocortical area (41) in Heschl's gyrus; however, also two [21, 35], three [86], eleven [20], or even 20 [4] different cytoarchitectonic areas have been distinguished in this region. Although there is no consensus regarding the cytoarchitecture of this region, there is agreement that the primary auditory cortex is located within the lateral fissure, on the supratemporal plane of the transverse temporal (Heschl) gyrus (Figure 1). The primary auditory cortex has been located in the medial two-thirds [73], in the posteromedial two-thirds [129] or in the mediolateral axis of the Heschl's gyrus [86]. Approximately 33% of the individuals have two Heschl's gyri [136, 134]; this occurs when the sulcus intermedius is extremely deep and cleaves the Heschl's gyrus along its entire length, otherwise this sulcus only produces a bifurcation in the Heschl's gyrus [134]. When two Heschl's gyri are present, the primary auditory cortex is mainly present in the most anterior gyrus [101]. The transverse temporal gyrus is difficult to identify in structural MRI (T1-weigthed images) [136] and it has lower signal intensity than surrounding gyri in functional MRI (T2-weigthed images) [134]. Moreover, the primary auditory cortex cannot be reliably identified with MRI because it has no macroanatomic landmarks [86]. Notwithstanding these technical difficulties, Penhune et al. [95] found in the MR images of 30 subjects that Heschl's gyrus is located 5 to 8 mm more anterior in the right than in the left hemisphere. Furthermore, these authors reported that the transverse temporal gyrus has a larger volume in the left than in the right hemisphere. To further study these differences, an additional analysis was computed on MR images to distinguish grey matter from white matter.

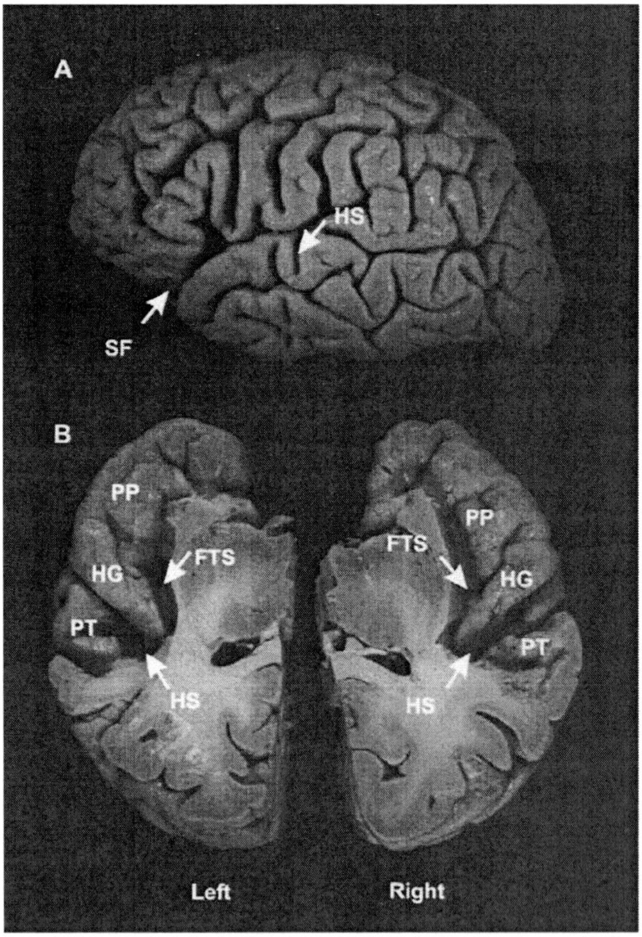

Figure 1. Human brain showing main macroanatomical landmarks of the primary auditory regions. Lateral view (A) and dorsal view (B) after removal of the frontal and parietal opercula. SF, Sylvian fissure; FTS, first transverse temporal sulcus; HS, Heschl's sulcus; HG, Heschl's gyrus; PP, planum polare; PT, planum temporale. The FTS marks the anterior border of the HG; while its posterior border is usually undefined. The HG divides the supratemporal plane into the planum polare (rostrally) and the planum temporale (caudally). Reprinted from *Neuroimage,* 13, Morosan, P., Rademacher, J., Schleicher, A., Amunts, K., Schormann, T. and Zilles, K. Human Primary Auditory Cortex: Cytoarchitectonic subdivisions and mapping into a spatial reference system, 684-701, Copyright 2001, with permission from Elesevier.

This examination revealed that volume differences between hemispheres were due to a larger amount of white matter and not of cortical tissue, which indicates the high affluence of afferent and efferent fibers in the primary auditory cortex. However, as pointed out by the authors [95], the MRI technique does not allow to distinguish which kind of fibers are more prevalent: thalamocortical or corticocortical; or whether the differences in white matter are due to a higher myelination of left hemisphere fibers than those of the right.

From a microscopic point of view, Nissl stains of the primary auditory cortex reveals that this region is characterized by high cell density on layers II to IV and by thick layers V and VI [35]. According to Wallace et al. [129], layers IV and VI constitute 40% of the entire cortical thickness in this area. Intense cytochrome oxidase activity confirms the existence of numerous granular cells in the base of layer III and layer IV, while layers V and VI show low activity [129]. By means of AChE staining, it has been confirmed that the primary auditory cortex has lower density of pyramidal cells than the surrounding areas [83]. Wallace et al. [129] also pointed out that pyramidal cells are almost absent in the anterior part of the primary auditory cortex; however, they identified a second auditory core in the lateral posterior area of Heschl's gyrus, which was characterized by high cytochrome oxidase activity, high parvalbumin immunoreactivity and high AChE activity in layer IV. Higher pyramidal cell density in layer IV of auditory core areas than most of the surrounding areas detected by AChE staining have been confirmed by other authors [104, 62]. Morosan et al. [86] identified three cytoarchitectonic areas within the primary auditory cortex with the use of an automated analysis to detect areal borders. These three areas have in common small granular cells across the ribbon, small pyramidal cells in layer III, thick layer IV and low cell density in layer V. These characteristics are similar to those described when two cytoarchitectonic areas have been identified within the primary auditory cortex [21, 35]. Because one of the three cytoarchitectonic areas detected by Morosan et al. [86] in the primary auditory cortex showed higher density of granular cells, more thalamocortical projections and more medium-sized pyramidal cells than the others, it was considered the koniocortical core field.

An objective measure to detect cytoarchitectonic differences between cortical areas consists in calculating the cell volume fraction or number of neurons per unit volume in brain images [115]. Morosan et al. [86] detected with this kind of analysis a great cell density variability in Heschl's gyrus among subjects without gender differences. In addition, they observed a higher number of neurons per unit volume in the left hemisphere than in the right in two of the three cytoarchitectonic areas that comprise the primary auditory cortex according with these authors, while the third area showed higher cell volume in the right hemisphere than in the left. Seldon [118] described similar results twenty years before employing Nissl staining: larger cortical columns in the left side than in the right with longer distances between columns and greater dendritic arborization.

Non-Primary Auditory Cortex

The exact number of non-primary auditory cortices is still unknown. Brodman [13] described that the primary auditory cortex (area 41) was surrounded by three secondary auditory areas: caudolaterally by area 42, rostrolaterally by area 22 and medially by area 52. In the lateral fissure on the upper surface of the temporal lobe lie the major human auditory areas identified by Galaburda and Sanides [35]: a double koniocortical core in the transverse gyrus surrounded by concentric parakoniocortical belts rostrally, laterally and caudally. The belt regions are characterized by the presence of granulated fields, and in layer III by the occurrence of pyramidal cells of medium and large size. The caudal parakoniocortical belt extends to the end of the lateral fissure around the insular region and then dorsally into the parietal operculum and inferior parietal lobe. Braak [11] also reported a belt area with less granular cells than the core, which is located anterior to the core and extends toward the insula and the superior temporal gyrus mainly in the region lateral to the core. In addition, Galaburda and Sanides [35] detected a parakoniocortical area in the superior temporal gyrus which corresponds to the anterior portion of Brodman's area 22; this region contains in layer III pyramid cells arranged in columns and probably receives inputs from the medial geniculate nucleus and adjacent parakoniocortical areas. This area, which extends above and slightly below the length of the superior temporal sulcus, has been identified as the auditory association cortex in humans [100, 16]. Recent studies have identified one [104] or two core areas [129] surrounded by at least six belt areas [104, 129]. A belt area was detected in the anterolateral third of Heschl's gyrus and was characterized by low cytochorme oxidase activity and high density of pyramidal cells as revealed by acetylcholinesterase stains [129]. Surrounding the primary cortex, Rivier and Clarke [104] identified a belt area across the supratemporal plane that extends into the insula.

Although the human auditory cortex has been studied for more than a century, at present there is no consensus yet about its anatomical organization. In contrast, the auditory cortex in the macaque monkey has been recently described with precision on the basis of its cytoarchitecture and connectivity [62, 102]. It has been divided into three areas: core, belt and parabelt. The core is characterized by koniocortical architecture, dense myelination, and high cytochrome oxidase, acetylcholinesterase and parvalbumin activity. Three fields have been identified in the core, which receives afferent fibers from the ventral division of the medial geniculate nucleus and projects efferent fibers ipsilateral and contralaterally to adjacent core areas and belt areas. The belt is constituted by seven fields that surround the core along the upper surface of the superior temporal gyrus. Larger pyramidal cells are observed in the belt than in the core; while cell density, columnar spacing and myelination are lesser in the belt than in the core area. The belt receives inputs from the core area and from the dorsal and medial division of the medial geniculate nucleus. The parabelt lies lateral to the belt fields along the surface of the superior temporal gyrus and has less cell density than the belt fields. Based on its connectivity two fields have been distinguished: the rostral parabelt, which receives inputs from the rostral belt field, and the caudal parabelt, which receives inputs from the caudal belt fields. In addition, the parabelt fields receive afferent inputs from the dorsal and medial divisions of the medial geniculate nucleus. The attempt to establish if the morphological organization of the auditory cortex found in non-human primates can be extended to explain the human auditory cortex have indicated so far, that the non-primary auditory areas described in humans are far from being similar to those found in non-human primates.

To conciliate the different descriptions of the non-primary human auditory areas it has been proposed to divide this region, based on gross morphological criteria, into the planum polare, which corresponds to the area anterior to the Heschl's gyrus, and the planum temporale, which comprises the area posterior to the Heschl's gyrus [47]. The auditory cortical system lies in one of the most folded regions of the human brain, consequently great variability between brains and between hemispheres of the same brain has complicated the identification of the auditory cortices. Galaburda and Sanides [35] emphasized the striking asymmetries between left and right hemispheres that they observed in the caudal area of the lateral fissure. Especially, they reported that the cytoarchitectonic volume was larger in the left hemisphere than in the right in the planum temporale. This hemisphere asymmetry has been consistently found in approximately 65% of the cases [138]. This finding has been considered to support the claim that this region of the left hemisphere is uncharged of linguistic processes. However, empirical evidence is still missing to confirm that this morphological distinction between hemispheres is due to linguistic functions or to other causes; for instance, handedness has also been related to this anatomical asymmetry [31].

Acoustic Parameters

This section attempts to provide a comprehensible understanding of the main acoustic parameters that have been manipulated in order to disentangle how the human auditory system processes and interprets our acoustic world. Vision is considered a synthetic sense since we are not able to distinguish the original colors once they are combined into a color mixture. In contrast, hearing is an analytic sense since we are capable of discriminating two different sounds even when they are played simultaneously. Probably because of this analytic characteristic of the auditory system, most of the research in this field has employed simple stimuli in which single acoustic parameters are modified. The exact manipulation of these acoustic features is essential to arrive to reliable and consistent results; and to allow comparison among different studies. This session may be skipped by readers specialized in these concepts. Basic acoustic parameters are reviewed, and not music or linguistic stimuli, because the research with this kind of stimulation will not be covered in the present chapter. However, the acoustic parameters that will be reviewed constitute basic sound concepts that can also be applied to appreciate or comprehend complex stimuli such as music or speech.

Frequency

Frequency has been the main acoustic parameter employed to determine the functional organization of the human auditory system. The number of cycles a sound wave completes in one second is called frequency. A pure tone is composed by a sine-wave of a particular frequency (Figure 2). Pitch corresponds to the psychological experience of frequency; however, frequency and pitch are not always closely related. For example, frequencies below (20 Hz) or above (20,000 Hz) the human audible range will produce no sense of pitch; or two frequencies too similar to be discriminated will be experienced as having the same pitch [43].

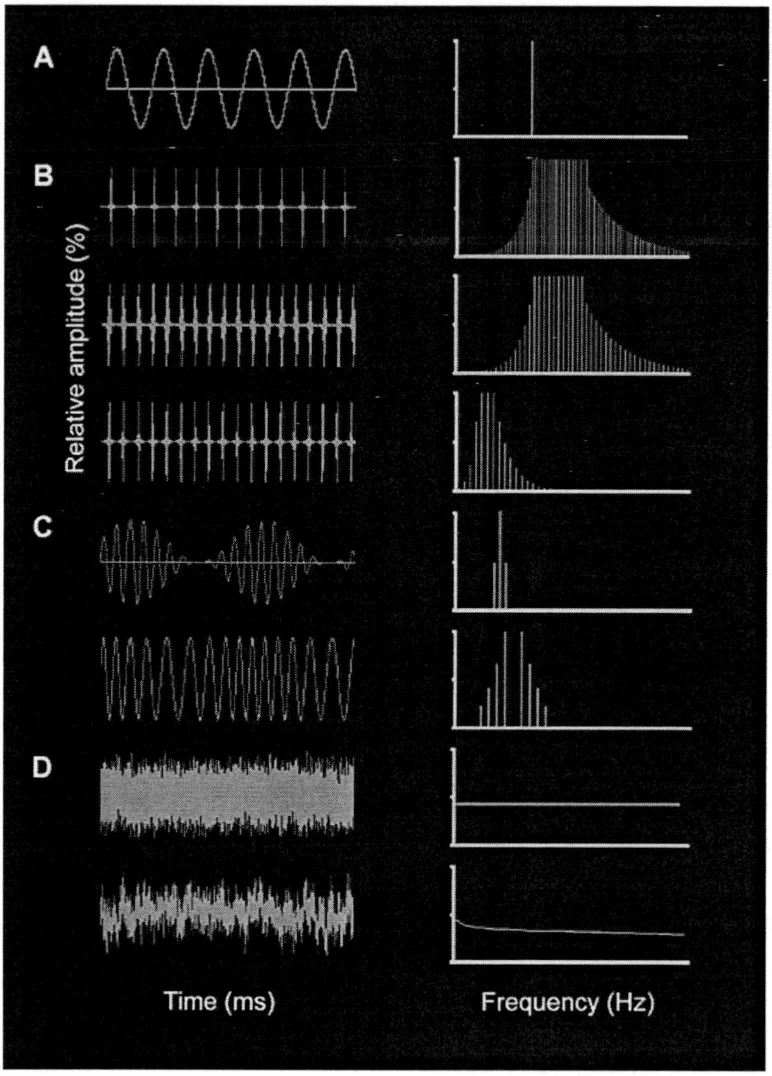

Figure 2. Waveform (left side) and spectral (right side) representations of different sounds. A, pure tone; B, three complex sounds, from top to bottom, the first and the second have the same central frequency (CF) but different fundamental frequency (Fo); whereas the second and the third have the same Fo but different CF; C, the first sound is amplitude-modulated and the second is frequency-modulated; D, white noise (top) and pink noise (bottom).

Besides, pitch perception of pure tones depends on the amplitude and duration of the sound. Pitch seems lower when the amplitude increases in pure tones below 200 Hz, and seems higher when it increases in sounds above 6,000 Hz [110]. Independently of the frequency, increasing the amplitude of short pure tones (below 40 ms) decreases the pitch [111]. Psychophysical studies have established that the absolute threshold, i.e. the smallest amount of a stimulus that can be detected 50% of the time, is lower for frequencies between 2,000 Hz and 5,000 Hz, with the highest sensitivity approximately at 3,000 Hz [114]. This range almost corresponds to speech frequencies, usually between 600 Hz and 4,000 Hz. The difference threshold, i.e. the smallest change in a stimulus that can produce a difference noticeable 50% of the time, expressed by the Weber fraction is of 0.3% for frequencies in the range of 500 Hz to 2,000 Hz [26]. The Weber fraction corresponds to the difference threshold divided by the frequency of the tone. Thus, a tone frequency has to be changed by only 0.3% in order to be detectable; for comparison, taste requires a stimulus change of 20% [81] and smell of 7% [14] to be noticeable. To evaluate the stimuli employed in the different experiments it is crucial to have some knowledge on the sensitivity and limits of the human auditory system. Pure tones are the type of stimulus most often used in acoustic experiments, despite the fact that they are extremely rare in the real world, probably because linear vibrations are easy to describe and generate by means of electroacoustical equipment; however, what we really hear every day are complex sounds.

Amplitude

The search for systematic variations in brain responses as a function of sound amplitude has also been investigated. A successive air-pressure change falling on our ears needs to displace our eardrum by only 1 billionth of a centimeter to be heard as a sound [38]. Amplitude is the maximum pressure variation usually from normal atmospheric pressure. If sound pressure is measured in terms of a standard force, as dyne per square centimeter, the range from a barely detectable sound (0.002 dynes/cm^2) to a painful sound (2000 dynes/cm^2) will be extremely wide to be manageable. Therefore, a logarithmic scale of sound pressure relative to the threshold pressure of 0.002 dynes /cm^2 is generally employed. The scale most often used is the sound pressure level (SPL) expressed in decibel units. A decibel (dB) of SPL is computed by means of the equation: Decibels = 20 log P_1 / P_0, where P_1 is the sound pressure level of the stimulus to be converted to decibels and P_0 is the reference level of 0.002 dynes /cm^2 [114]. In the SPL scale, the sound pressure doubles every 6 dB. With this scale, a painful pressure of 2,000 dynes /cm^2 will be 140 dB, a sound intensity that can cause permanent hearing loss [53]. Loudness corresponds to the psychological experience of amplitude; however, loudness and amplitude are not entirely correlated. Loudness perception depends on the frequency and the duration of the sound. Fletcher and Munson [28] elaborated the curves, which show that low frequencies require more amplitude to be audible. Short duration sounds (below 150 ms) are less loud than longer sounds [43]. Frequencies between 1,000 and 5,000 Hz have the lowest amplitude threshold [28]. For pure tones of almost all frequencies, the amplitude difference threshold expressed in Wever fractions is of 0.3 to produce a noticeable perception of a change in loudness [43].

Spectrum

The waveforms generated by natural physical vibrations or by movement patterns occurring in mechanical objects are usually complex tones and not sinusoidal. A complex sound, such as the human voice or music, is composed of many simple sounds. Fourier's theorem [32] stipulates that a complex sound is equivalent to a series of sine-waves. This series is made up of a fundamental frequency and of harmonics. The fundamental frequency corresponds to the component of a complex tone with the lowest frequency, and the harmonics are multiples of the fundamental frequency, hence they have higher frequencies than the fundamental. The fundamental frequency reflects the periodicity pitch of the wave and it is perceived as the musical note, the harmonics account for the wave-shaped complexity of the sound. The spectrum corresponds to the distribution of harmonic amplitude and frequency, and it can be modified if some frequencies are made to be predominant. The central frequency (CF) is referred to as the main resonant frequencies in a complex sound or where harmonics are emphasized and can be defined by the equation: CF = sqrt (f1 x f2), where f1 and f2 are the region between two frequencies where harmonic are emphasized [15]. The central frequency allows vowels to be differentiated, independently from the periodicity pitch at which the vocal cords vibrate, or permits to discriminate among different musical instruments when they play the same note, because even though they will produce the same fundamental frequency, each of them emphasizes different harmonics. Timbre corresponds to the psychological experience of spectrum. Two sounds may have the same pitch and loudness but differ in timbre quality. Timbre is the acoustic quality that allows us to distinguish someone's voice, whereas pitch and loudness will not provide sufficient information for this detection.

A sound signal can be amplitude- or frequency-modulated for transmission or sound synthesis purposes (Figure 2). In acoustic experiments, modulated sounds are often used because these stimuli can be accurately controlled and defined. Amplitude modulation consists in varying systematically the amplitude of a carrier signal by means of a modulated signal. Two tones of different frequency, initially in phase, will move gradually out of phase until they reach a moment of interference, which will reduce loudness; when they move back into phase, the loudness will increase. This phenomenon is known as beat frequency and is a form of amplitude modulation, which occurs at a rate equal to the difference between the two frequencies [67]. When the carrier and the modulating signals are sine waves they produce a spectrum composed of the carrier frequency and a pair of sidebands at each side of the carrier at a distance equal to the modulating frequency [98]. The amplitude of this spectrum will be controlled by the amplitude of the modulating signal. Depth modulation expresses the strength of this modulation and is defined as $100*(A - B)/(A + B)$, where A and B are the maximum and minimum amplitudes of the modulated signal, respectively. The amplitude of the sidebands will be 50% that of the carrier when depth modulation is of 100 %, and as this percentage decreases, the spectral energy at the carrier frequency increases, and decreases at the sidebands [98]. In contrast, frequency modulation consists in systematically changing the frequency of the carrier instead of the amplitude through a modulation frequency. The percentage of frequency modulation can be expressed by the total range of frequency change divided by the carrier frequency [17].

Temporality

Time is an inherent attribute of any acoustic stimulation, therefore it is in fact impossible to segregate temporal features from any wave sound. However, it is possible to maintain the same temporal pattern among stimuli to study other acoustic parameters, or to maintain other acoustic traits constant while temporal attributes of the sound are manipulated in order to study how the brain decodes this information. Periodicity pitch is one of the temporal parameters more extensively studied. The harmonics of a complex sound are characterized by periodic envelope modulations, the periodicity of which corresponds to the fundamental frequency. The envelope of a wave serves to describe temporal characteristics of a sound and is refereed to as the curve connecting successive peaks in the waveform [114]. The periodic envelope elicits the perception of periodic pitch, which endures as long as the periodicity of the sound is the same independently of the harmonic composition [116]. In a complex sound, two or more contiguous harmonics will have an envelope period similar to the fundamental frequency and will elicit the same periodicity pitch because their frequencies are multiples of the fundamental frequency [68]. This property of complex sounds explains the phenomenon of the missing fundamental: a complex sound that elicits the same pitch as the fundamental frequency even though it is only composed of harmonics and the fundamental frequency is absent. The periodic pitch of complex sounds might be modified by changing their periodic envelopes while maintaining the same spectrum signal or timbre; on the contrary, the spectrum might be changed while conserving the same envelope period or pitch (Figure 2).

Another temporal parameter of sounds is the phase angle, which is the position of the pressure change throughout one complete cycle. Phase indicates the temporal relation between two or more sinusoids in a complex sound or the relation between one sinusoid with its onset or with another fixed event [114]. Phase angle is expressed in degrees at each position of the cycle: 0° and 180° represent normal air pressure, which depends on the altitude, at higher altitude the pressure is lower; while 90° and 270° correspond to the maximum and minimum pressure, respectively. If two identical waves are perfectly out of phase they will cancel each other and no sound will be produced. Conversely, if two waves are in phase they will be added. Two complex tones will sound extremely dissimilar if each of them has a different phase relation among its harmonic components.

Although noise is considered an undesired complex sound produced by improper handling of signals or by nature sources, it has proved to be useful as stimulus in auditory experiments. White noise, like the color white, contains all frequencies within the range of human hearing randomized so they will not correlate. Since the energy is equivalent at all frequencies, this noise might produce the perception that it is composed by high frequencies more than by low frequencies. This occurs because the frequency increases twice at each successive octave increment; the term octave represents a doubling of frequency. White noise lacks frequency specificity; however, it is useful to generate high amplitude brain responses in a large range of frequencies; it is also used as a masking stimulus. By contrast, pink noise has equal energy per octave instead of equal energy per frequency as white noise. Thus each increasing octave contains half the power of the preceding one. This noise is usually used as a masking sound (Figure 2). Noise has been recently employed to generate a stimulus in which it is possible to manipulate pitch on a temporal basis, maintaining the same noise spectrum for all frequencies. This is achieved by adding a noise wave to itself with a delay of a few milliseconds. If this delay and adding process is repeated, the sound will have a pitch with a frequency equal to the inverse of the delay in time, but it will maintain its same noise spectrum [135]. The strength of the salient pitch depends on the number of iterations or repetitions of the delay and adding process. This stimulus allows to study the brain responses associated to the extraction of pitch information based on the perception of regular intervals of a few milliseconds without spectral cues.

Functional Auditory Cortical Maps

In the present context, the term mapping refers to the examination of the auditory cortical brain areas with the aim of discovering brain activity spatially distributed for functional purpose. The empirical research conducted to achieve this objective will be analyzed. One of the main difficulties in this research field is the great anatomical variability observed in the regions devoted to auditory stimulation. The unevenness of this region is complicated to overcome by techniques that rely on the analysis of brain activity averaged across several subjects, such as event-related potentials (ERP), magnetoencephalography (MEG), positron emission tomography (PET) and functional magnetic resonance imaging (fMRI). Even though inter- and intra-subject anatomical variability might mitigate the strength of the averaged brain activity, functional cortical maps have been described with these techniques. However, the exact spatial locations of the sources that give rise to the activity recorded outside the head by means of ERP or MEG have been subjected to debate due to the difficulty to disentangle how many sources are responsible for such activity. On the other hand, most research with PET and fMRI have revealed broad maps associated to functional properties of the auditory cortex. Notwithstanding these obstacles, the knowledge on this topic has advanced substantially as will be described below.

Tonotopic Maps

The term "tonotopy" describes the topographical organization of neural populations according to their sensitivity to respond to specific frequencies of an acoustic stimulus. In humans, empirical evidence supports the existence of tonotopy in the cochlea [5] and in the auditory cortex [e.g. 105, 73]. The first evidence of a tonotopic map in the human primary auditory cortex across the supratemporal surface was reported by Romani et al. [105] with MEG. In this study a steady-state paradigm was employed, which consisted of a continuous tone amplitude modulated in a sinewave fashion at a rate of 32 Hz, with carrier frequencies of 100 Hz, 200 Hz, 600 Hz, 2,000 Hz and 5,000 Hz. Since the stimuli are presented at high rates in a steady-state paradigm, the brain responses to a single stimulus is still present when the next stimulus is delivered, thus recordings might include superimposed activity of the auditory system. This stimulation elicited a latency response of approximately 50 ms with sources lying deeper in the lateral sulcus with increasing frequency. Moreover, the depth progression increased with the logarithm of stimulus frequency (Figure 3). Subsequent research [e.g. 23, 125, 94, 91, 65, 132, 16] tested transient stimulation in which long interval interstimulus allows brain responses to return to their initial state before the next stimulus is delivered. The most prominent response elicited by this kind of stimulation is a 100 ms latency component, denoted 100m, where the "m" indicates its magnetic origin, the equivalent electrical response is designated as N100 or N1. The sources for this component have been located approximately 1 cm more posterior than those for the steady state responses [94, 93].

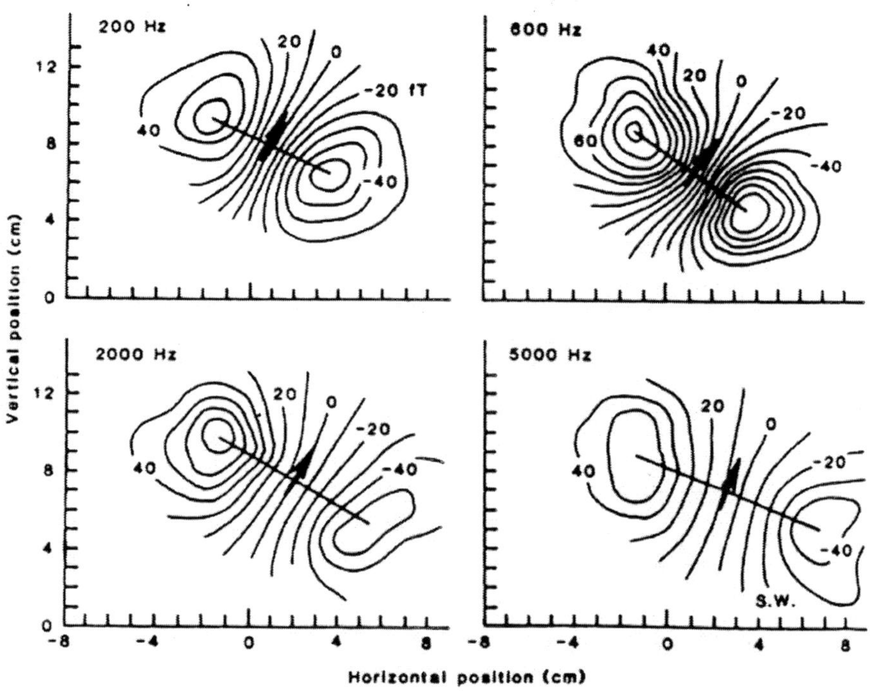

Figure 3. The first human cortical tonotopic map detected by neuromagnetic measurements in the right hemisphere of one subject. The images represent isofield contours of the evoked magnetic field elicited by 200, 600, 2,000 and 5,000 Hz tones. The arrows denote the position and orientation of the equivalent current dipole. For each tone, two maximum fields were recorded, one emerging and one reentering, which signifies that the sources lie beneath the scalp midway between the two maximum fields. As stimuli frequency increased, the distance between the two extremes augmented, indicating a deeper source position. The horizontal axis originates at the ear canal, position (0,9) corresponds to the corner of the eye, and the vertical axis points to the vertex. Reprinted with permission from Romani, G. L., Williamson, S. J. and Kaufman, L. Tonotopic organization of the human auditory cortex. *Science, 216,* 1339-1340. Copyright 1982 AAAS.

Elberling et al. [23] found that the sources for the 100m component were progressively located more anterior as the frequency of the tone burst decreased from 4,000 Hz to 1,000 Hz, and from 1,000 Hz to 500 Hz; the distance between the most extreme sources was 9 mm. Similar results were reported by Pantev et al. [91] with stimuli that ranged from 250 Hz to 4,000 Hz. In this study, the sources for the 100m component, located in the transverse temporal gyri, showed deeper positions as tone frequency increased. Pantev et al. [91] observed that the source for the 500 Hz tone was positioned 6 mm anterior to that for the 4,000 Hz, which is a distance similar to that reported by Elberling et al. [23]. Kuriki and Murase [65] found a deeper source for the 100m response elicited by a 1,000 Hz tone than for that elicited by a 170 Hz tone; while Yamamoto et al. [132] arrived to analogous results testing 1,500 Hz and 750 Hz tone bursts. The study by Cansino et al. [16] also revealed that high frequency tones evoked responses lying deeper within the primary auditory cortex. Single subject studies have also provided evidence of deeper source displacement with frequency increment [78, 72, 77]. Tonotopic maps have also been studied with microelectrode recordings in humans; with this technique, 73% (19 of 26) units showed sharply mean best frequency responses, which increased as the recording site position shifted more posterior and medially [56]. Intracerebral recordings in 45 adult patients showed tonotopic maps with high frequency responses recorded more medially than laterally, predominantly in the right hemisphere [71]. The increase of the dipole depth as a function of frequency varied from 6 mm /decade [65], 7 mm /decade [105, 91], to 10 mm /decade [16] according with MEG studies.

The scenario in this research field is not as clear as it seems from the studies described above, since concurrently a series of studies have arrived to different results. Tuomisto et al. [125] reported an anterior shift of position with increasing tone frequency for one of three subjects; while Hari and Mäkelä [49] reported the same direction shift with continuous tones of 500 Hz and 1,000 Hz, and frequency modulated at intervals of 2.3 s. These two studies showed the opposite direction reported by Elberling et al. [23] and by Pantev et al. [91]. Several studies have been unable to detect a frequency-depth tonotopic organization in the lateral-medial axis. Using frequency glides of continuous short tones (20 ms), which changed by 20% of the base frequency, Arlinger et al. [3] found a tonotopic organization in the right hemisphere of their subjects, but not in the left hemisphere. This asymmetrical result may be explained by the specific stimulus employed in this study, which clearly differed from the classic steady state and transient paradigms. In an experiment with three subjects, Pelizzone et al. [94] did not find any evident dipole depth shift increasing tone burst frequency. May et al. [80] did not report any dipole location displacement associated with frequency increment, however, dipole orientation varied as a function of frequency. The source of the 100m response elicited by a 5,000 Hz tone burst was located about 3 mm more posterior and more superior than that elicited by a 1,000 Hz tone in the left hemisphere [106] and in both hemispheres in a follow-up study by the same research group [107]. Fujioka et al. [33] developed a study to test the 100m responses to pure tones at very high frequencies (from 400 Hz to 40,000 Hz) and observed no neurophysiological response above 20,000 Hz, which corresponds to the upper limit of the human audible frequency range. Although in this study dipole positions showed a tendency to lie more medially for higher frequencies, this displacement was not significant. Moreover, in an experiment [76] in which the 100m response to pure tones between 250 Hz and 5,000 Hz was tested in four consecutive sessions in the same subjects, high intra- and inter-individual variability was observed. Only five out of 19 hemispheres exhibited a tonotopic organization map; however, the axis where the dipole location was dependent on frequency varied among subjects.

The main explanation for the inconsistent results found in MEG tonotopic studies is that the 100m response is actually the manifestation of more than one source. Näätänen and Picton [87] provided an extensive review about the 100 ms auditory response and its multiple structure. Therefore, single dipole models may fail to demonstrate a tonotopic cortical map arrangement when the different sources responsible for the 100m response intervene in an unpredictable and variable fashion. However, when one of these sources predominates, it is possible to observe a dipole location alignment as a function of frequency. Some evidence accounts for the existence of multiple sources underlying the 100m response and probably the must direct proof arrives from intracortical recordings. Liégeois-Chauvel et al. [73] described at least two generators for the 100 ms response with intracerebral recordings: one in the lateral part of the Heschl's gyrus and one in the planum temporale. In a follow up study by this same group [37], which attempted to provide evidence for the correspondence between intracerebral and neuromagnetic recordings in the same subjects, it was concluded that three overlapping sources account for the neuromagnetic response observed between 70 and 150 ms, which make up the 100m component. The generator of the first part of the 100m response seemed to be located in the intermediate part of the Heschl's gyrus, the source for the central part of the 100m response was located in the lateral part of the Heschl's gyrus; while the source for the last part of this component was positioned in the planum temporale. Even though different sources were identified for the different latencies of the 100m component, this component appeared as a single wave in surface recordings. It is worth noting that there was high correspondence between the MEG dipole localizations and the intracerebral recordings in this study. ERP studies have been able to detect two dipoles for the N100 component: one of them derived from the early latencies of the N100 response and the other from the latest latencies, but only the orientation of the first tilted as frequency increased [7, 127]. The tilt in dipole orientation has been related to the folding geometry of the Heschl's gyrus. A distinction between ERP and MEG tonotopic experiments is that the former technique is more sensitive for detecting dipole orientation variations related to sound frequency than dipole position changes. Moreover, MEG studies have also been able to provide evidence of multiple sources for the 100m responses. Cansino et al. [16] detected two dipoles, one in the primary auditory cortex (Heschl's gyrus) and the other in the association auditory cortex within the superior temporal sulcus by means of a short (1 sec) and a long (10 sec) interstimulus interval, respectively. The dipoles for both cortices lay deeper beneath the scalp for progressively high frequencies (Figure 4).

The study by Cansino et al. [16] reveals that it is possible to segregate different sources for the 100m responses by manipulating stimulus parameters. Huotilainen et al. [58] were also able to detect two sources for the 100m response as a result of employing two types of stimuli: constant frequency tones and constant frequency glides of 250 Hz and 4,000 Hz tones. Both stimuli showed dipole depth and orientation variations as a function of frequency; however, these variations were dissimilar between them, which indicated that different sources are responsible for each type of stimulation. Tonotopic experiments have mostly concentrated on the analysis of the 100m or N100 component because it is the major neurophysiological manifestation after auditory stimulation. However, there is evidence that the sources of other components also show tonotopic organization. This is the case of the Pam (magnetic) or Pa (electric) component, which has a 30 ms latency. In a study by Pantev et al. [89], the sources of this response were located more superficially as sound frequency increased while the sources for the classic 100m and N100 component were located deeper for high frequency tones than for low frequency tones. Thus, the responses exhibited a mirrored tonotopic organization. Longer latency components, such as a 150 ms latency response, recorded with the ERP technique, showed an amplitude frequency dependency that has been interpreted as probable evidence that its sources are tonotopically organized [128].

However, in a MEG study the sources of a 160 ms latency component did not show any position shift as tone frequency increased [91].

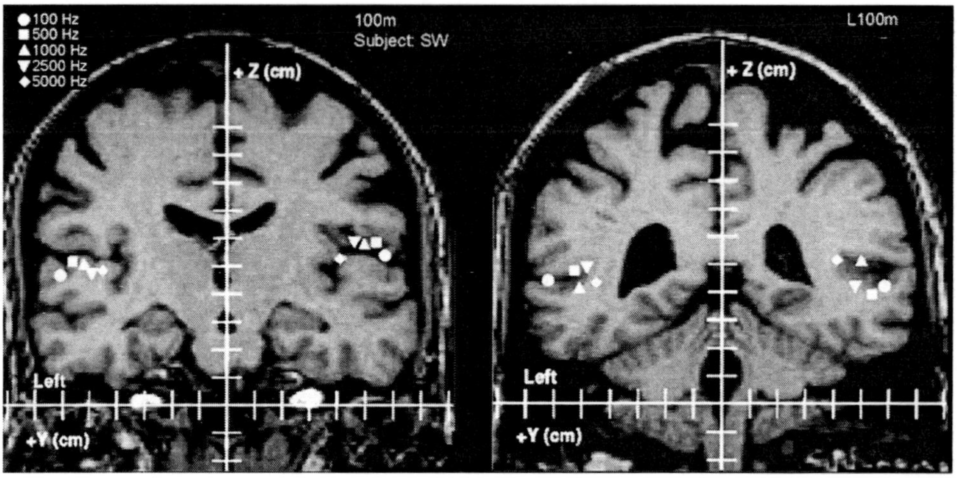

Figure 4. Tonotopic maps recorded in the primary (100m) and association (L100m) auditory cortices with neuromagnetic measurements for tones of the indicating frequencies. Source positions and magnetic resonance images (MRI), which correspond to the same subject, were co-registered with the same coordinate system. Sources in both cortices showed a progressively lateral to medial shift as frequency increased. The coronal MRI slices lie closest to loci of the 100m and L100m sources, the latter lying several centimeters posterior to the former. Coronal positions are X = 1.9 cm for the left MRI slice and X = -1.6 for the right one. Reprinted from *Brain Research,* 663, Cansino, S., Williamson, S. J. and Karron, D. Tonotopic organization of human auditory association cortex, 38-50, Copyright 1994, with permission from Elesevier.

Studies with non-human primates have demonstrated that several tonotopic maps coexist in the auditory cortex [82, 85, 62]. Consequently, they provide the most compelling indication that similar findings should be expected in the human auditory cortex. Moreover, ERP, MEG and intracerebral recording experiments have illustrated that diverse tonotopic maps are manifested through different components or even within the same component. The knowledge on human auditory cortical organization has substantially progressed with findings from fMRI studies, which have demonstrated to some extent, the existence of multiple tonotopic maps in the human auditory cortex. Nevertheless, the first experiments with neuroimaging techniques were only able to identify frequency-dependent activation in broad cortical areas. A 500 Hz tone activated a more laterally located region than a 4,000 Hz tone in two PET studies [70, 74]; however, the exact location of these activations were indecipherable due to the low spatial resolution of this technique. In a single photon emission tomography (SPET) study it was observed that a 500 Hz tone activated a more narrow sagital region than a multi-frequency stimulation [88]. As in PET experiments, when two frequency tones are compared in fMRI studies, different wide brain activations have been observed for each of the frequency tones. Separated region activations against a base line without stimulation have been distinguishable between 500 Hz and 4,000 Hz [8] and between 55 Hz and 880 Hz [130]. Multiple types of stimuli, including instrumental music, amplitude modulated white noise and tone bursts of 650 Hz and 2,500 Hz were tested by Talavage et al.

[122] and their results led them to the conclusion that at least four tonotopic areas exist in the human auditory cortex.

The fMRI studies employing three or more different frequency tones have also reported separate activation regions for the distinct frequencies suggesting the existence of tonotopic maps. Shönwiesner et al. [120] detected different activation regions as a function of frequency, however, they considered that these activation regions belong to different cytoarchitectonic areas, instead of reflecting endpoints of the same tonotopic map. In a recent experiment by Talavage et al. [123], subjects listened to narrow bandwidth, amplitude-modulated noise that changed its center frequency every 64 s between 125 Hz and 8,000 Hz. The slow sweeping of the center frequency served to identify the location of the active regions in the auditory cortex. The areas where the hemodynamic response latency varied progressively of position with the systematic change in frequency over time were considered tonotopically organized regions. With this approach, Talavage et al. [123] identified six tonotopic maps in the superior temporal plane: two frequency progressions were located in the koniocortical primary auditory cortex, one along the anterior-medial portion of the Heschl's gyrus and the other in the postero-lateral portion of the Heschl's gyrus; and four were positioned in parakoniocortical areas of the superior temporal plane.

One of the difficulties faced by acoustic fMRI studies is that experiments are performed in a noisy environment due to the intrinsic noise generated by the scanner. This problem has been partially solved by employing headphones that mitigate the environmental noise by 30 dB or by increasing SPL. The latter solution introduces another difficulty, which is that high intensity stimulation may activate more extensive areas, and hence obscure the fine resolution required to detect tonotopic maps. More recent fMRI acoustic studies have improved their experimental design by introducing silent paradigms [6, 133]. Yang et al. [133] proposed a silent paradigm consisting in measuring the activations only during the expected peak hemodynamic response for stimulus-locked trials, which guarantees a silent period of at least 12 sec before and of 4 sec after each stimulus is presented. In this study, a more lateral activation was observed for high frequencies than for low frequencies in the most lateral portion of the Heschl's gyrus, a region that was considered to be located outside the primary auditory cortex. In a subsequent experiment by this research group [25], in which the same silent paradigm was employed, two mirroring tonotopic maps in the Heschl's gyrus were identified, both of which probably correspond to the primary auditory cortex. It is worth noting that high spatial resolution was achieved in this study by focusing the scanning slices on the primary auditory cortices. Likewise, Formissano et al. [29] conducted a high resolution fMRI study not only by limiting their scanning slices to auditory areas but also by employing a 7 Tesla magnet. This study provided evidence of two mirroring and symmetrical representations of sound frequency in a region which was identified as the primary auditory cortex (Figure 5).

Frequency and its cortical representation have been the more exhaustively examined acoustic parameters as can be judged from the numerous experiments reviewed. Empirical evidence suggests that multiple tonotopic maps coexist in the human auditory cortex as in non-human primates; however, the exact number is still unknown. At least two tonotopic maps have been consistently observed in experiments carried out with MEG, ERP, fMRI and intracerebral recordings. The existence of more than two frequency-dependent maps, as reported by a few studies, requires more empirical examination in order to be confirmed.

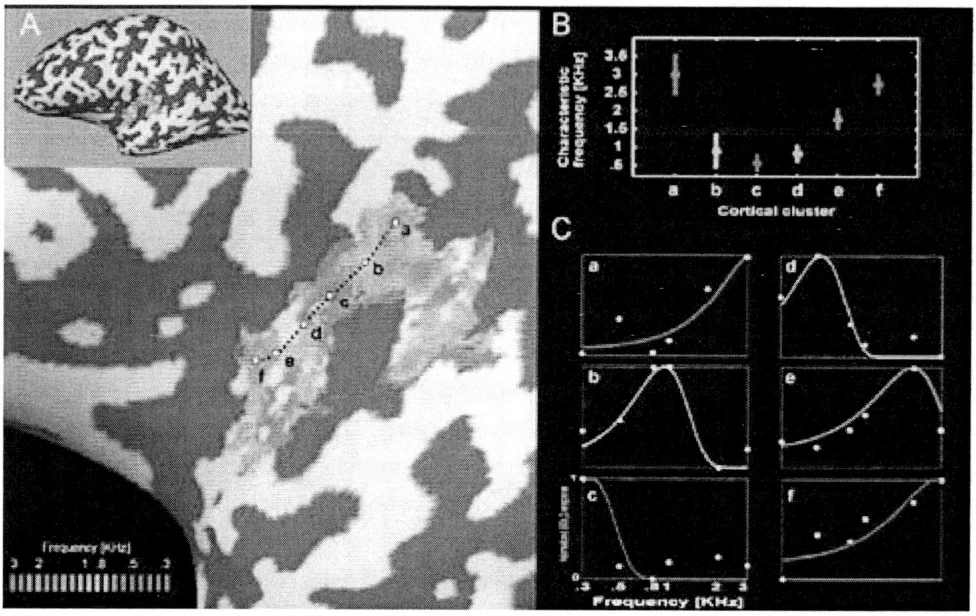

Figure 5. Mirror tonotopic maps in primary auditory cortex recorded in one subject with fMRI. A, best frequency maps along the rostral-caudal direction for 300, 500, 800, 1,000, 2,000 and 3,000 Hz tones; frequencies are represented by different colors on an inflated image of the subject's cortex. B, average best frequency in approximately 5 mm^2 cortical clusters (a, b, c, d, e and f) located in the primary auditory cortex. Clusters a to c are located in the caudal to medial region while clusters c to f in the most rostral region. These two sets of clusters have inverse best frequency gradients and share low best frequency responses at cluster c; lines represent the standard deviation. C, frequency tuning curves for selected voxels in clusters (a, b, c, d, e and f), the curves represent normalized amplitude data of the event-related average BOLD responses to each frequency. Reprinted from *Neuron,* 40, Formissano, E., Kim, D.-S., Di Salle, F., van de Moortele, P.-F., Ugurbil, K. and Goebel, R. Mirror-symmetric tonotopic maps in human primary auditory cortex, 859-869, Copyright 2003, with permission from Elesevier.

Amplitopic Maps

The topographical organization of neuronal populations as a function of their sensitivity to respond to stimuli of specific intensities is termed amplitopy. Few experiments have questioned if there is an amplitopic representation in the human auditory cortex; although amplitopic maps have been described in bats [121], guinea pigs [124] and cats [54]. Microelectrode recordings in cats have revealed two distinctive neural response patterns depending on stimulus intensity. When a pure tone is presented from low (10-20 dB SPL) to moderate (40-60 dB SPL) sound pressure levels the neural activity along the entire isofrequency strip increases with the sound intensity but its spatial pattern reminds stable; while for higher intensities (80 dB SPL), the neural activation reminds constant along the isofrequency contour but spreads across the primary cortex when sound intensity rises; this activity expansion is bi-directional and orthogonal to the isofrequency strip [97]. In other words, neural populations employ two different processes to encode intensity: place and discharge rate. The first is dealt with by non-monotonic neurons that respond to specific intensities and are characterized by narrow dynamic ranges; while the latter is accomplished by monotonic neurons, which increase their discharge rate with higher intensities and are distinguished by their wide dynamic ranges. In cats [96] and in macaque monkeys [103] the distribution of monotonic and non-monotonic neurons varies in primary and non-primary auditory cortices. These findings have influenced human experiments searching for amplitopic maps.

Pantev et al. [90] reported the first amplitopic experiment in humans conducted with MEG. They found that the dipole sources for the 100m response shifted their position from medial to lateral locations as stimulus intensity increased. Source depth decreased about 1 cm when stimulus intensity varied from 30 to 80 dB HL (hearing level). The HL is the level relative to the mean standard threshold of normal listeners according to the American National Standards Institute [2] and the International Standards Organization [59]. Hence, this amplitopic representation was perpendicular and in opposite direction to the typical tonotopic map found in the medial-lateral axis. Two subsequent MEG studies failed to find any amplitopic organization in the human auditory cortex [57, 126]. In the experiment by Vasama et al. [126], six subjects listened to a 200 ms tone burst of 1,000 Hz, with intensity that varied randomly among 40, 50, 60 and 65 dB HL. Even though source strength values were similar to those reported by Pantev et al. [90], no clear amplitopy was observed. The only intensity effect reported was a decrease in latency and an increase in amplitude of the 100m response as stimulus intensity augmented. A more recent MEG experiment [44] attempted to investigate the auditory magnetic field in response to regular and irregular click trains presented at three sound intensities (23, 43 and 53 dB HL). This study did not aim to identify an amplitopic gradient in the human auditory cortex, but to distinguish the sources of the sustained magnetic field sensitive to changes in temporal regularity from those sensitive to variations in sound level. The sustained auditory field is a response to sounds longer than 100 ms, that builds up over 50 and 200 ms after stimulus onset and lasts until stimulus offset [99]. The 100m and 200m components overlap this sustained response. Gutschalk et al. [44] identified that the source for the sustained response sensitive to regularity lay in the lateral portion of the Heschl's gyrus; while the source sensitive to sound level was located posterior to the first in the planum temporale. Interestingly, the first source was completely insensitive to sound level, while the second was unaffected by regularity, which suggests that each region is devoted exclusively to a specific acoustic parameter.

The lack of consistent results in MEG amplitopic studies contrasts with the findings reported with neuroimaging techniques. Lockwood et al. [74] investigated with PET whether there are tonotopic and amplitopic representations in the human auditory cortex. Two tones of 500 Hz and 4,000 Hz were presented to their subjects at 30, 50, 70 and 90 dB HL. Activation in the right temporal lobe varied as a function of stimulus intensity while the left temporal lobe was sensitive to tone frequency. Acoustic stimulation was always presented to the right ear so it was not possible to distinguish the role of ipsilateral and contralateral stimulation on these brain activations. All fMRI studies have been able to detect brain activity variations as a function of stimulus intensity [61, 46, 9, 12, 51] except one [84]. The amplitopic study by Millen et al. [84] was the first to employ fMRI, consequently, some of the methodological procedures used in this study may explain their difficulty to detect brain activation related to sound intensity. At present, it has been observed that some of these procedures diminish the sensitivity of the technique. Specifically, Millen et al. [84] did not implement any control to avoid the brain activation associated with the noise emitted by the scanner. Moreover, the stimulus intensity they employed ranged from 20 to 50 dB SPL; these low intensity stimuli may have been masked by the scanner noise. Besides, the thickness of their slices was 15 mm, probably a resolution beyond that required to detect amplitopic maps.

Pure tones of different frequencies and consonant-vowel syllables were used as stimuli by Jäncke et al. [61] to test the effect of sound level on the blood oxygen level dependent (BOLD) response in the auditory cortex. Stimuli were presented at three different sound intensities (75, 85 and 95 dB SPL). The spatial extent of the activation in the superior temporal gyrus increased as a function of stimulus intensity in an area that comprised primary and non-primary auditory cortices. Thus, intensity changes were associated with the increment in cerebral blood flow but not with the magnitude of the BOLD response. In this study, the noise generated by the scanner was controlled to some extent by employing a repetition time (TR) of 5 s, which resulted in 60% of stimuli not masked by the scanner noise, since silence intervals were 3 s and scans lasted about 2 s. Subsequent studies [46, 9, 12] have employed more sparse imaging paradigms with silent periods of about 10 s. Hall et al. [46] presented two kinds of stimuli to their subjects: a pure tone of 300 Hz at intensities that increased by 5 dB from 66 to 91 dB SPL, and a harmonic complex tone at 65 and 85 dB SPL. An increase in spatial extent, as in Jäncke et al. [61] was associated to intensity increments of pure tones but not of harmonic sounds, in both primary and non-primary auditory areas. In addition, an enhancement of the response magnitude was observed as a function of intensity increments for both kinds of stimuli. A more precise description of brain areas showing amplitopic maps was provided by Bilecen et al. [9] in a study where subjects listened to a 1,000 Hz tone burst presented at 70, 82 and 90 dB SPL. Two cortical areas in the transverse temporal gyrus showed spatial expansion of activation with intensity increments: one from the ventral to the dorsal edge and the other from the lateral to the medial regions. This last one mimics in position and direction the classic tonotopic map described in this axis (Figure 6). The study by Brechmann et al. [12] examined four auditory areas identified by anatomical landmarks and activation patterns: the primary auditory cortex, and three non-primary auditory areas, one located caudally to Heschl's gyrus, another rostrally to Heschl's gyrus and a region on the planum temporale. These experiments were conducted under reduced scanner noise conditions (48 dB), which allowed testing frequency-modulated and pure tones from 36 to 102 dB SPL. The scanner noise usually exceeds 100 dB SPL [46]. An increase in spatial extension and BOLD signal intensity was observed in the primary auditory cortex of both hemispheres as sound level augmented. The caudal region to Heschl's gyrus showed an increased in spatial activation as a function of sound intensity only in the left hemisphere and the other examined regions did not show any sound level dependence. Hart et al. [51] also investigated the dependence of specific auditory regions to sound intensity (from 42 to 96 dB SPL), and their results showed that the primary auditory cortex expands its activation more as a function of sound intensity, followed by the planum temporale and then by the antero-lateral portion of Heschl's gyrus. This activity expansion was more pronounced in the hemisphere contralateral to the stimulated ear.

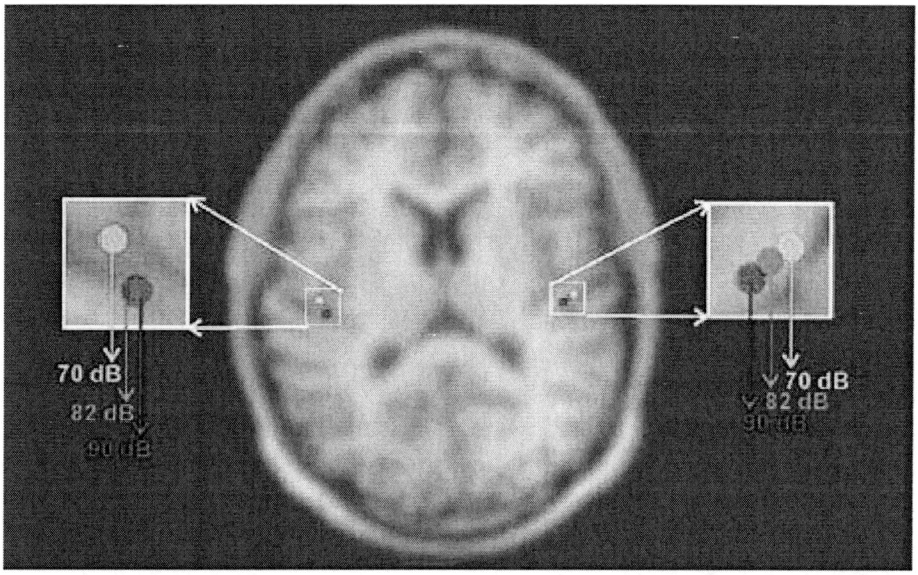

Figure 6. Centers of activation recorded with fMRI for the three stimulus intensities indicated in different colors. Data are from nine subjects and only clusters containing more than 200 activated voxels were considered. The activation gradient from high to low SLP dB showed a medial to lateral and a dorsal to ventral directions across the Heschl's gyrus. The underlying MRI axial slice is located in Tailairach space at z = 10. Reprinted from *Neuroimage,* 17, Bilecen, D., Seifritz, E., Schffler, K., Henning, J. and Schulte, A.-C. Amplitopicity of the human auditory cortex: An fMRI study, 710-718, Copyright 2002, with permission from Elesevier.

The employment of neuroimaging techniques to study amplitopic maps and the improvement of their experimental paradigms have expanded our knowledge on this topic; however, many questions still remain open. The most consistent amplitopic map described in the majority of the experiments reviewed was located in the primary auditory cortex but its exact direction cannot be established since it is reported to be from the medial to the lateral [90], from the lateral to the medial [9] and from the ventral to the dorsal portions of the Heschl's gyrus [9]. It is also possible that these activation patterns correspond to different amplitopic maps in this area. The non-primary auditory areas showing intensity dependence either varied among studies or the resolution of the experiments did not allow to establish the exact region of the activation. Some studies report sound level sensitivity activation in the planum temporale [44, 51], while others do not [12], or report it in the region caudal to Heschl's gyrus [12] or in the antero-lateral portion of Heschl's gyrus [51]. Moreover, some studies report spatial expansion activation [61, 46, 9, 12, 51] while others response magnitude activation [46, 12] associated to increments in sound intensity, even though both kinds of activations are expected to be closely related. As pointed out by Hall et al. [46], both the magnitude and the spatial extension of the BOLD response depend on the metabolic demands of the underlying neural population. The magnitude of the response is related to an enhancement in blood oxygenation; while the spatial extent activation may be the result of an increase in the underlying neuronal population, or may be produced by the increment of the draining veins due to the metabolic demands of the same amount of neurons. The exact meaning of these two types of activation are still unknown. They are not related to specific ranges of stimuli intensities because the studies which employed a wide range of sound intensities report both kinds of activations [74, 46, 12]. Furthermore, different activation patterns related to low and high intensity stimuli as in cats, has not been observed in humans.

Tonotopic Maps of Complex Sounds

Most of the sounds that are biologically relevant are complex periodic sounds, therefore in the auditory research field, one of the main interests is to understand how the auditory cortex processes the acoustic parameters of these stimuli. As described previously, the spectrum of a complex sound corresponds to the distribution of its components as a function of time in terms of frequency, amplitude and phase. The spectrum can be defined by its central frequency (CF), which corresponds to the frequencies that are emphasized in a complex sound. In a simple sine-wave stimulus, the frequency spectrum is limited to a single spectral line that corresponds to the fundamental frequency (Fo) or pitch itself, and therefore the pitch and spectrum dimensions are confounded (Figure 2). In other words, in a pure tone the Fo and the CF are the same. Because of this, pure tones cannot reveal whether neural tonotopy represents the actual fundamental component (periodicity) or the spectrum of complex tones. Consequently, classical tonotopic studies, which usually employed sine waves, were unable to disentangle whether the frequency map on the cortex represents the Fo or the CF of the sounds. However, as will be described, recent experiments have been able to address this question by employing complex tones in which the spectrum and the periodicity pitch of stimuli are varied independently.

One of the first MEG studies [92] employing a complex sound tested whether the tonotopic organization of the primary auditory cortex represented the pitch of a complex sound or the fundamental frequency of pure tones. The complex sound was composed of the fourth to the seventh harmonic of 250 Hz, which produced a virtual pitch of 250 Hz. The spectrum of this complex sound ranged between 1,000 Hz and 1,750 Hz. The pure tones have a fundamental frequency of 250 Hz and 1,000 Hz, which also correspond to their spectrum frequency, respectively. Their results revealed that the depth of the 250 Hz pure tone and the complex tone did not differ, but the dipole depth of these two tones differed significantly from the 1,000 Hz pure tone. This finding confirmed that the neural populations uncharged to encode the fundamental frequency and the periodic pitch are the same. A more recent experiment arrived to an identical conclusion [34] employing the same type of stimuli. Conversely, in another MEG study [75], this result was not replicated, and this was attributed to the inadequacy of using single dipole models. Langner et al. [69] observed a periodicity pitch map lying orthogonal to the classic tonotopic map for frequency. The sources of the 100m component elicited by pure tones of 50 Hz, 100 Hz, 200 Hz and 400 Hz showed a lateral-medial shift as has been previously described; while the sources for the 100m response to complex sounds with the same periodicity as the pure tones and a spectrum between 400 Hz and 5,000 Hz shifted from posterior to anterior positions as periodicity pitch increased.

Subsequent studies [15, 34] have been unable to reproduce an orthogonal map for periodicity pitch.

The question of whether the tonotopic organization of the human auditory cortex represents the pitch or the spectrum of a complex sound was tackled by Crottaz-Herbette and Ragot [18] in an ERP study. The aim of this study was achieved by means of nine complex auditory stimuli, for which the pitch and spectrum dimensions were independently varied: three different fundamental frequencies (62.5 Hz, 125 Hz and 250 Hz) were combined with three different central frequencies (low, mid and high). Their results demonstrated that these sounds were represented on the cortex according to their spectral CF structure, since it was observed that dipole source orientations varied as a function of CF, while their fundamental pitch was reflected by N100 latency variations. Cansino et al. [15] addressed this same question with the MEG technique, by setting an experimental paradigm in which spectrum and periodicity were directly compared, as in Crottaz-Herbette and Ragot [18]. Subjects listened to nine complex auditory stimuli, in which the pitch (Fos: 62.5 Hz, 125 Hz and 250 Hz) and the spectrum (CFs: 280 Hz, 1,600 Hz and 4,600 Hz) dimensions were independently varied. The sources for the 100m component showed an orderly progression along the lateral-medial axis for both hemispheres, with higher CFs represented more medially. In the right hemisphere, sources for higher CFs were more posterior, while in the left hemisphere they were more inferior (Figure 7). Dipole orientations, as in Crottaz-Herbette and Ragot [18], also varied as a function of the sound CF. Their results demonstrated that the spectral content CF of the complex sounds predominated over a concurrent mapping of their periodic frequency Fo. A similar approach was implemented by another MEG study published in the same year [34], in which the stimuli were pure tones of 250 Hz, 500 Hz and 1,000 Hz, complex sounds composed by different harmonics of each of the Fo of the pure tones (2nd to 5th, 6th to 9th and 10th to 13th harmonics), and three pure tones with Fos equal to the lowest component of each complex sound. Their main results are in agreement with Cansino et al. [15], since they also found in both hemispheres that high central frequencies of their complex sounds were more medially located than low central frequencies. However, some results differ in the two studies; Fujioka et al. [34] reported that in the inferior-superior and anterior-posterior directions, the tonotopic maps were different between pure tones and complex tones; and based on the more pronounced tonotopic representation observed for complex sounds in the right hemisphere, they suggested that this hemisphere has preference for processing spectral information while the left hemisphere for processing temporal information. In contrast, in the study by Cansino et al. [15], the representation of spectral content was completely predominant hiding from view a possible concurrent representation based on sound periodicity. Moreover, these tonotopic representations did not predominate in one of the hemispheres; although the tonotopic maps of each of them showed different directions: an anterior-posterior shift in the right hemisphere and a superior-inferior shift in the left hemispheres for higher CFs. Together, these studies provide evidence for a tonotopic organization in the auditory cortex based on the spectral content of sounds (CF). It is important to mention that these findings do not preclude topographical organization of the auditory cortex based on the fundamental frequency, since there is evidence that multiple maps coexist in the auditory cortices. Furthermore, these findings do not contradict results reported by classic tonotopic experiments with pure tones, because these stimuli simply do not allow to distinguish the effect of the two acoustic dimensions.

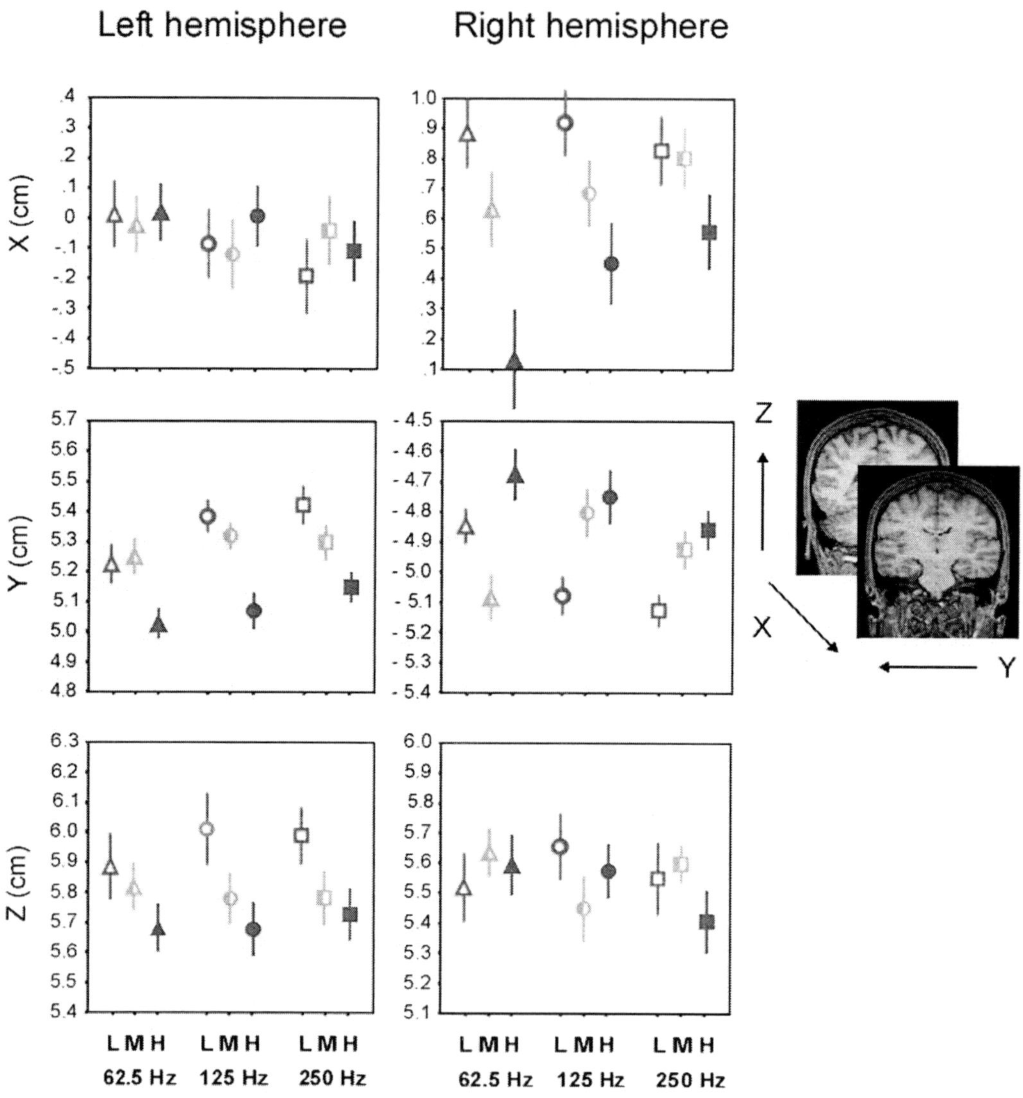

Figure 7. Source locations for the 100m response averaged across 12 subjects as a function of stimulus spectrum (orange bullets for low (L), green bullets for mid (M) and blue bullets for high (H)) and stimulus pitch (triangles for 62.5 Hz, circles for 125 Hz, and squares for 250 Hz). Along the y axis, sources increased in depth as CF augmented in both hemispheres. In the left hemisphere, a superior-inferior shift was observed with increasing CF of complex sounds, whereas in the right hemisphere, a posterior-anterior shift was detected. Source positions did not vary as a function of stimulus pitch in any axis. Positive x values for anterior positions, positive y values for left positions, and positive z values for superior positions; lines represent the standard error. Reprinted from *Human Brain Mapping,* 20, Cansino, S., Ducorps, A. and Ragot, R. Tonotopic cortical representation of periodic complex sounds, 71-81, Copyright 2003, with permission from John Wiley and Sons Inc.

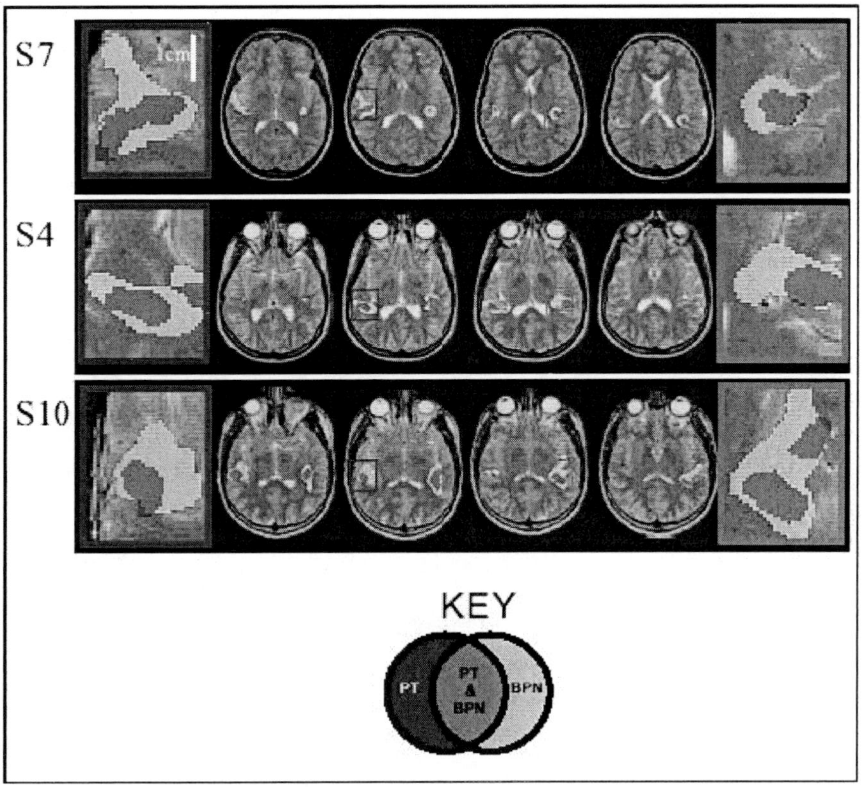

Figure 8. Activations recorded with the fMRI technique to pure tones (PT) of 500, 2,000 and 8,000 Hz and to band pass noise (BPN) bursts with central frequencies separated logarithmically and bandwidths of one octave (from 350 to 700 Hz, from 1,400 to 2,800 Hz and from 5,600 to 11,200 Hz). Data from three different subjects are depicted in each row. Blue areas are activated by PT, yellow areas by BPN bursts and green areas were activated by both kinds of stimuli. PT activated only the core region of the auditory cortex, while BPN activated surrounding belt areas. Activated regions are enlarged in red and green frames for the right and left hemispheres, respectively. The four slices arranged from left to right for each subject increased from inferior to superior positions. Reprinted from *Journal of Cognitive Neuroscience,* 13, Wessinger, C. M., van Meter, J., Tian, B., van Lare, J., Pekar, J. and Rauschecker, J. P. Hierarchical organization of the human auditory cortex revealed by functional magnetic resonance imaging, 1-7, Copyright 2001, with permission from The MIT Press.

Few neuroimaging studies have concentrated on identifying the auditory cortical areas responsible for processing temporal and spectral properties of complex sounds. In a PET study [137], the temporal and spectral patterns of a sequence of two pure tones (500 Hz and 1,000 Hz) were varied systematically. In one condition the spectral information remained constant, while the speed of alternation was doubled at different levels; in another condition the speed was constant, while the number of tones within the octave was double at different levels. Their results showed that in both hemispheres, the core auditory areas were more sensitive to temporal variations; while the anterior superior temporal areas responded more to spectral variations. In addition, they reported hemisphere asymmetries: the right hemisphere was more activated during spectral processing and the left during temporal processing. Dynamic ripples based on pink noise were used in an fMRI experiment [66] to identify auditory cortical regions related to spectral and temporal acoustic parameters. The spectral modulation density was defined by the number of spectral peaks present in a frequency band of one octave, whereas the temporal modulation frequency was equal to the number of spectral peaks that passed per second. These stimuli produced a broad bilateral activation in the superior surface of the temporal lobe that includes the Heschl's gyrus, the planum temporale and a portion anterior to the planum temporale. Interestingly, opposite to amplitopic map experiments, the extent and the level of activation were strongly correlated (R^2 = 0.97). The rise of the spectral density was associated to an activation from posterolateral to anteromedial regions; while the increase in frequency was related to an activation from lateral to medial positions. Contrary to Zatorre and Belin [137], no hemisphere differences were observed in this study.

FMRI studies have also attempted to test whether the human auditory cortex is hierarchically organized as demonstrated in non-human primates. In the session dedicated to the "non-primary auditory cortex", it was described that in the macaque, the core areas receive direct inputs from the thalamus and then send inputs to the belt areas, which, in turn, send inputs to the parabelt regions. This hierarchical processing has been tested in humans by comparing the activation elicited by pure tones with that generated by complex sounds [131, 48, 52]. Wessinger et al. [131] observed that pure tones activated mainly core areas; while narrow band noise burst of one octave with different central frequencies activated belt areas (Figure 8). A finer anatomical activation was described by Hall et al. [48] for static and modulated harmonic sounds. Their results demonstrated that harmonic sounds produced more activation than single tones in the right Heschl's gyrus and bilaterally in the lateral supratemporal plane. Additionally, frequency modulated sounds produced an activation in the lateral portion of the primary auditory cortex and in the non-primary auditory cortex anterior and posterior to Heschl's gyrus. In a subsequent study by this same group [52], frequency and amplitude-modulated sounds generated overlapping activations in the lateral portion of Heschl's gyrus and in the planum temporale. Except for Wessinger et al. [131], the findings of these studies do not provide consistent evidence for a hierarchical organization of the human auditory cortices, since both primary and non-primary auditory areas have been sensitive to complex sounds. Further research is required to investigate this hypothesis, and probably a more sophisticated experimental paradigm than employing sounds of different complexity to test such a complicated functional organization.

Temporal Maps

The term temporal map was adopted in this review to include the research focused on identifying auditory brain areas responsive to changes in temporal acoustic parameters, such as gaps of different duration, stimulus rate, sound duration, temporal envelope, time structure in sound or temporal regularity of sounds. The tonotopic maps for pitch, which is also a temporal sound feature, either generated by sinusoidal sounds or complex sounds, were reviewed before in this chapter, because, presumably, pitch perception in the previously revised studies have been based on analysis of the frequency composition or spectrum of the sound, rather than on the temporal analysis of its structure, due to the difficulty to manipulate each parameter separately. Spectral models of pitch perception proposed that the temporal information is averaged out by the neural activity in order to construe the auditory spectrum [40]; whereas temporal models of pitch perception derive from single-unit recordings in non-human primates [108], in which phase-locked responses to tones in single auditory nerve fibers showed a sub-millisecond temporal precision following stimulation. The examination of temporal models is currently feasible mainly by means of stimulus based on noise delayed and added to itself, described above, since these stimuli have the same energy and auditory spectra throughout but their temporal regularity can be varied [135]. Therefore, pitch perception has to be extracted from these stimuli by perceiving the regular intervals of few milliseconds without spectral information.

Human accuracy to detect fast temporal changes in acoustic stimuli is crucial to appreciate speech and music. Psychophysical studies have ascertained the temporal acuity of the human auditory system by exploring the threshold to detect silent gaps in a continuous sound. Gap detection threshold in broadband noise of equal intensity is between 2 and 3 ms [30]. Few neurophysiological experiments [113, 112, 109] have been performed to investigate the shortest gap that produces an observable brain response. These studies have employed the MEG technique, but different brain responses have been examined: magnetic middle latency fields [113, 112] and auditory steady state responses [109]. In the study by Rupp et al. [113], subjects listened to gaps of 1, 4, 8 and 14 ms inserted in pairs of sounds with the same or different spectrum; their results showed that gaps longer than 4 ms increased the amplitude of a 40 ms latency response. This same group tested in a later study [112], gaps of 3, 6 and 9 ms introduced in broadband noise bursts. Under these conditions, the 3 ms gap elicited an amplitude enhancement of the 40m response, which confirms that the physiological and perceptual thresholds are equivalent. The sources for this early component were located in the primary auditory cortex in both studies. The auditory steady state response, recorded by Ross and Pantev [109], was chosen by these authors because it follows the temporal structure of the stimulus closely. In this study, sequences of tone bursts of 500 Hz and 300-ms duration were fully amplitude-modulated with a frequency of 40 Hz; gap duration was 3, 12.5 and 25 ms, and they were inserted in the sequences avoiding any phase change in the unaffected remaining tone bursts. Additionally, the 100m component to a 500 Hz tone burst was recorded as a reference measurement. The sources for the auditory steady state response were considered to be located in the primary auditory cortex, given that they were more anterior, more medial and more inferior than the sources for the 100m component, as previously described [94, 93]. Gaps as short as 3 ms elicited long-lasting perturbations in the steady state response, indicating that the physiological threshold was analogous to the behavioral threshold. It is noteworthy that in these three studies, the data for the gaps of different silence periods were analyzed together to determine the source locations, so the question whether different neural populations are dedicated to detect specific temporal silence periods still remains open.

The ability of the human auditory system to encode temporal parameters as the rate at which a stimulus appears was explored by May and Tiitinen [79] in a MEG study. They proposed that multiple rebound responses occur when a sequence of stimuli presented at a specific rate ends, and that the cells responsible for these tuning responses as a function of stimulus rate contribute to the 100m component. To test this hypothesis, they presented to their subjects stimulus sequences of 2 s duration separated by 10 s of silent periods. The sequences comprised 4 to 10 sinusoidal tones of 1,000 Hz and 50-ms duration. Hence, presentation stimulus rates varied between 2 and 10 Hz, which corresponded to onset intervals between 103 ms and 650 ms. The rebound responses were observed as predicted, and their sources did not differ from those of the 100m response, which lead them to the conclusion that the generator of both kinds of responses lay in the supratemporal plane, in the vicinity of the auditory cortex. In addition, they reported that the positions of the sources did not differ across the diverse stimulus rates. This may be an indication that the cells uncharged to discriminate stimulus rates are not organized topographically; however, more research should test this possibility. The question of whether the BOLD response varied as a function of stimulus duration was addressed by Jäncke et al. [60], employing pure tones of 1,000 Hz with 200, 400, 600 and 800 ms duration. Their study allowed them to conclude that neither the intensity nor the spatial extent of the hemodynamic response in the auditory cortices varied as a function of stimulus duration, at least for the kind of stimuli they specifically tested. These stimuli generated a broad and indistinguishable activation in primary and non-primary auditory cortices.

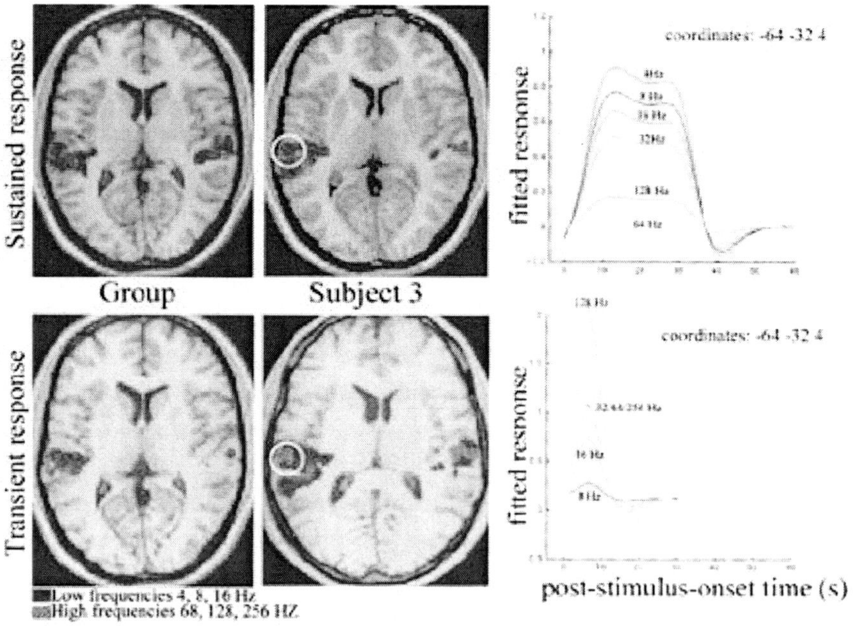

Figure 9. fMRI activations to white noise amplitude modulated (AM) at different frequencies. The group activation corresponds to 5 subjects. The BOLD responses were modeled as a sustained response (top) and as a transient response (bottom). Responses to low AM frequencies (4, 8 and 16 Hz) are shown in red, and responses to high AM frequencies (68, 128 and 256 Hz) in green. In the right, fitted responses in the same voxel. Low AM frequencies were best modeled by sustained responses; while high AM frequencies activations were detectable only when modeled by a transient response. Reprinted from Giraud, A.-L., Lorenzi, C., Ashburner, J., Wable, J., Johnsrude, I., Frackowiak, R. and Kleinschmidt, A. Representation of the temporal envelope of sounds in the human brain. *Journal of Neurophysiology,* 2000, 84, 1588-1598. Used with permission from the American Physiological Society.

The interest to determine how and where in the auditory human system the temporal attributes of an acoustic stimulus are processed has attracted the attention of researchers due to the extremely high temporal resolution of the auditory system. It is considered to be at least an order of magnitude higher than the resolution of any other system [41]. Indeed, this high resolution is a basic quality for understanding speech. Some experiments [50, 36] have been conducted with stimuli that resemble some of the attributes that characterize speech. In view of the fact that low frequencies predominate in speech, amplitude-modulated in their temporal envelopes by modulation frequencies below 50 Hz [19], Giraud et al. [36] carried out an fMRI study with unmodulated and sinusoidally modulated white noise in amplitudes of 4, 8, 16, 32, 64, 128 and 256 Hz; with a modulation depth of 100 %. Their experiment allowed them to record activity even at subcortical structures of the human auditory system. The sound amplitude modulated at frequencies above 8 Hz, elicited activity predominantly at the lower brainstem, inferior colliculus and medial geniculate body; while the amplitude modulated at frequencies between 8 Hz and 4 Hz activated preferentially the primary auditory cortex, and the amplitude modulated by frequencies below 4 Hz, activated the non-primary auditory areas lateral and posterior to Heschl's gyrus, specifically the association cortex situated in the superior temporal sulcus (Brodman area 22) and the lateral surface of the superior temporal gyrus (Brodman area 42). Similar results were reported by Harms et al. [50]. Moreover, Giraud et al. [36] observed two types of responses at the same cortical locus according with the amplitude-modulated frequency: low frequencies below 16 Hz elicited sustained BOLD responses, while high frequencies above 128 Hz were associated to transient BOLD responses (Figure 9). However, none of these responses showed spatial gradients related to amplitude modulation frequencies. The authors concluded that the temporal envelope is hierarchically processed in the auditory system as information travels from subcortical to cortical areas, since, at each level, the system applied an orderly lower amplitude modulated frequency filter; besides, it is processed in parallel at cortical levels, since the same neural populations were differently activated at specific amplitude-modulated frequencies.

Pitch perception models have guided the development of studies [40, 41, 64, 45] in which the energy spectrum of a sound is held constant while the temporal regularity of the sound is manipulated in order to produce the perception of pitch. Gustschalk et al. [45] employed regular click trains that generate a sustained temporal pitch perception and irregular click trains that do not have a pitch, but both kinds of stimuli have the same energy and average click rates. These stimuli were chosen because in a previous MEG study by this same group [44], it was observed that regular click trains elicited a stronger sustained field response than irregular click trains. Gutschalk et al. [45] observed that the regular click trains elicited two responses: a sustained field starting 70 ms after pitch onset and lasting 70 ms after pitch offset, and a transient field with a latency between 130 and 190 ms after pitch onset. Sources for both responses were located in the lateral Heschl's gyrus, a non-primary auditory area. Two additional sources for both the sustained and transient field were located posterior to Heschl's gyrus in the planum temporale; the responses related to these sources were insensitive to temporal regularity. Noise delayed and added to itself has proved to be a reliable method to introduce a pitch into the perception of the sound without changing the spectral energy [10]. This type of stimulus has been employed to search brain activity related to pitch perception with MEG [64], PET [40] and fMRI [41]. The study by Krumbholz et al. [64], attempted to isolate the pitch onset response from other responses of the 100m component, which are known to be sensitive to other acoustic parameters such as spectrum and amplitude [87]. Their results showed that the sources for the 100m component and the pitch onset response are not the same, the sources for the latter being located in the medial Heschl's gyrus, adjacent to the antero-lateral portion of Heschl's gyrus. Because the latency and the amplitude of the pitch onset response varied with the pitch of the sound, the authors concluded that the neural populations underlying this component are involved in extracting an initial estimate of the pitch of a sound. Neuroimaging studies have reported that the activity in the primary auditory cortex varied with the temporal regularity of the sound at a millisecond level, independently of its spectrum; while the activity in the anterior and posterior temporal lobes varied with the presentation of a melody delayed and added to itself, which requires a temporal resolution in the order of seconds to extract the regularity of the sound [40]. Moreover, the extracting process of temporal regularity of a sound starts in an early structure of the auditory pathway, the cochlear nucleus, and continues up to the primary auditory cortex and non-primary auditory areas, specifically in the lateral Heschl's gyrus and the region posterior to Heschl's gyrus in the planum temporale [41]. Both MEG and neuroimaging studies have consistently observed an activation related to pitch perception in the anterior, medial or lateral to primary areas of the auditory cortex; whereas only PET and fMRI experiments have reported that the primary auditory cortex and a region posterior to the primary auditory cortex in the planum temporale are related to pitch perception. The different results may be due to the dissimilar spatial resolution provided by these techniques.

Conclusion

To provide an integral portrait of the functional organization of the human auditory cortices is an elaborate task in view of the fact that research in this field is characterized by being extremely segregated and specialized in discovering how and where the auditory system processes a specific acoustic parameter, not to mention that real acoustic stimulation arrives at our ears as a composite sound with all these acoustic parameters combined. Next is an attempt to highlight the findings that have proved to be more consistent by different techniques or in various experiments with the same technique, in order to propose a more integral view of the function of the auditory cortical regions.

Some consensus can be outlined about the anatomy of the human auditory cortices. The primary auditory cortex is located in the medial portion of the Heschl's gyrus and at least two core areas have been clearly delineated in several cytoarchitectonic [21, 35] and histochemical [129] studies. The core areas are characterized by their high granular cell density, which provide them with their koniocortical cytoarchitecture. In addition, three non-primary cortical areas have been consistently observed in cytoarchitectonic examinations: rostrally, laterally and caudally to the Heschl's gyrus [13, 35]. These areas are characterized by their parakoniocortical cytoarchitecture. Furthermore, there is strong evidence that auditory cortical areas in the left hemisphere comprise a more spatially extended region than in the right hemisphere [118, 95, 138, 86]. Moreover, some of the main characteristics of the human auditory cortices are their extreme anatomical inter- and intra-subject variability and their lack of macroanatomical landmarks. These features of the auditory cortices are to some extent the reason why the knowledge of the human auditory system is clearly behind that of other systems, such as the visual.

Two tonotopic maps for pure tones have been consistently observed in MEG [89] and in fMRI [25, 29] studies. The MEG technique allowed to distinguish the temporal characteristics of each of these topographical representations and their specific directions: one of them corresponds to a 30 ms latency component with sources lying more laterally for higher frequencies, and the other corresponds to the 100m component with sources lying deeper for higher frequencies. While there is consensus that the sources for the early component are located in the primary auditory cortex, the sources for the 100m response vary because it is composed by at least three components and the sources of some of them lie in non-primary auditory areas [87]. Both fMRI studies located these mirror maps in the primary auditory cortex. Amplitopic maps have been repeatedly observed in MEG [90, 44], PET [74] and fMRI [61, 46, 9, 12, 51] experiments, in both primary and non-primary auditory cortices. Experiments with complex sounds in which pitch and spectrum were varied independently [18, 15, 34] showed that tonotopic maps are based on the spectral content of sounds rather than on their periodicity pitch, at least for the mapping of electrical and magnetic sources eliciting maximum responses at the latencies surrounding the 100m component. This finding in humans closely agrees with results from non-human primates [27, 117]. When spectrum is held constant and no other parameter but temporal regularity varies in the sound, it is possible to observe activation in primary and non-primary auditory cortices [40, 41, 64, 45]. Hence, the human auditory system is capable of discerning pitch by perception of both spectrum and temporal parameters.

The activity in primary and non-primary auditory cortical areas has been related to frequency, amplitude, spectrum and temporal acoustic parameters. This lack of specificity only creates a puzzling representation of the functional organization of the human auditory cortices. Nevertheless, it is possible to delineate some reasons for these findings. One possibility could be that the brain responses recorded in some of the experiments may not reflect the underlying organization of the cortical auditory areas but be a sign of the lower spatial resolution of the different techniques. For example, several PET and fMRI experiments searching for tonotopic, amplitopic and temporal maps have regularly reported activity in both primary and non-primary cortices. This lack of detail consistently observed in most of the neuroimaging experiments may be due to the spatial smoothing of images, which blurs and expands the activity across the region of interest removing possible functional differences between cortical areas. Indeed, experiments that have reached a more detailed description of their activation regions have implemented sophisticated experimental paradigms or data analyses, which indicate that spatial resolution can be improved to obtain more sensitive results. For instance, by varying the acoustic parameter of interest systematically and along a broad range of values [123], by determining the activated regions through analysis of the frequency-dependent responses [122, 123, 36], by performing the analysis on separate auditory brain regions selected by their anatomical landmarks or by spatial activation criteria [12] or by identifying the location of the activations comparing the fMRI data with cytoarchitectonic data [48]. Similarly, MEG and ERP studies have had difficulties to isolate the different sources underlying the 100m or N100 component, respectively, which are the more prominent responses after almost any kind of acoustic stimulation. As a result, several studies only provide information of a single map underlying this 100 ms component for almost any acoustic parameter. Nevertheless, at present it has been demonstrated that several responses and sources can be distinguished surrounding the 100 ms latency component and some of them are related to specific acoustic parameters [44].

Another explanation is that this lack of specificity, which has predominated in most of the experiments, is actually reflecting how the auditory cortices are functionally organized. It has been suggested that the auditory system, as other systems, is hierarchically [36, 131] and probably also parallel [36] organized. If this proposal turns out to be true, the undefined activity observed in extensive cortical areas may be due to the fact that the stimulation generated by a specific acoustic parameter travels in a hierarchical fashion from one core area of the primary auditory cortex to another, and from there to non-primary auditory areas in a sequentially or parallel manner in order to be further processed. This performance will certainly reflect a wide activation pattern, since several auditory maps are acting serially and simultaneously; furthermore, this manifestation will be more evident if no temporal resolution is provided by the technique. Moreover, since auditory stimulation is composed of several acoustic parameters, it is expected that several maps specialized in each of them concurrently intervene to decipher and to interpret the sound, or that a number of maps are specialized in more than one acoustic parameter. This multiple mapping representation and intricate view of the functional organization of the human auditory cortices seems definitely more realistic.

Acknowledgements

This review was supported by a grant from CONACyT (36203-H) and from the National Autonomous University of Mexico (DGAPA PAPIIT IN304202). I am grateful to I. Pérez Montfort for revising the manuscript.

References

[1] Allison, T. (1984) Recording and interpreting event-related potentials. In E. Donchin (Ed.), *Cognitive psychophysiology: Event related potentials and the study of cognition. The Carmel Conferences, Volume I* (pp. 1-36). New Jersey, PA: Lawrence Erlbaum Associates, Inc.

[2] American National Standards Institute. (1969). *American National Standard Specifications for Audiometers S3.6.* New York, NY: American National Standards Institute.

[3] Arlinger, S., Elberling, C., Bak, C., Kofoed, B., Lebech, J. and Saermark, K. (1982). Cortical magnetic fields evoked by frequency glides of a continuous tone. *Electroencephalography and Clinical Neurophysiology, 54,* 642-653.

[4] Beck, E. (1928). Die myeloarchitektonische felderung des in der sylvischen furche gelegenen teiles des menschlichen schläfenlappens. *Journal fur Psychologie Neurologie, 36,* 1-21.

[5] Békésy, G. V. (1960). *Experiments in Hearing*. New York, NY: McGraw Hill.

[6] Belin, P., Zatorre, R. J., Hoge, R., Evans, A. C. and Pike, B. (1999). Event-related fMRI of the auditory cortex. *NeuroImage, 10,* 417-429.

[7] Bertrand, O., Perrin, F. and Pernier, J. (1991). Evidence for a tonotopic organization of the auditory cortex observed with auditory evoked potentials. *Acta Oto-laryngologica. Supplementum, 49,* 116-123.

[8] Bilecen, D., Scheffler, K., Schmid, N., Tschopp, K. and Seelig, J. (1998). Tonotopic organization of the human auditory cortex as detected by BOLD-fMRI. *Hearing Research, 126,* 19-27.

[9] Bilecen, D., Seifritz, E., Schffler, K., Henning, J. and Schulte, A.-C. (2002). Amplitopicity of the human auditory cortex: An fMRI study. *Neuroimage, 17,* 710-718.

[10] Bilsen, F. A. (1966). Repetition pitch: Monoaural interaction of sound with the repetition of the same, but phase-shifted sound. *Acustica, 17,* 295-300.

[11] Braak, H. (1978). The pigment architecture of the human temporal lobe. *Anatomy and Embryology, 154,* 213-240.

[12] Brechmann, A., Baumgart, F. and Scheich, H. (2002). Sound-level-dependent representation of frequency modulations in human auditory cortex: A low-noise fMRI study. *Journal of Neurophysiology, 87,* 423-433.

[13] Brodmann, K. (1909). *Brodmann's "Localisation in the cerebral cortex".* Translated by L. J. Garey. London: Smith-Gordon.

[14] Cain, W. S. (1977). Differential sensitivity for smell: Noise at the nose. *Science, 195,* 796-798.

[15] Cansino, S., Ducorps, A. and Ragot, R. (2003). Tonotopic cortical representation of periodic complex sounds. *Human Brain Mapping, 20,* 71-81.

[16] Cansino, S., Williamson, S. J. and Karron, D. (1994). Tonotopic organization of human auditory association cortex. *Brain Research, 663,* 38-50.

[17] Cohen, L. T., Rickards, F. W., and Clark, M. G. (1991). A comparison of steady-state evoked potentials to modulated tones in awake and sleeping humans. *Journal Acoustic Society American, 90,* 2467-2479.

[18] Crottaz-Herbette, S. and Ragot, R. (2000). Perception of complex sounds: N1 latency codes pitch and topography codes spectra. *Clinical Neurophysiology, 111,* 1759-1766.

[19] Drullman, R., Festen, J. M. and Plomp, R. (1994). Effect of temporal envelope smearing on speech repetition. *Journal Acoustic Society American, 95,* 1053-1064.

[20] Economo, C. and Horn, L. (1930). Über windungsrelief, masse und rindenarchitectonik der supratemporalfläche, ihre individuellen und ihre seitenunterschiede. *Zeitschrift fur Neurologie und Psychiatrie, 130,* 678-757.

[21] Economo, C. and Koskinas, G. N. (1925). *Die cytoarchitektonik der hirnrinde des erwachsenen menschen.* Berlin: Springer-Verlag.

[22] Ehret, G. (1997). The auditory cortex. *Journal of Comparative Physiology A, 181,* 547-557.

[23] Elberling, C., Bak, C., Kofoed, B., Lebech, J. and Saermark, K. (1982). Auditory magnetic fields: Source location and tonotopical organization in the right hemisphere of the human brain. *Scandinavian Audiology, 11,* 61-65.

[24] Elliott, D. N. and Trahiotis, C. (1972). Cortical lesions and auditory discrimination. *Psychological Bulletin, 77,* 198-222.

[25] Engelien, A., Yang Y., Engelien, W., Zonana, J., Stern, E. and Silbersweig, D. A. (2002). Physiological mapping of human auditory cortices with a silent Event-Related fMRI Technique. *Neuroimage, 16,* 944-953.

[26] Evans, E. F. (1982). Functions of the auditory system. In H. B. Barlow, and D. J. Mollon (Eds.), *The Senses* (pp. 307-322). Cambridge: Cambridge University Press.

[27] Fishman, Y. I., Reser, D. H., Arezzo, J. C. and Steinschneider, M. (1998). Pitch vs. spectral encoding of harmonic complex tones in primary auditory cortex of the awake monkey. *Brain Research, 786,* 18-30.

[28] Fletcher, H. and Munson, W. A. (1933). Loudness, its definition, measurement and calculation. *Journal Acoustic Society American, 5,* 82-108.

[29] Formissano, E., Kim, D.-S., Di Salle, F., van de Moortele, P.-F., Ugurbil, K. and Goebel, R. (2003). Mirror-symmetric tonotopic maps in human primary auditory cortex. *Neuron, 40,* 859-869.

[30] Forrest, T. G. and Green, D. M. (1987). *Journal Acoustic Society American, 82,* 1933-1943.

[31] Foundas, A. L., Leonard, C. M. and Heilman, K. M. (1995). Morphologic cerebral asymmetries and handedness. *Archives of Neurology, 52,* 501-508.

[32] Fourier, J. B. (1822). *Théorie Analytique de la Chaleur.* Paris: Didot.

[33] Fujioka, T., Kakigi, R., Gunji, A. and Takeshima, Y. (2002). The auditory evoked magnetic fields to very high frequency tones. *Neuroscience, 112,* 367-381.

[34] Fujioka, T., Ross, B., Okamoto, H., Takeshima, Y., Kakigi, R. and Pantev, C. (2003). Tonotopic representation of missing fundamental complex sounds in the human auditory cortex. *European Journal of Neuroscience, 18,* 432-440.

[35] Galaburda, A. and Sanides, F. (1980). Cytoarchitectonic organization of the human auditory cortex. *The Journal of Comparative Neurology, 190,* 597-610.

[36] Giraud, A.-L., Lorenzi, C., Ashburner, J., Wable, J., Johnsrude, I., Frackowiak, R. and Kleinschmidt, A. (2000). Representation of the temporal envelope of sounds in the human brain. *Journal of Neurophysiology, 84,* 1588-1598.

[37] Godey, B., Schwartz, D., Graaf, J. B., Chauvel, P. and Liégeois-Chauvel, C. (2001). Neuromagnetic source localization of auditory evoked fields and intracerebral evoked potentials: A comparison of data in the same patients. *Clinical Neurophysiology, 112,* 1850-1859.

[38] Green, D. M. (1976). *An introduction to hearing.* New Jersey, PA: Lawrence Erlbaum Associates, Inc.

[39] Griffiths, T. D. (1999). Human complex sound analysis. *Clinical Science, 96,* 231-234.

[40] Griffiths, T. D., Büchel, C., Frackowiak, R. S. J. and Patterson, R. D. (1998). Analysis of temporal structure in sound by the human brain. *Nature Neuroscience, 1,* 422-427.

[41] Griffiths, T. D., Uppenkamp, S., Johnsrude, I., Josephs, O. and Patterson, R. D. (2001). Encoding of the temporal regularity of sound in the human brainstem. *Nature Neuroscience, 4,* 633-637.

[42] Griffiths, T. T., Warren, J. D., Scott, S. K., Nelken, I. and King, A. J. (2004). Cortical processing of complex sound: A way forward?. *Trends in Neurosciences, 27,* 181-185.

[43] Gulick, W. L., Geschneider, W. L., and Frisina, R. D. (1989). *Hearing: Physiological acoustics, neural coding, and psychoacoustics.* New York: Oxford University Press.

[44] Gutschalk, A., Patterson, R. D., Rupp, A., Uppenkamp, S. and Scherg, M. (2002). Sustained magnetic fields reveal separate sites for sound level and temporal regularity in human auditory cortex. *Neuroimage, 15,* 207-216.

[45] Gutschalk, A., Patterson, R. D., Scherg, M., Uppenkamp, S. and Rupp, A. (2004). Temporal dynamics of pitch in human auditory cortex. *Neuroimage, 22,* 755-766.

[46] Hall, D. A., Haggard, M. P., Summerfield, A. Q., Akeroyd, M. A. and Palmer, A. R. (2001). Functional magnetic resonance imaging measurements of sound-level encoding in the absence of background scanner noise. *Journal Acoustic Society American, 109,* 1559-1570.

[47] Hall, D. A., Hart, H. C. and Johnsrude, I. S. (2003). Relationships between human auditory cortical structure and function. *Audiology and Neuro-Otology, 8,* 1-18.

[48] Hall, D. A., Johnsrude, I. S., Haggard, M. P., Palmer, A. R., Akeroyd, M. A. and Summerfield, A. Q. (2002). Spectral and temporal processing in human auditory cortex. *Cerebral Cortex, 12,* 140-149.

[49] Hari, R., and Mäkelä, J. P. (1986). Neuromagnetic responses to frequency modulation of a continuous tone. *Acta Oto-laryngologica, 432,* 26-32.

[50] Harms, M. P., Melcher, J. R. and Weisskoff, R. M. (1998). Time courses of the fMRI signals in the inferior colliculus, medial geniculate body, and auditory cortex show different dependencies on noise burst rate. *Neuroimage, 7,* S365.

[51] Hart, H. C., Palmer, A. R. and Hall, D. A. (2002). Heschl's gyrus is more sensitive to tone level than non-primary auditory cortex. *Hearing Research, 171,* 177-190.

[52] Hart, H. C., Palmer, A. R. and Hall, D. A. (2003). Amplitude and frequency-modulated stimuli activate common regions of human auditory cortex. *Cerebral Cortex, 13,* 773-781.

[53] Hartman, B. J. (1982). An exploratory study of the effects of disco music on the auditory and vestibular systems. *Journal of Auditory Research, 22,* 271-274.

[54] Heil, P., Rajan, R. and Irvine, D. R. F. (1994). Topographic representation of tone intensity along the isofrequency axis of cat primary auditory cortex. *Hearing Research, 76,* 188-202.

[55] Henderson, G., Tomlison, B. E. and Gibson, P. H. (1980). Cell counts in human cerebral cortex in normal adults throughout life using an image analysing machine. *Journal of the Neurological Sciences, 27,* 389-405.

[56] Howard III, M. A, Volkov, I. O., Abbas, P. J., Damasio, H., Ollendieck, M. C. and Granner, M. A. (1996). A chronic microelectrode investigation of the tonotopic organization of human auditory cortex. *Brain Research, 724,* 260-264.

[57] Huotilainen, M., Sinkkonen, J., Tiitinen, H., Ilmoniemi, R. J., Pekkonen, E., Parkkonen, L. and Näätänen, R. (1997). Intensity representation in the human auditory

cortex. TKK Report Series of the Laboratory of Acoustics and Audio Signal Processing, *42,* 1-4.

[58] Huotilainen, M., Tiitinen, H., Lavikainen, J., Ilmoniemi, R. J., Pekkonen, E., Sinkkonen, J., Laine, P. and Näätänen, R. (1995). Sustained fields of tones and glides reflect tonotopy of the auditory cortex. *NeuroReport, 6,* 841-844.

[59] International Standards Organization. (1975). *Standard reference zero for the calibration of pure-tone audiometers 389.* New York: International Standards Organization.

[60] Jäncke, L., Buchanan, T., Lutz, K., Specht, K., Mirzazade, S. and Shah, N. J. S. (1999). The time course of the BOLD response in the human auditory cortex to acoustic stimuli of different duration. *Cognitive Brain Research, 8,* 117-124.

[61] Jäncke, L., Shah, N. J., Posse, S., Grosse-Ryuken, M. and Müller-Gärtner, H.-W. (1998). Intensity coding of auditory stimuli: an fMRI study. *Neuropsychologia, 36,* 875-883.

[62] Kaas, J. H. and Hackett, T. A. (2000). Subdivisions of auditory cortex and processing streams in primates. *Proceedings of the National Academy of Sciences, 97,* 11793-11799.

[63] Kaas, J. H., Hackett, T. A. and Tramo, M. K. (1999). Auditory processing in primate cerebral cortex. *Current Opinion in Neurobiology, 9,* 164-170.

[64] Krumbholz, K., Patterson, R. D., Seither-Preisler, A., Lammertmann, C. and Lütkenhöner, B. (2003). Neuromagnetic evidence for a pitch processing center in Heschl's gyrus. *Cerebral Cortex, 13,* 765-772.

[65] Kuriki, S. and Murase, M. (1989). Neuromagnetic study of the auditory responses in right and left hemispheres of the human brain evoked by pure tones and speech sounds. *Experimental Brain Research, 77,* 127-134.

[66] Langers, D. R. M., Backes, W. H. and Van Dijk, P. (2003). Spectrotemporal features of the auditory cortex: The activation in response to dynamic ripples. *Neuroimage, 20,* 265-275.

[67] Langner, G. (1992). Periodicity coding in the auditory system. *Hearing Research, 60,* 115-142.

[68] Langner, G. (1997). Neural processing and representation of periodicity pitch. *Acta Oto-laryngologica, 532,* 68-76.

[69] Langner, G., Sams, M., Heil, P. and Schulze, H. (1997). Frequency and periodicity are represented in orthogonal maps in the human auditory cortex: Evidence from magnetoencephalography. *Journal of Comparative Physiology A, 181,* 665-676.

[70] Lauter, J. L., Herscovitch, P., Formby, C. and Raichle, M. E. (1985). Tonotopic organization in human auditory cortex revealed by positron emission tomography. *Hearing Research, 20,* 199-205.

[71] Liégeois-Chauvel, C., Giraud, K., Badier, J.-M., Marquis, P. and Chauvel, P. (2001). Intracerebral evoked potentials in pitch perception reveal a functional asymmetry of the human auditory cortex. In: R. J. Zatorre, and I. Peretz (Eds.), *The Biological Foundation of Music. Annals of the New York Academy of Sciences, vol. 930* (pp. 117-132). New York, NY: New York Academy of Sciences.

[72] Liégeois-Chauvel, C., Laguitton, V., Badier, J. M., Schwartz, D. and Chauvel, P. (1995). Étude des mécanismes corticaux de la perception auditive chez l'homme: Apport des potentiels intracérébraux et des champs magnétiques évoqués par les stimulations auditives. *Revue Neurologique, 151,* 495-504.

[73] Liégeois-Chauvel, C., Musolino, A. and Chauvel, P. (1991). Localization of primary auditory area in man. *Brain, 114,* 139-151.

[74] Lockwood, A. H., Salvi, R. J., Coad, M. L., Arnold, S. A.., Wack, D. S., Murphy, B. W. and Burkard, R. F. (1999). The functional anatomy of the normal human auditory sytem: Responses to 0.5 and 4.0 KHz tones at varied intensities. *Cerebral Cortex, 9,* 65-76.

[75] Lütkenhöner, B. (2003). Single-dipole analyses of the N100m are not suitable for characterizing the cortical representation of pitch. *Audiology Neuro-Otology, 8,* 222-233.

[76] Lütkenhöner, B., Krumbholz, K. and Seither-Preisler, A. (2003). Studies of tonotopy based on wave N100 of the auditory evoked field are problematic. *NeuroImage, 19,* 935-949.

[77] Lütkenhöner, B. and Steinsträter, O. (1998). High-Precision neuromagnetic study of the functional organization of the human auditory cortex. *Audiology and Neuro-otology, 3,* 191-213.

[78] Mäkelä, J. P. and Hari, R. (1994). Neuromagnetic cortical signals in a patient with hydrocephalus. *Neuroreport, 5,* 1125-1128.

[79] May, P. and Tiitinen, H. (2001). Human cortical processing of auditory events over time. *NeuroReport, 12,* 573-577.

[80] May, P. Tiitinen, H., Ilmoniemi, R. J., Nyman, G., Taylor J. G., and Näätänen, R. (1999). Frequency change detection in human auditory cortex. *Journal of Computational Neuroscience, 6,* 99-120.

[81] McBurney, D. H. (1978). Psychological dimensions and perceptual analysis of taste. In E. C. Carterette, and M. P. Friedman (Eds.), *Handbook of Perception* (pp. 125-155). New York, NY: Academic Press.

[82] Merzenich, M. M. and Brugge, J. F. (1973). Representation of the cochlear partition on the superior temporal plane of the macaque monkey. *Brain Research, 50,* 275-296.

[83] Mesulam, M. M. and Geula, C. (1991). Acetylcholinesterase-rich neurons of the human cerebral cortex: Cytoarchitectonic and ontogenetic patterns of distribution. *The Journal of Comparative Neurology, 306,* 193-220.

[84] Millen, S. J, Haughton, V. M. and Yetkin, Z. (1995). Functional magnetic resonance imaging of the central auditory pathway following speech and pure-tone stimuli. *Laryngoscope, 105,* 1305-1310.

[85] Morel, A., Garraghty, P. E. and Kaas, J. H. (1993). Tonotopic organization, architectonic fields, and connections of auditory cortex in macaque monkeys. *The Journal of Comparative Neurology, 335,* 437-459.

[86] Morosan, P., Rademacher, J., Schleicher, A., Amunts, K., Schormann, T. and Zilles, K. (2001). Human Primary Auditory Cortex: Cytoarchitectonic subdivisions and mapping into a spatial reference system. *Neuroimage, 13,* 684-701.

[87] Näätänen, R. and Picton, T. W. (1987). The N1 wave of the human electric and magnetic response to sound: A review and an analysis of the component structure. *Psychophysiology, 24,* 375-425.

[88] Ottaviani, F., Di Girolamo, S., Briglia, G., De Rossi, G., Di Giuda, D. and Di Nardo, W. (1997). Tonotopic organization of human auditory cortex analyzed by SPET. *Audiology, 36,* 241-248.

[89] Pantev, C., Bertrand, O., Eylitz, C., Verkindt, C., Hampson, S., Shuierer, G. and Elbert, T. (1995). Specific tonotopic organizations of different areas of the human auditory cortex reveled by simultaneous magnetic and electric recordings. *Electroencephalography and Clinical Neurophysiology, 94,* 26-40.

[90] Pantev, C., Hoke, M., Lehnertz, K. and Lütkenhöner, B. (1989). Neuromagnetic evidence of an amplitopic organization of the human auditory cortex. *Electroencephalography and Clinical Neurophysiology, 72,* 225-231.

[91] Pantev, C., Hoke, M., Lehnertz, K., Lütkenhöner, B., Anogianakis, G. and Wittkowski, W. (1988). Tonotopic organization of the human auditory cortex revealed by transient auditory evoked magnetic fields. *Electroencephalography and Clinical Neurophysiology, 69,* 160-170.

[92] Pantev, C., Hoke, M., Lütkenhöner, B. and Lehnertz, K. (1989). Tonotopic organization of the auditory cortex: Pitch versus frequency representation. *Science, 246,* 486-488.

[93] Pantev, C., Roberts, L. E., Elbert, T., Ross, B., and Wienbruch, C. (1996). Tonotopic organization of the sources of human steady–state responses. *Hearing Research,* 101, 62-74.

[94] Pelizzone, M., Williamson, S. J., Kaufman, L. and Schafer, K. L. (1984). Different sources of transient and steady state responses in human auditory cortex revealed by neuromagnetic fields. *Annals of the New York Academy of Sciences, 435,* 570-571.

[95] Penhune, V. B., Zatorre, R. J., MacDonald, J. D., and Evans, A. C. (1996). Interhemispheric anatomical differences in human primary auditory cortex: Probabilistic mapping and volume measurement from magnetic resonance scans. *Cerebral Cortex, 6,* 661-672.

[96] Phillips, D. P. and Orman, S. S. (1984). Responses of single neurons in posterior field of cat auditory cortex to tonal stimulation. *Journal of Neurophysiology, 51,* 147-163.

[97] Phillips, D. P., Semple, M. N., Caldford, M. B. and Kitzes, L. M. (1994). Level-dependent representation of stimulus frequency in cat primary auditory cortex. *Experimental Brain Research, 102,* 210-226.

[98] Picton, T. W., John, M. S., Dimitrijevic, A. and Purcell, D. (2003). Human auditory steady-state responses. *International Journal of Audiology, 42,* 177-219.

[99] Picton, T. W., Woods, D. L. and Proulx, G. B. (1978). Human auditory sustained potentials I. The nature of the response. *Electroencephalography and Clinical Neurophysiology, 45,* 186-197.

[100] Poritsky, R. (1992). *Neuroanatomy: A functional atlas of parts and pathways.* Philadelphia: Hanley and Belfus.

[101] Rademacher, J., Morosan, P., Schormann, T., Schleicher, A., Werner, C., Freund, H. J. and Zilles, K. (2001). Probabilistic mapping and volume measurement of human primary auditory cortex. *Neuroimage, 13,* 669-683.
[102] Rauschecker, J. P. and Tian, B. (2000). Mechanisms and streams for processing of "what" and "where" in auditory cortex. *Proceedings of the National Academy of Sciences, 97,* 11800-11806.
[103] Rencanzone, G. H., Guard, D. C. and Phan, M. L. (2000). Frequency and intensity response properties of single neurons in the auditory cortex of the behaving macaque monkey. *Journal of Neurophysiology, 83,* 2315-2331.
[104] Rivier, F. and Clarke, S. (1997). Cytochrome oxidase, acetylcholinesterase, and NADPH-diaphorase staining in human supratemporal and insular cortex: Evidence for multiple auditory areas. *NeuroImage, 6,* 288-304.
[105] Romani, G. L., Williamson, S. J. and Kaufman, L. (1982). Tonotopic organization of the human auditory cortex. *Science, 216,* 1339-1340.
[106] Rosburg, T., Kreitschmann-Andermahr, I., Emmerich, E., Nowak, H. and Sauer, H. (1998). Hemispheric differences in frequency dependent dipole orientation of the human auditory evoked field component N100m. *Neuroscience Letters, 258,* 105-108.
[107] Rosburg, T., Kreitschmann-Andermahr, I., Ugur, T., Nestmann, H., Nowak H. and Sauer, H. (2000). Tonotopy of the auditory–evoked field component N100m in patients with schizophrenia. *Journal Psychopysiology, 14,* 131-141.
[108] Rose, J. E., Brugge, J. F., Anderson, D. J. and Hind, J. E. (1967). Phase-locked response to low-frequency tones in single auditory nerve fibers of the squirrel monkey. *Journal of Neurophysiology, 30,* 769-793.
[109] Ross, B. and Pantev, C. (2004). Auditory steady-state responses reveal amplitude modulation gap detection thresholds. *Journal Acoustic Society American, 115,* 2193-2206.
[110] Rossing, T. D. (1990). *The science of sound.* Reading, MA: Addison-Wesley.
[111] Rossing, T. D. and Houstsma, A. J. M. (1986). Effects of signal envelope on the pitch of short sinusoidal tones. *Journal of the Acoustical Society of America, 79,* 1926-1933.
[112] Rupp, A., Gutschalk, A., Hack, S. and Scherg, M. (2002). Temporal resolution of the human primary auditory cortex in gap detection. *Neuroreport, 13,* 2203-2207.
[113] Rupp, A., Hack, S., Gutschalk, A., Schneider, P., Picton, T. W., Stippich, C. and Scherg, M. (2000). Fast temporal interactions in human auditory cortex. *Neuroreport, 11,* 3731-3736.
[114] Scharf, B. and Buss, S. (1986). Audition I: Stimulus, physiology, thresholds. In K. R. Boff, L. Kaufman, and J. P. Thomas (Eds.). *Handbook of Perception and Human Performance, Volume I* (pp. 14-1 to 14-71). New York, NY: John Wiley and Sons, Inc.
[115] Schleicher, A. and Zilles, K. (1990). A quantitative approach to cytoarchitectonics: Analysis of structural inhomogeneities in nervous tissue using an image analyser. *Journal of Microscopy, 157,* 367-381.
[116] Schouten, J. F. (1940). The perception of pitch. *Philips Technical Review, 5,* 286-294.
[117] Schwarz, D. W. F. and Tomlinson, R. W. W. (1990). Spectral response patterns of auditory cortex neurons to harmonic complex tones in alert monkey (macaca mulatta). *Journal of Neurophysiology, 64,* 282-298.

[118] Seldon, H. L. (1981). Structure of human auditory cortex I:. Cytoarchitectonics and dendritic distributions. *Brain Research, 229,* 277-294.

[119] Semple, M. N. and Scotte, B. H. (2003). Cortical mechanisms in hearing. *Current Opinion in Neurobiology, 13,* 1-7.

[120] Shönwiesner, M., von Cramon, D. Y. and Rübsamen, R. (2002). Is it tonotopy after all? *Neuroimage, 17,* 1144-1161.

[121] Suga, N. and Manabe, T. (1982). Neural basis of amplitude-spectrum representation in auditory cortex of the mustached bat. *Journal of Neurophysiology, 47,* 225-255.

[122] Talavage, T. M., Ledden, P. J., Benson, R. R., Rosen, B. R. and Melcher, J. R. (2000). Frequency-dependent responses exhibited by multiple regions in human auditory cortex. *Hearing Research, 150,* 225-244.

[123] Talavage, T. M., Sereno, M. I., Melcher, J. R., Ledden, P. J., Rosen, B. R. and Dale, A. M. (2004). Tonotopic organization in human auditory cortex revealed by progressions of frequency sensitivity. *Journal of Neurophysiology, 91,* 1282-1296.

[124] Taniguchi, I. and Nasu, M. (1993) Spatio-temporal representation of sound intensity in the guinea pig auditory cortex observed by optical recording. *Neuroscience Letters, 151,* 178-181.

[125] Tuomisto, T., Hari, R., Katila, T., Poutanen, T. and Varpula, T. (1983). Studies of auditory evoked magnetic and electric responses: Modality specificity and modelling. *Il Nuovo Cimento, 2D,* 471-483.

[126] Vasama, J.-P., Mäkelä, J. P., Tissari, S. O. and Hämäläinen, M. S. (1995). Effects of intensity variation on human auditory evoked magnetic fields. *Acta Oto-Laryngologica, 155,* 616-621.

[127] Verkindt, C., Bertrand, O., Perrin, F., Echallier, J. F. and Pernier, J. (1995). Tonotopic organization of the human auditory cortex: N100 topography and multiple dipole model analysis. *Electroencephalography and Clinical Neurophysiology, 96,* 143-156.

[128] Verkindt, C., Bertrand, O., Thevenet, M. and Pernir, J. (1994). Two auditory components in the 130-230 ms range disclosed by their stimulus frequency dependence. *NeuroReport, 5,* 1189-1192.

[129] Wallace, M. N., Johnston, P. W. and Palmer, A. R. (2002). Histochemical identification of cortical areas in the auditory region of the human brain. *Experimental Brain Research, 143,* 499-508.

[130] Wessinger, C. M., Buonocore, M. H., Kussmaul, C. L. and Mangun, G. R. (1997). Tonotopy in human auditory cortex examined with functional magnetic resonance imaging. *Human Brain Mapping, 5,* 18-25.

[131] Wessinger, C. M., van Meter, J., Tian, B., van Lare, J., Pekar, J. and Rauschecker, J. P. (2001). Hierarchical organization of the human auditory cortex revealed by functional magnetic resonance imaging. *Journal of Cognitive Neuroscience, 13,* 1-7.

[132] Yamamoto, T., Uemura, T. and Llinás, R. (1992). Tonotopic organization of human auditory cortex revealed by multi-channel SQUID system. *Acta Oto-Laryngologica,112*, 201-204.

[133] Yang, Y., Engelien, A., Engelien, W., Xu, S., Stern, E. and Silbersweig, D. A. (2000) A silent event-related functional MRI technique for brain activation studies without interference of scanner acoustic noise. *Magnetic Resonance in Medicine, 43,* 185-190.

[134] Yoshiura, T., Higano, S., Rubio, A., Shrier, D. A., Kwok, W. E., Iwanaga, S. and Numaguchi, Y. (2000). Heschl and superior temporal gyri: Low signal intensity of the cortex on T2-weighted MR Images of the normal brain. *Radiology, 214,* 217-221.

[135] Yost, W. A., Patterson, R. D. and Sheft, S. (1996). A time domain description for the pitch strength of iterated rippled noise. *Journal Acoustic Society American, 99,* 1066-1078.

[136] Yousry, T. A., Fesl, G., Büttner, A., Noachtar, S. and Schmid, U. D. (1997). Heschl's gyrus: Anatomic description and method of identification on magnetic resonance imaging. *International Journal of Neuroradiology, 3,* 3-12.

[137] Zatorre, R. J. and Belin, P. (2001). Spectral and temporal processing in human auditory cortex. *Cerebral Cortex, 11,* 946-953.

[138] Zattorre, R. J. and Binder, J. R. (2000). Functional and structural imaging of the human auditory system. In A. W. Toga, and J. C. Mazziotta (Eds.), *Brain Mapping. The systems* (pp. 365-402). San Diego: Academic Press.

In: Progress in Brain Mapping Research
Editor: F. J. Chen, pp. 123-157
ISBN 1-59454-580-4

Chapter 3

Modelling Time-Series in Neuroimaging

Olivier David*[*], *Stefan J. Kiebel and Karl J. Friston
The Wellcome Dept. of Cognitive Neurology,
University College London

Abstract

Inferences about brain function, using neuroimaging data, rest on models of how the data are caused. These models can be quite diverse, ranging from conceptual models of functional anatomy to nonlinear mathematical models of neuronal and hemodynamic responses. The aim of this review is to introduce the key models used in imaging neuroscience, focussing on functional magnetic resonance imaging (fMRI) and electroencephalography (EEG), and how they relate to each other. In particular, we consider how the analysis of neuronal dynamics can be used to infer functional segregation and integration. We start with anatomical models of functional brain architectures, which motivate some of the fundaments of neuroimaging. We then turn to basic statistical models (*e.g.* the general linear model) used for making classical and Bayesian inferences about *where* neuronal responses are expressed (regionally specific responses). By incorporating biophysical constraints, these basic models can be finessed and, in a dynamic setting, rendered causal. This allows us to infer *how* interactions among brain regions are mediated. The latter models afford mechanistic inferences about how evoked responses are caused, at the level of neuronal subpopulations and the coupling among them.

Keywords: Models, Dynamic, Inference, Causal, and Neuroimaging

[*] The Wellcome Dept. of Cognitive Neurology, University College London Queen Square, London, UK WC1N 3BG; Tel (44) 020 7833 7456; Fax (44) 020 7813 1445; Email odavid@fil.ion.ucl.ac.uk

I. Introduction

Neuroscience depends on conceptual, anatomical, statistical and causal models that link ideas about how the brain works to observed neuronal responses. The brain appears to adhere to two key principles of functional organisation, *functional specialisation* and *functional integration,* where the integration within and among specialised areas is mediated by effective connectivity due to neuronal interactions. These two concepts are cornerstones of modern system neuroscience and emerged from early theories about functional localisation.

Since the nineteenth century, the identification of a particular brain region with a specific function has become a central theme in neuroscience. However, functional localisation *per se* was not easy to demonstrate given the dependence of cerebral activity on underlying connections. Early attempts to localise brain functions used electrical stimulation in dog and monkey cortex (Goltz 1881) but were considered inconclusive because localisationism discounted interactions, or functional integration among different brain areas. It was proposed that lesion studies could supplement excitation experiments. Observations on patients with brain lesions (Absher and Benson 1993) led to the concept of *disconnection syndromes* and the refutation of localisationism as a complete or sufficient explanation of cortical organisation. Therefore, *functional localisation*, which implies that a function can be localised in a cortical area, has been supplemented by the concept of functional specialisation. Functional segregation suggests that a cortical area is specialised for some aspect of perceptual or motor processing, and that this specialisation is anatomically *segregated* within the cortex. The cortical infrastructure supporting a single function may then involve many specialised areas whose union is mediated by the functional integration among them. In this view functional specialisation is only meaningful in the context of functional integration and *vice versa*.

The functional role of any component (*e.g.* cortical area, sub-area or neuronal population) of the brain is defined largely by its connections. Certain patterns of cortical projections are so common that they could amount to rules of cortical connectivity. Functional segregation demands that cells with common functional properties be grouped together. This architectural constraint necessitates both convergence and divergence of cortical connections. Extrinsic connections among cortical regions are not continuous but occur in patches or clusters. This patchiness has, in some instances, a clear relationship to functional segregation. For example, V2 has a distinctive cytochrome oxidase architecture, consisting of thick stripes, thin stripes and inter-stripes. When recordings are made in V2, directionally selective (but not wavelength or colour selective) cells are found exclusively in the thick stripes. Retrograde (*i.e.* backward) labelling of cells in V5 is limited to these thick stripes. All the available physiological evidence suggests that V5 is a functionally homogeneous area that is specialised for visual motion. Evidence of this nature supports the notion that patchy connectivity is the anatomical infrastructure that mediates functional segregation and specialisation. If it is the case that neurons in a given cortical area share a common responsiveness, by virtue of their extrinsic connectivity, to some sensorimotor or cognitive attribute, then this functional segregation is also an anatomical one.

The aim of this review is to highlight the relationships among the sorts of models that are employed in imaging, with an emphasis on dynamical processes. We will show how simple statistical models, used to identify *where* evoked brain responses are expressed can be elaborated to provide models of *how* neuronal responses are caused. These successive elaborations rely, increasingly, on biological mechanisms. We will review a series of models that cover conceptual models, motivating experimental design, to detailed biophysical models of coupled neuronal ensembles that enable questions to be asked, at a physiological and computational level. In section II, we start with models of functional segregation; namely simple statistical models (*e.g.* the general linear model) used for making classical and Bayesian inferences about functional specialisation, in terms of *where* neuronal responses are expressed. Characterising a region-specific effect rests on estimation and inference. Inferences in neuroimaging may be about differences seen when comparing one group of subjects to another or, within subjects, changes over a sequence of observations. They may pertain to structural differences (*e.g.* in voxel-based morphometry - Ashburner and Friston 2000) or neurophysiological indices of brain functions (*e.g.* fMRI or EEG). The principles of data analysis are very similar for all these applications. We will focus on the analysis of fMRI and EEG time-series, because this covers most of the issues encountered in other modalities. By incorporating biological constraints, simple observation models can be made more realistic and, in a dynamic framework, causal. This section concludes by considering some of the recent advances in biophysical modelling of hemodynamic responses. All the models considered in this section pertain to regional responses. In the next section (section III), we focus on models of distributed responses (functional integration), where the interactions among cortical areas or neuronal subpopulations are modelled explicitly. This section covers the distinction between *functional* and *effective* connectivity and reviews dynamic causal modelling of functional integration, using fMRI and EEG. The models introduced in this section deal explicitly with neuronal modelling and how parameters of neural networks can be inferred from macroscopic data such as fMRI and EEG. These modelling initiatives should be extended in the near future to enable the conjoint modelling, or fusion, of different modalities and the marriage of computational neuroscience with the modelling of brain responses. We will deal first with models of regionally specific responses and return to models of functional integration later.

II. Models of Functional Segregation

Functional segregation is studied by modelling regional responses. The first approach is to detect where significant effects are expressed in the brain by testing the null hypothesis that the effect is zero at each location. This is the goal of *Statistical Parametric Mapping* (SPM) which uses classical inference. Later we will consider the Bayesian alternative. This rests on conditional inferences about an effect, given the data, as opposed to classical inferences about the data, given the effect is zero. Bayesian inference can be used to construct *Posterior Probability Maps* (PPMs). Although less established than *Statistical Parametric Maps* (SPMs), PPMs are potentially very useful, not least because they do not have to contend with the multiple-comparisons problem induced by classical inference (Berry and Hochberg 1999). In contradistinction to SPM, this means that inferences about a given regional response do not depend on inferences about responses elsewhere. Both classical and

Bayesian inferences will be introduced in the framework of the general linear model (GLM). We will then turn to dynamic systems and show how they can be formulated as GLMs. These dynamic models, which account explicitly for the time dimension, take us closer to how brain responses are actually caused by experimental manipulations. These models represent the next step towards causal models of brain responses and rest on biophysical models of interacting neuronal populations. Examples will be introduced when dealing with functional integration in the next section.

II.1. Statistical Parametric Mapping

Functional mapping studies are usually analysed with some form of SPM. SPM entails the construction of spatially extended statistical processes to test hypotheses about regionally specific effects (Friston *et al* 1991). SPMs are image processes with voxel values that are, under the null hypothesis, distributed according to a known probability density function, usually the Student's T or F distributions. These are known colloquially as T- or F-maps. The success of statistical parametric mapping is due largely to the simplicity of the idea. Namely, one analyses each and every voxel using any standard (univariate) statistical test. These usually test for activation, or regression on some explanatory variable. The resulting statistical parameters are assembled into an image - the SPM. SPMs are interpreted as statistical processes that are continuous in space (or sometimes time) by referring to the probabilistic behaviour of random fields (Adler 1981, Friston *et al* 1991, Worsley *et al* 1992, Worsley *et al* 1996). Random fields model both the univariate probabilistic characteristics of a SPM and any non-stationary spatial covariance structure under the null hypothesis. 'Unlikely' excursions of the SPM are interpreted as regionally specific effects, attributable to the sensorimotor or cognitive process that has been manipulated experimentally.

Over the years SPM has come to refer to the conjoint use of the *General Linear Model* (GLM) and *Random Field Theory* (RFT) to analyse and make classical inferences about spatially extended data through SPMs (Friston *et al* 1995a). The GLM is used to *estimate* some parameters that could explain continuous data in exactly the same way as in conventional analysis of discrete data. RFT is used to resolve the multiple-comparisons problem that ensues when making *inferences* over a volume of the brain. RFT provides a method for adjusting p values for the search volume of an SPM to control false positive rates. It plays the same role for *continuous* data (*i.e.* images or time-series) as the Bonferroni correction for a family of discontinuous or *discrete* statistical tests.

II.2. The General Linear Model

II.2.1. The Design Matrix

Statistical analysis of imaging data corresponds to (i) modelling the data to partition observed neurophysiological responses into components of interest, confounds and error and (ii) making inferences, about interesting effects, using the variances of the partitions. A brief review of the literature may give the impression that there are numerous ways to analyse fMRI and EEG time-series, with a diversity of statistical and conceptual approaches. This is not the case. With very few exceptions, every analysis is a variant of the general linear model. These include; (i) Simple T-tests on signal intensity assigned to one condition or another. (ii) Correlation coefficients between observed responses and boxcar stimulus functions in fMRI (Bandettini *et al* 1993). (iii) Inferences made using multiple linear regression. (iv) Evoked responses estimated using linear time invariant models and (v) Selective averaging to estimate event-related responses. Mathematically, they are all identical and can be implemented with the same equations and algorithms. The only thing that distinguishes among them is the *design matrix X* encoding the experimental design.

The general linear model is an equation

$$y = X\beta + \varepsilon \tag{1}$$

expressing the observed response y in terms of a linear combination of explanatory variables (*e.g.* designed effects or confounds) in the design matrix X (β are the weights assigned to each explanatory variable) plus a well-behaved error term ε. The general linear model is variously known as 'analysis of [co]variance' or 'multiple regression ' and subsumes simpler variants, like the 'T-test' for a difference in means, to more elaborate linear convolution models such as *Finite Impulse Response* (FIR) models. Each column of the design matrix corresponds to some effect one has built into the experiment or that may confound the results. These are referred to as explanatory variables, covariates or regressors. Sometimes the design matrix contains covariates or indicator variables that take values of 0 or 1, to indicate the presence of a particular level of an experimental factor (*c.f.* analysis of variance - ANOVA). The example in Figure 1 relates to an fMRI study of visual stimulation under four conditions. The effects on the response variable are modelled in terms of functions of the presence of these conditions (*i.e.* box or stick functions smoothed with components of a hemodynamic response function). Note that this is more complicated than a simple ANOVA, because the design matrix is modelling a time-series, as opposed to discrete observations. The relative contribution of each of these columns to the response is controlled by the parameters β. These are estimated using standard least squares. Inferences about the parameter estimates are made using T or F statistics, depending upon whether one is looking at one (T statistic), or more, linear combinations of them (F statistic).

In simple analyses the design matrix contains indicator variables or parametric variables encoding the experimental manipulations. These are formally identical to classical ANOVA or multiple linear regression models. However, when the observations correspond to time-series, convolution models are often used: An important instance of the GLM, from the perspective of fMRI and EEG, is the *Linear Time Invariant* (LTI) convolution model. Mathematically this is no different from any other GLM. However, it treats the data-sequence explicitly as an ordered time-series and enables a signal processing perspective that can be useful.

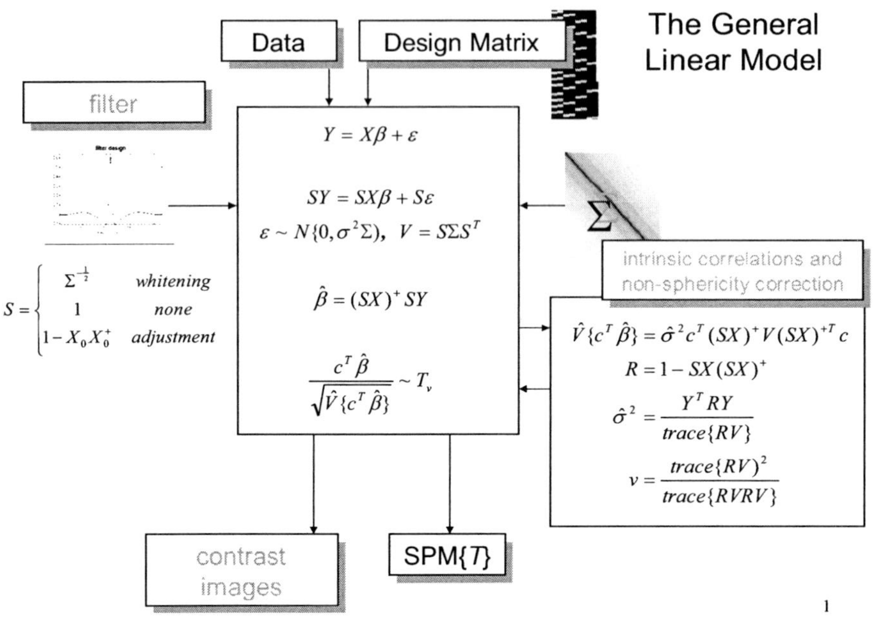

Figure 1. The general linear model is an equation expressing the response variable Y in terms of a linear combination of explanatory variables in a design matrix X and an error term with assumed or known autocorrelation Σ. In fMRI the data can be filtered with a convolution or residual forming matrix (or a combination) S, leading to a generalised linear model that includes [intrinsic] serial correlations and applied [extrinsic] filtering. Different choices of S correspond to different estimation schemes as indicated on the upper left. The parameter estimates obtain in a least squares sense using the pseudoinverse (denoted by +) of the filtered design matrix. An effect of interest is specified by a vector of contrast weights c that give a weighted sum or compound of parameter estimates, referred to as a *contrast*. The T statistic is simply this contrast divided by the standard error (*i.e.* square root of its estimated variance). The ensuing T statistic is distributed with v degrees of freedom. The equations for estimating the variance of the contrast and the degrees of freedom are provided in the right-hand panel and accommodate the non-sphericity implied by Σ.

II.2.2. Contrasts, T and F Statistics

Each column of X has an associated but unknown parameter β. Some of these parameters will be of interest (*e.g.* the effect of a sensorimotor or cognitive condition or the regression coefficient of hemodynamic responses on reaction time). The remaining parameters will be of no interest and pertain to nuisance or confounding effects (*e.g.* the effect of being a particular subject or the regression slope of regional activity on global activity). The statistical test is directed to interesting effects by specifying the null hypothesis with a *contrast*. A contrast is simply a linear mixture of parameter estimates. The T statistic allows one to test the null hypothesis that some contrast (*e.g.* a subtraction) of the estimates is zero. The T statistic obtains by dividing the contrast (specified by contrast weights) of the parameter estimates, by its standard error. Sometimes, several contrasts are tested jointly, for example when using polynomial (Büchel *et al* 1996) or basis function expansions of some experimental factor. In these instances, the SPM{F} is used and is specified with a *matrix* of contrast weights that can be thought of as a collection of 'T contrasts' that one wants to test *en masse*.

Having computed the statistic, RFT is used to assign adjusted p-values to topological features of the SPM, such as the height of peaks or the spatial extent of regions above a threshold. This p-value is a function of the search volume and smoothness of the residuals (see Figure 1).

The intuition behind RFT is that it allows one to control the false positive rate of peaks or 'blobs' corresponding to regional effects. A Bonferroni correction would control the false positive rate of voxels, which is inexact and unnecessarily severe. The p-value is the probability of getting a peak in the SPM, or higher, by chance over the search volume. If sufficiently small (usually less than 0.05) the regional effect can be declared significant.

II.2.3. Experimental Designs

The equations summarised in Figure 1 can be used to implement a vast range of statistical analyses. The issue is therefore not so much the mathematics but the formulation of an appropriate design matrix X. This is the device to specify the experimental design, where explanatory variables encode treatment effects that we assume are expressed in a linear and instantaneous fashion in the data, without reference to any particular mechanism. Experimental designs employed in neuroimaging studies can be classified as *single factor* or *multifactorial* designs; within this classification the levels of each factor can be *categorical* or *parametric*.

The simplest *categorical design* is cognitive subtraction where one assumes the difference between two tasks can be formulated as a separable cognitive or sensorimotor component. Consequently, regionally specific differences, in the responses evoked by the two tasks, identify the corresponding functionally specialised area. Early applications of subtraction range from the functional anatomy of word processing (Petersen *et al* 1989) to functional specialisation in extrastriate cortex (Lueck *et al* 1989). The latter studies involved presenting visual stimuli with and without some sensory attribute (*e.g.* colour, motion *etc*). Cognitive conjunctions (Price and Friston 1997) can be thought of as an extension of the subtraction technique, in the sense that they combine a series of subtractions. In subtraction one tests a *single* hypothesis pertaining to the activation in one task relative to another. In conjunction analyses *several* contrasts are tested, asking whether all the activations, in a series of task pairs, are expressed conjointly. Consider the problem of identifying regionally specific activations due to a particular cognitive component (*e.g.* object recognition). If one can identify a series of task pairs whose differences have only that component in common, then the region which activates, in all the corresponding subtractions, can be associated with the common component. In short, conjunction analyses allow one to disclose context-invariant regional responses.

The premise behind *parametric designs* is that regional physiology will vary systematically with the degree of cognitive or sensorimotor processing or deficits thereof. Examples of this approach include the PET experiments of Grafton *et al* (1992) that demonstrated significant correlations between hemodynamic responses and the performance of a visually guided motor tracking task. In sensory studies Price *et al* (1992) demonstrated a remarkable linear relationship between perfusion in peri-auditory regions and frequency of aural word presentation. This correlation was not observed in Wernicke's area, where perfusion appeared to correlate, not with the discriminative attributes of the stimulus, but with the presence or absence of semantic content. These relationships or *neurometric functions* may be linear or nonlinear. Using polynomial regression, in the context of the GLM, one can identify nonlinear relationships between stimulus parameters (*e.g.* stimulus duration or presentation rate) and evoked responses. To do this one usually uses a SPM{F} (see Büchel *et al* 1996).

Factorial designs, where two or more factors are combined in the same experiment, are more prevalent than single factor designs because they enable inferences about interactions. At its simplest, an interaction represents a change in a change, thus referring to second order behaviour. These interaction effects can sometimes be interpreted as (i) the integration of the two or more [cognitive] processes or (ii) the modulation of one [perceptual] process by another. Factorial designs have a wide range of applications. An early application, in neuroimaging, examined physiological adaptation and plasticity during motor performance, by assessing time by condition interactions (Friston *et al* 1992). Factorial designs have an important role in the context of cognitive subtraction and additive factor logic by virtue of being able to test for context-sensitive activations (*i.e.* to demonstrate the fallacy of 'pure insertion'. See Friston *et al* 1996a).

In summary, the design matrix encodes the causes of observed data and, in particular, treatment effects caused by changes in the level of various experimental factors. These factors can have categorical or parametric levels and most experiments nowadays use multiple factors to test for both main effects and interactions. Before turning to mechanistically more informed formulations of the GLM we will consider briefly the two sorts of inferences that can be made about the parameter estimates.

II.3. Classical and Bayesian Inference

To date, inference in neuroimaging has been restricted largely to classical inferences based upon statistical parametric maps. The statistics that comprise these SPMs are essentially functions of the data. The probability distribution of the chosen statistic, under the null hypothesis (*i.e.* the null distribution) is used to compute a *p*-value. This *p*-value is the probability of obtaining the statistic, or the data, given that the null hypothesis is true. If sufficiently small, the null hypothesis can be rejected and an inference is made. The alternative approach is to use Bayesian or conditional inference based upon the posterior distribution of the activation given the data (Holmes and Ford, 1993). This necessitates the specification of priors (*i.e.* the probability distribution of the activation). Bayesian inference requires the posterior distribution and therefore rests upon a posterior density analysis. A useful way to summarise this posterior density is to compute the probability that the activation exceeds some threshold. This represents a Bayesian inference about the effect, in relation to the specified threshold. By computing posterior probability for each voxel we can construct posterior probability maps or PPMs that are a useful complement to classical SPMs.

II.3.1.The Multiple-Comparisons Problem

The motivation for using conditional or Bayesian inference is that it has high face validity. This is because the inference is about an effect, or activation, being greater than some specified size that has some meaning in relation to underlying neurophysiology. This contrasts with classical inference, in which the inference is about the effect being significantly different than zero. The problem for classical inference is that trivial departures from the null hypothesis can be declared significant, with sufficient data or sensitivity.

In classical inference, one tries to ensure that the probability of rejecting the null hypothesis incorrectly is maintained at a small rate, despite making inferences over large volumes of the brain. This induces a multiple-comparisons problem that, for spatially continuous data, requires an adjustment or correction to the *p*-value using RFT as mentioned above. This correction means that classical inference becomes less sensitive or powerful with large search volumes. In contradistinction, posterior inference does not have to contend with the multiple-comparisons problem because there are no false-positives. The probability that activation has occurred, given the data, at any particular voxel is the same, irrespective of whether one has analysed that voxel or the entire brain. For this reason, posterior inference using PPMs represents a relatively more powerful approach than classical inference in neuroimaging.

II.3.2. Hierarchical Models and Empirical Bayes

PPMs require the posterior distribution or conditional distribution of the activation (a contrast of conditional parameter estimates) given the data. This posterior density can be computed, under Gaussian assumptions, using Bayes rule. Bayes rule requires the specification of a likelihood function and the prior density of the model's parameters. The models used to form PPMs and the likelihood functions are exactly the same as in classical SPM analyses, namely the GLM. The only extra information that is required is the prior probability distribution of the parameters. Although it would be possible to specify priors, using independent data or some plausible physiological constraints, there is an alternative to this *fully* Bayesian approach. The alternative is *empirical Bayes* in which the prior distributions are estimated from the data. Empirical Bayes requires a *hierarchical observation model* where the parameters and hyper-parameters at any particular level can be treated as priors on the level below. There are numerous examples of hierarchical observation models in neuroimaging. For example, the distinction between fixed- and mixed-effects analyses of multi-subject studies relies upon a two-level hierarchical model. However, in neuroimaging there is a natural hierarchical observation model that is common to all brain mapping experiments. This is the hierarchy induced by looking for the same effects at every voxel within the brain (or grey matter). The first level of the hierarchy corresponds to the experimental effects at any particular voxel and the second level comprises the effects over voxels. Put simply, the variation in a contrast, over voxels, can be used as the prior variance of that contrast at any particular voxel.

Hierarchical linear models have the following form:

$$y = X^{(1)}\beta^{(1)} + \varepsilon^{(1)}$$
$$\beta^{(1)} = X^{(2)}\beta^{(2)} + \varepsilon^{(2)}$$
$$\beta^{(2)} = \ldots \tag{2}$$

This is exactly the same as Eq(1) but now the parameters of the first level are generated by a supraordinate linear model and so on to any hierarchical depth required. These hierarchical observation models are an important extension of the GLM and are usually estimated using Expectation Maximisation (EM) (Dempster *et al* 1977). In the present context, the response variables comprise the responses at all voxels and $\beta^{(1)}$ are the treatment effects we want to make an inference about. Because we have invoked a second level the first-level parameters embody random effects and are generated by a second level linear model. At the second level $\beta^{(2)}$ is the average effect over voxels and $\varepsilon^{(2)}$ its voxel-to-voxel variation. By estimating the variance of $\varepsilon^{(2)}$ one is implicitly estimating an empirical prior on the first-level parameters at each voxel. This prior can then be used to estimate the posterior probability of $\beta^{(1)}$ being greater than some threshold at each voxel. An example of the ensuing PPM is provided in Figure 2 along with the classical SPM.

In this section we have seen how the GLM can be used to test hypotheses about brain responses and how, in a hierarchical form, it enables empirical Bayesian or conditional inference. In the next section we will deal with dynamic systems and how they can be formulated as GLMs. These dynamic models take us closer to how brain responses are actually caused by experimental manipulations and represent the next step in working toward causal models of brain responses.

II.4. Dynamic Models

Dynamic models rest upon the fact that time samples are not independent. Indeed measured responses in fMRI and EEG represent continuous and smooth processes. This can be modelled efficiently in the context of the GLM using convolution models that are constructed from a known stimulus function and a set of temporal basis functions. Temporal basis functions do model the biophysical mechanisms of measured responses, but can capture the input-output relationships of a system. The basic idea behind temporal basis functions is that the hemodynamic and electrical responses, induced by any given trial type, can be expressed as a linear combination of several [basis] functions of peristimulus time.

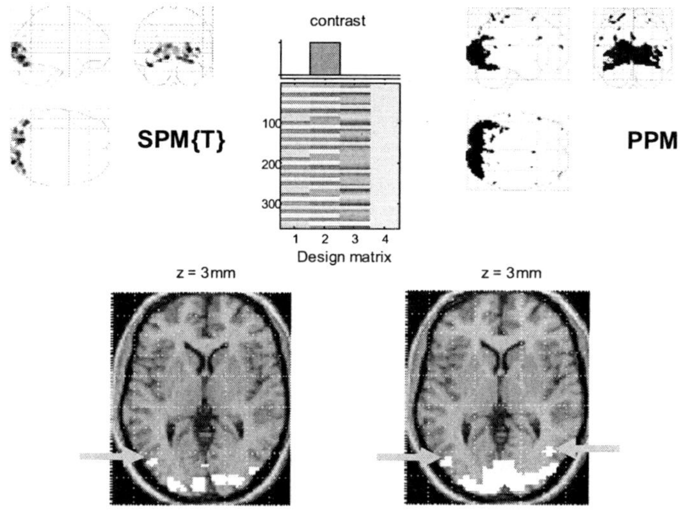

Figure 2. SPM and PPM for an fMRI study of attention to visual motion. The display format in the lower panel uses an axial slice through extrastriate regions but the thresholds are the same as employed in maximum intensity projections (upper panels). Upper right: The activation threshold for the PPM was 0.7 a.u., meaning that all voxels shown had a 90% chance of an activation of 0.7% or more. Upper left: The corresponding SPM using an adjusted threshold at $p = 0.05$. Note the bilateral foci of motion-related responses in the PPM that are not seen in the SPM (grey arrows). As can be imputed from the design matrix (upper middle panel), the statistical model of evoked responses comprised boxcar regressors convolved with a canonical hemodynamic response function. The middle column corresponds to the presentation of moving dots and was the stimulus property tested by the contrast.

II.4.1.The Convolution Model

The convolution model for both fMRI responses and event-related potentials (ERPs) takes a stimulus function, encoding neuronal input, and *convolves* or smoothes it with a basis function (defined below) to give a regressor that enters the design matrix. When using basis functions, the stimulus function is convolved with all the basis functions to give a series of regressors (in Figure 1 we used four stimulus functions and two basis functions to give eight regressors). Mathematically we can express this model as

$$\begin{array}{lcl} y(t) = X\beta + \varepsilon & & y(t) = u(t) \otimes h(t) \\ X_i = T_i(t) \otimes u(t) & \Leftrightarrow & h(t) = \beta_1 T_1(t) + \beta_2 T_2(t) + \ldots \end{array} \tag{3}$$

where $\otimes$ means convolution. This equivalence illustrates how temporal basis functions allow one to take any convolution model (right) and convert it into a GLM (left). The parameter estimates β_i are the coefficients or weights that determine the mixture of basis functions of time $T_i(t)$ that best model $h(t)$, the evoked response for the trial type and voxel in question. Temporal basis functions are important because they enable a graceful transition between conventional multi-linear regression models with one stimulus function per condition and FIR models with a parameter for each time point following the onset of a condition or trial type. Figure 3 illustrates this graphically (see Figure legend). In short, temporal basis functions offer useful constraints on the form of the estimated response that retain the flexibility of FIR models and the efficiency of single regressor models.

We now to consider fMRI and ERP separately, as the temporal basis functions required by both modalities are very different. This reflects fundamental differences in the biophysical generation of these signals.

II.4.2. Temporal Basis Functions for fMRI

In Friston *et al* (1994) the form of the hemodynamic impulse response function (HRF) was estimated using a least squares deconvolution and a time invariant model, where evoked neuronal responses are convolved with an HRF to give the measured hemodynamic response (see also Boynton *et al* 1996). This simple linear convolution model is the cornerstone for making statistical inferences about activations in fMRI with the GLM. An impulse response function is the response to a single impulse, measured at a series of times after the input. It characterises the input-output behaviour of the system (*i.e.* voxel) and places important constraints on the sorts of inputs that will excite a response.

Knowing the form that the HRF can take is important for several reasons, not least because it allows for better statistical models of the data. The HRF may vary from voxel to voxel and this has to be accommodated in the GLM. To allow for different HRFs in different brain regions the notion of temporal basis functions, to model evoked responses in fMRI, was introduced (Friston *et al* 1995b) and applied to event-related responses in Josephs *et al* (1997) (see also Lange and Zeger 1997). We find the most useful basis set to be a canonical HRF and its derivatives with respect to the key parameters that determine its form (onset and width).

II.4.3. Temporal Basis Functions for EEG

In contradistinction to fMRI, in which the HRF adopts a fairly stereotyped form, the impulse response function in EEG, *i.e.* the ERP, exhibits high variability between subjects and conditions, although standard waveforms (N20, N100, P300, *etc.*) are commonly used to describe its components. The most common technique to analyse epoched EEG data is to compute the average within a user-specified peristimulus time window and compare these averages among conditions and groups. Typically, one would choose the averaging window such that it covers the area around a peak of a specific component (*e.g.* the N100). This [averaging] analysis is equivalent to saying that one does not have an informed model for the ERP, because, in the context of the general linear model, the corresponding design matrix is simply a finite impulse response model (Kiebel and Friston 2004a; Kiebel and Friston 2004b). An alternative is to choose a generic basis that can capture the important features of ERPs. One such set comprise discrete wavelets. The key feature of wavelets is that they partition the time-frequency domain of an ERP. If one knows a-priori, which of these partitions contain the ERP, it is possible to specify a wavelet set that captures the signal (Kiebel and Friston 2004b). Selecting the appropriate wavelet subspace can be based on the assumptions that (i) noise is mainly expressed at high frequencies, (ii) there is no signal in pre-stimulus times, and (iii) high-frequency signal components are found early in peristimulus time.

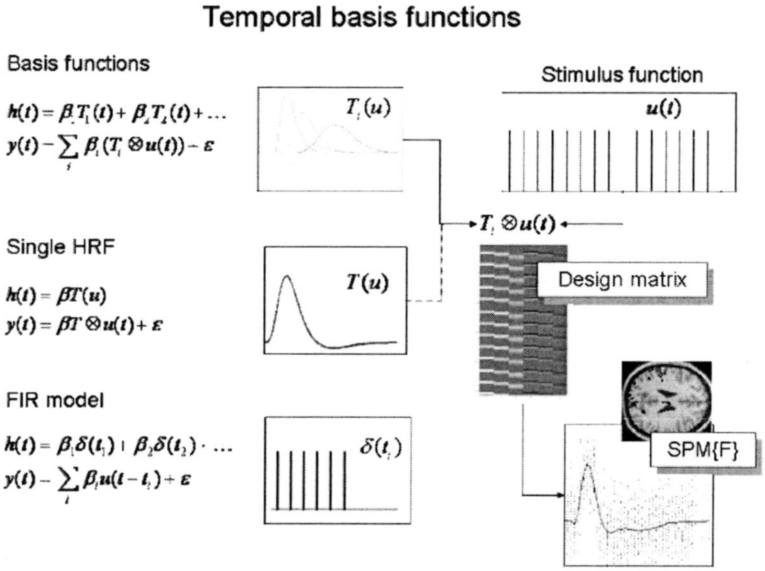

Figure 3. Temporal basis functions offer useful constraints on the form of the estimated response that retain the flexibility of FIR models and the efficiency of single regressor models. The specification of these constrained FIR models involves setting up stimulus functions $u(t)$ that model expected neuronal changes [*e.g.* boxcars of epoch-related responses or spikes (delta functions) at the onset of specific events or trials]. These stimulus functions are then convolved with a set of basis functions $T_i(t)$ of peri-stimulus time that, in some linear combination, model the impulse response. The ensuing regressors are assembled into the design matrix. In the case of fMRI, in this figure, the basis functions can be as simple as a single canonical HRF (middle), through to a series of delayed delta functions (bottom). The latter case corresponds to a FIR model and the coefficients constitute estimates of the impulse response function at a finite number of discrete sampling times. Selective averaging in event-related fMRI (Dale and Buckner 1997) is mathematically equivalent to this limiting case.

An alternative approach to EEG analysis is to make inferences after nonlinear transformations of the data. For example, instead of modelling the EEG in the temporal domain, one can model the data in the time-frequency domain. Such an analysis is based on time-frequency transforms like the short-term Fourier transform (Makeig 1993), the (continuous) Morlet wavelet transform (Tallon-Baudry *et al* 1996) or the band-pass Hilbert-transform (Tass *et al* 1998). These transforms are almost mathematically equivalent (Kiebel *et al* submitted) and are designed to disclose changes in power and phase in the time-frequency domain. Two different kinds of power transforms analysis have been proposed. The first models power in one or more frequency bands as a function of time, using a general linear model (Brookes *et al* 2004). However, with this approach, one returns to the same issue of selecting a suitable temporal basis set. The second approach eschews this issue by modelling every time-frequency bin separately and solving the implicit multiple comparison problem through *post hoc* adjustments to the *p*-values, *e.g.* by using results from the Gaussian Random Field theory (Kilner *et al* in press). With this approach one can assess the significance (*p*-value) of an observed difference in power at some peristimulus time and frequency. This *p*-value is corrected so that the false positive rate is controlled for the search volume over time and frequency. In other words, one does not need a prior hypothesis about where in the time-frequency domain a power difference exists, but can search for it while controlling for false positives.

Hitherto, we have described EEG analysis schemes that are largely uninformed about the fundamental features of the evoked response. However, in principle, these features can be learned from the data. One way of doing this is to use an over-complete wavelet transform and learn from the data which coefficients are relevant (Durka 2003). An alternative is to construct a generative or forward model of EEG responses that embodies the underlying neuronal and biophysical mechanisms. We can then learn the parameters of this dynamic causal model from the data. A following example of such a model is provided.

II.5. Biophysical Models

II.5.1. Input-State-Output Systems

By adopting a convolution model for brain responses in fMRI and EEG we are implicitly positing some underlying dynamic system that converts neuronal inputs into observed hemodynamic and electrical responses. Our understanding of the biophysical and physiological mechanisms that underpin the HRF has grown considerably in the past few years (*e.g.* Buxton and Frank 1997, Mandeville *et al* 1999, Hoge *et al* 1999). Figure 5 shows some simulations based on the hemodynamic model described in Friston *et al* (2000). Here, neuronal activity induces some auto-regulated vasoactive signal that causes transient increases in regional cerebral blood flow (rCBF). The resulting flow increases dilate a venous balloon, increasing its volume (v) and diluting venous blood to decrease deoxyhemoglobin content (q). The blood oxygenation-level-dependent (BOLD) signal is roughly proportional to the concentration of deoxyhemoglobin (q/v) and follows the rCBF response with about a one second delay. The model is framed in terms of differential equations, examples of which are provided in Figure 4.

EEG responses have been modelled since the 1970s using neural mass models (Freeman 1978; Lopes da Silva et al. 1974; Wilson and Cowan 1972). These models use a small number of variables to represent the expected states of large neuronal populations, *i.e.* neural masses. Many neural mass models have been proposed. They differ largely in terms of how the neuronal populations are coupled. However, they all rely upon the same basic principles of how the activity of a neuronal population evolves (Figure 5): a neuronal population receives inputs modelled as a mean firing rate (m) which in turn elicits a post synaptic potential (v), obtained by convolving the input with a kernel h. This kernel is the impulse response function of the neuronal population in terms of mean depolarisation. The output is the mean firing rate (m), which is usually an instantaneous nonlinear function S of the mean membrane potential of the source population. This nonlinear function, usually a sigmoid, reflects the fact that neuronal firing saturates (because of refractory periods) and cannot be

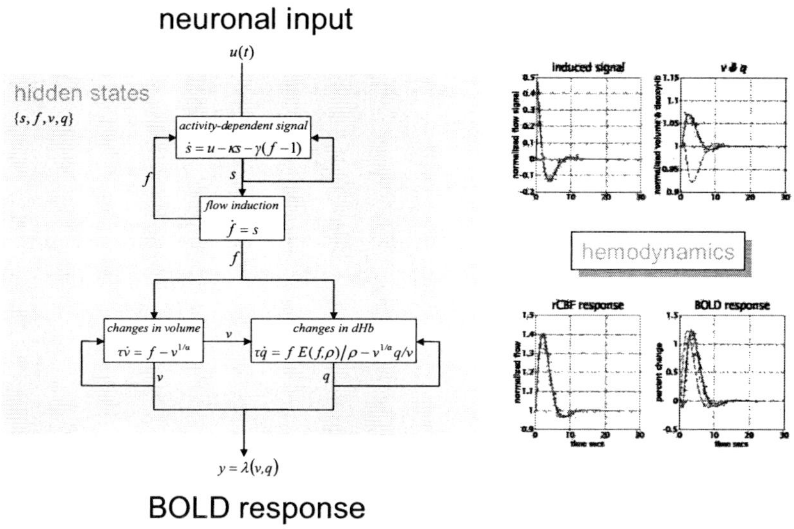

Figure 4.Right: Hemodynamics elicited by an impulse of neuronal activity as predicted by a dynamical biophysical model (left). A burst of neuronal activity causes an increase in flow-inducing signal that decays with first order kinetics and is down regulated by local flow. This signal increases rCBF, which dilates the venous capillaries, increasing volume (v). Concurrently, venous blood is expelled from the venous pool decreasing deoxyhemoglobin content (q). The resulting fall in deoxyhemoglobin concentration leads to a transient increases in BOLD (blood oxygenation level dependent) signal and a subsequent undershoot. Left: Hemodynamic model on which these simulations were based (see Friston *et al* 2000 for details).

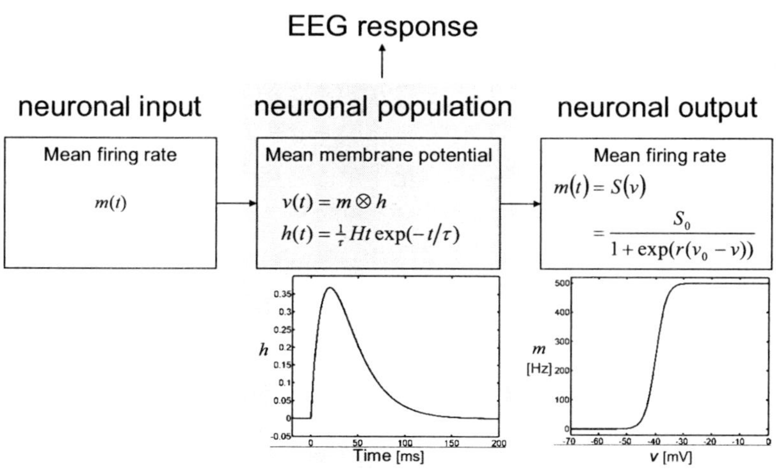

Figure 5. Neural mass model of a neuronal population. A neuronal population receives a neuronal input modelled as mean firing rate (m) which in turn elicits a post synaptic potential (v) obtained by convolving the input with a kernel (h). This kernel is the impulse response function of the population's depolarisation. It is parameterised by H and τ. H controls the maximum post-synaptic potential and τ represents a lumped rate constant. The output of the neuronal population is a mean firing rate that is assumed to be an instantaneous nonlinear function S of the mean membrane potential v. This nonlinear function, usually a sigmoid (here parameterised by S_0, r and v_0), reflects the fact that neuronal firing saturates because of the refractory period and cannot be negative.

negative. The EEG signal, either measured on the scalp or reconstructed in the cortex, is assumed to be proportional to the mean depolarisation of pyramidal cells. A complete model for EEG obtains by coupling several neuronal populations, either through excitatory (pyramidal and stellate cells) or inhibitory (interneurons) subpopulations (see David and Friston 2003 for details).

Notice that we have introduced variables, like volume and deoxyhemoglobin concentrations or mean firing rates, which are not actually observed. These are referred to as the *hidden states* of input-state-output models. The state and output equations of any analytic dynamical system are

$$\begin{aligned} \dot{x}(t) &= f(x,u,\theta) \\ y(t) &= g(x,u,\theta)+\varepsilon \end{aligned} \tag{4}$$

where $\dot{x} = \partial x / \partial t$. The first line is an ordinary differential equation and expresses the rate of change of the states as a function (with parameters θ) of the states x and inputs u. Typically the inputs $u(t)$ correspond to designed experimental effects (*e.g.* the stimulus function in fMRI or an impulse for EEG). There is a fundamental and causal relationship (Fliess *et al* 1983) between the outputs and the history of the inputs in Eq(4). This relationship conforms to a Volterra series, which expresses the output $y(t)$ as a generalised convolution of the input $u(t)$, critically without reference to the hidden states $x(t)$. This series is simply a functional Taylor expansion of the outputs with respect to the inputs (Bendat 1990). The reason it is a *functional* expansion is that the inputs are a function of time[2].

$$\begin{aligned} y(t) &= \sum_i \int_0^t \ldots \int_0^t \kappa_i(\sigma_1,\ldots,\sigma_i) u(t-\sigma_1),\ldots,u(t-\sigma_i)d\sigma_1,\ldots,d\sigma_i \\ \kappa_i(\sigma_1,\ldots,\sigma_i) &= \frac{\partial^i y(t)}{\partial u(t-\sigma_1),\ldots,\partial u(t-\sigma_i)} \end{aligned} \tag{5}$$

where $\kappa_i(\sigma_1,\ldots\sigma_i)$ is the ith order kernel. In Eq(5) the integrals are restricted to the past. This renders Eq(5) causal, hence dynamic *causal* modelling. The key thing here is that Eq(5) is simply a convolution and can be expressed as a GLM as in Eq(3). This means that we can take a neurophysiologically realistic model of brain responses and use it as an observation model to estimate parameters using observed data. Here the model is parameterised in terms of kernels that have a direct analytic relation to the original parameters θ of the biophysical system through Eq(5). In fMRI the first-order kernel is simply the conventional HRF. High-order kernels correspond to high-order HRFs and can be estimated using basis functions as described above. In fact, by choosing basis functions according to

[2] For simplicity, here and in and Eq(7), we deal with only one experimental input.

$$A(\sigma)_i = \frac{\partial \kappa(\sigma)_1}{\partial \theta_i} \tag{6}$$

one can estimate the biophysical parameters because, to a first order approximation, $\beta_i = \theta_i$. The critical step we have taken here is to start with a dynamic causal model of how responses are generated and construct a general linear observation model that allows us to estimate and infer the parameters of that model. This is in contrast to the conventional use of the GLM with design matrices that are not informed by a forward model of how data are caused. This approach to modelling brain responses has a much more direct connection with underlying physiology and rests upon an understanding of the underlying system.

II.5.2. Nonlinear System Identification

Once a suitable causal model has been established (*e.g.* Figure 4 or Figure 5), we can estimate second-order kernels. These kernels represent a nonlinear characterisation of brain responses that can model interactions among stimuli in causing responses. One important manifestation, of nonlinear effects captured by the second order kernels, is a modulation of stimulus-specific responses by preceding stimuli that are proximate in time. This means that responses at high stimulus presentation rates saturate and, in some instances, show an inverted 'U' behaviour. In fMRI, this behaviour appears to be specific to BOLD effects (as distinct from evoked changes in cerebral blood flow) and may represent a *hemodynamic refractoriness*. This effect has important implications for event-related fMRI, where one may want to present trials in quick succession. Such adaptation effects are also commonly expressed in ERPs: the amplitude of ERPs estimated from the first few trials of an experimental session are usually larger that the amplitude of ERPs estimated from trials at the end. This could reflect some short-term plasticity (*e.g.* calcium-dependent effects) that induces a change in synaptic efficacy. At the level of a single ERP, compound stimuli may also interact to shape the evoked response.

The results of a typical nonlinear analysis from fMRI are given in Figure 6. The right panel shows the average response, integrated over a 32-second train of stimuli as a function of stimulus onset asynchrony (SOA). These responses are based on the kernel estimates (left hand panels) using data from a voxel in the left posterior temporal region of a subject obtained during the presentation of single words at different rates. The solid line represents the estimated response and shows a clear maximum at just less than one second. The dots are responses based on empirical data from the same experiment. The broken line shows the expected response in the absence of nonlinear effects (*i.e.* that predicted by setting the second order kernel to zero). It is clear that nonlinearities become important at around two seconds, leading to an actual diminution of the integrated response at sub-second SOAs. The implication of this sort of result is that the assumptions of the linear convolution models discussed above are violated with sub-second SOAs (see also Buckner *et al* 1996 and Burock *et al* 1998)

In summary, we started with models of regionally specific responses, framed in terms of the general linear model, in which responses were modelled as linear mixtures of designed changes in explanatory variables. Hierarchical extensions to linear observation models enable random-effects analyses and, in particular an empirical Bayesian approach. The mechanistic utility of these models is realised through the use of forward models that embody causal dynamics. Simple variants of these are the linear convolution models used to construct explanatory variables in conventional analyses of fMRI and EEG data. These are a special case of generalised convolution models that are mathematically equivalent to input-state-output systems comprising hidden states. Estimation and inference with these dynamic models tell us something about *how* the response was caused, but only at the level of a single voxel, channel or source. The next section retains the same perspective on models, but in the context of distributed responses and functional integration.

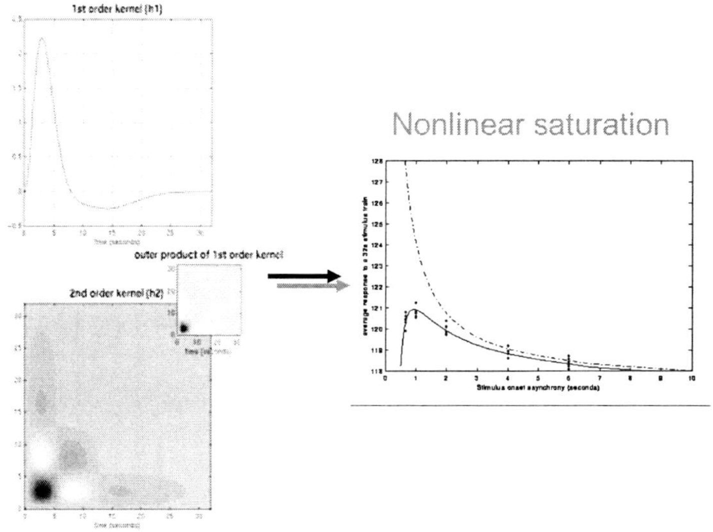

Figure 6. Nonlinearity analysis of fMRI responses. Left panels: Volterra kernels (fMRI) from a voxel in the left superior temporal gyrus at -56, -28, 12mm. These kernel estimates were based on a single-subject study of aural word presentation at different rates (from 0 to 90 words per minute) using a second order approximation to a Volterra series expansion modelling the observed hemodynamic response to stimulus input (a delta function for each word). These kernels can be thought of as a characterisation of the second-order hemodynamic response function. The first order kernel κ_1 (upper panel) represents the (first-order) component usually presented in linear analyses. The second-order kernel (lower panel) is presented in image format. The colour scale is arbitrary; white is positive and black is negative. The insert on the right represents $\kappa_1\kappa_1^T$, the second-order kernel predicted by a simple model that involved a linear convolution with κ_1 followed by some static nonlinearity. Right panel: Integrated responses over a 32-second stimulus train as a function of SOA. Solid line: Estimates based on the nonlinear convolution model parameterised by the kernels on the left. Broken line: The responses expected in the absence of second-order effects (*i.e.* in a truly linear system). Dots: Empirical averages based on the presentation of actual stimulus trains.

III. Models of Functional Integration

III.1. Functional and Effective Connectivity

III.I.1 Functional Connectivity

Imaging neuroscience has firmly established functional specialisation as a principle of brain organisation in man. The integration of specialised areas has proven more difficult to assess. Functional integration is usually inferred on the basis of correlations among measurements of neuronal activity. *Functional connectivity* has been defined as statistical dependencies or correlations *among remote neurophysiological events*. However correlations can arise in a variety of ways. For example in multi-unit electrode recordings they can result from stimulus-locked transients evoked by a common input or reflect stimulus-induced oscillations mediated by synaptic connections (Gerstein and Perkel 1969).

In EEG there is an uncertain consensus about the best method to characterise functional connectivity. Dependencies can be synchronous or asynchronous, linear or nonlinear, and so forth, engendering many different types of synchronisation, *i.e.* a common behaviour of at least one property of EEG generators (Pikovsky et al., 2001). This may be why different dependency measures appear in the EEG literature: these include linear (cross-correlation, coherence) or nonlinear (mutual information, nonlinear correlation, mutual dimension, nonlinear interdependencies or generalised synchronisation), or are based upon the quantification of phase-locking of oscillations (phase synchronisation). This battery of measures has been assembled during the last decade, making research in this area exciting but quite confusing. Recently, an attempt has been made to evaluate the performance of some of these measures in a case study of EEG signals (Quian Quiroga et al 2002) and using a neural mass model of EEG oscillations (David et al 2004a).

The classical analysis of cross-correlation (CC), *i.e.* normalised covariance, is the most widely used approach to quantify interactions. However, it only enables one to extract interdependences under linear assumptions. Statistical dependencies can be better assessed with the broader concept of generalised synchronisation (Rulkov *et al* 1995). By definition, generalised synchronisation (GS) exists between two dynamical systems X and Y when the state of the response system Y is a function of the state of the driving system X: Y=F(X). If F is continuous, two close points on the attractor of X should correspond to two close points on the attractor of Y. An important feature of GS is that synchronised time series can look very dissimilar. This is in contradistinction to other measures, which require some similarity between time courses to detect interactions. Let us illustrate differences between CC and GS with a toy example. Le X be the Henon map ($x_n = 1 - 1.4x_{n-1}^2 + 0.3x_{n-2}$) and Y be either a random permutation of X (representing the absence of coupling) or is given by $y_n = \sin(wx_n)$. The scalar w controls the degree of nonlinear coupling between Y and X: When w is sufficiently small, y_n is approximately equal to wx_n, i.e. a linear transform of x_n. Figure 7 shows performances of CC and GS in detecting the coupling between X and Y (see figure caption for further details). Clearly, GS is much more robust than CC. In principle GS encompasses all the dependences that can be measured with CC. However, GS is computationally more expensive and precludes the use classical statistics to infer the significance of the coupling. This usually calls for non-parametric approaches, through the use of surrogate data (*e.g.* Schreiber and Schmitz 2000).

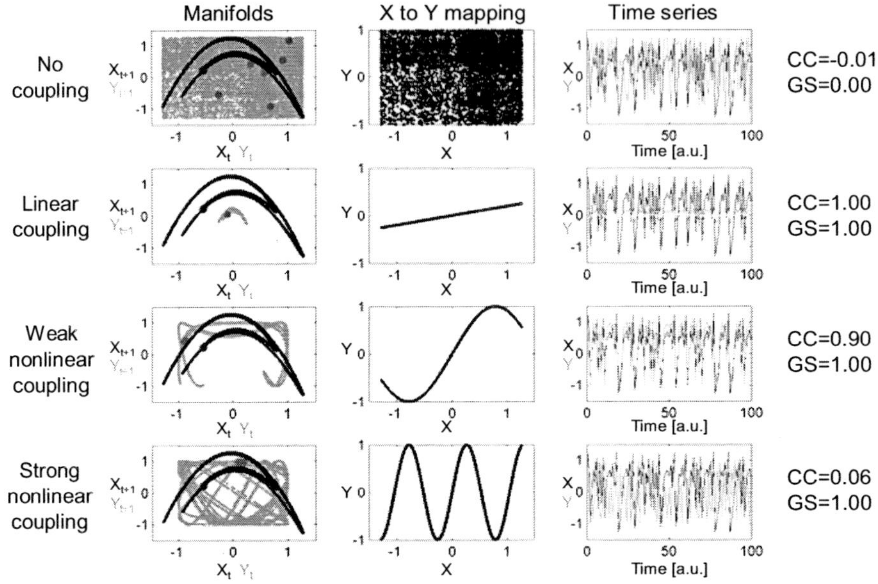

7

Figure 7.Cross-correlation (CC) and generalised synchronisation (GS) compared. *X* is the classical Henon map ($x_n = 1 - 1.4x_{n-1}^2 + 0.3x_{n-2}$), here using 10000 samples (the time-series shown in right column comprise the first one hundred samples,). This dynamical system can be portrayed with a one-return map (left column, black dots). *Y*, shown in grey, is a second time-series created from *X*. The cross-correlation (0<|CC|<1) and a measure of generalised synchronisation (0<GS<1) are used to quantify the interactions between *X* and *Y*. When there is no dependency (first line; where *Y* is simply a random permutation of the elements of *X*) no coupling is detected by either method. In the last three lines, *Y* is given by $y_n = \sin(wx_n)$. The scalar *w* controls the degree of nonlinearity in the coupling between Y and X (second column of the Figure): When *w* is sufficiently small, y_n is approximately equal to wx_n, *i.e.* a linear transform of x_n (second line: *w*=0.2). When *w* is increased (third line: *w*=2, fourth line: *w*=6), the relationship between *X* and *Y* becomes increasingly nonlinear, which results in a progressive deformation of the manifold of *Y*, compared to *X*. As shown by the values on the right, CC is very sensitive to this nonlinear effect, whereas GS is not because the local neighbourhood relationships within the attractor (red for X, blue for Y) are conserved by the nonlinear mapping. Clearly, GS is much more robust than CC in detecting interactions, especially when time-series do not resemble each other (see bottom right). In principle, GS encompasses all the dependences that can be measured with CC.

III.I.1 Effective Connectivity

Integration within a distributed system is usually better understood in terms of effective connectivity: *Effective connectivity* refers explicitly to *the influence that one neural system exerts over another*, either at a synaptic (*i.e.* synaptic efficacy) or population level. It has been proposed that "the [electrophysiological] notion of effective connectivity should be understood as the experiment- and time-dependent, simplest possible circuit diagram that would replicate the observed timing relationships between the recorded neurons" (Aertsen and Preißl 1991). This speaks to two important points: (i) Effective connectivity is dynamic, *i.e.* activity- and time-dependent and (ii) it depends upon a model of the interactions. The estimation procedures employed in functional neuroimaging can be divided into those based on (i) linear regression models (*e.g.* McIntosh and Gonzalez-Lima 1994) or (ii) nonlinear dynamic causal models.

There is a necessary link between functional integration and multivariate analyses because the latter are necessary to model interactions among brain regions. Multivariate approaches can be divided into those that are inferential in nature and those that are data-led or exploratory. We will first consider multivariate approaches that are generally based on functional connectivity or covariance patterns (and are generally exploratory) and then turn to models of effective connectivity (that allow for some form of inference).

III.2. Eigenimage Analysis and Related Approaches

In Friston *et al* (1993) we introduced voxel-based principal component analysis (PCA) of neuroimaging time-series to characterise distributed brain systems implicated in sensorimotor, perceptual or cognitive processes. These distributed systems are identified with principal components or *eigenimages* that correspond to spatial modes of coherent brain activity. This approach represents one of the simplest multivariate characterisations of functional neuroimaging time-series and falls into the class of exploratory analyses. Principal component or eigenimage analysis generally uses singular value decomposition (SVD) to identify a set of orthogonal spatial modes that capture the greatest amount of variance expressed over time. As such the ensuing modes embody the most prominent aspects of the variance-covariance structure of a given time-series. Noting that covariance among brain regions is equivalent to functional connectivity renders eigenimage analysis particularly interesting because it was among the first ways of addressing functional integration (*i.e.* connectivity) with neuroimaging data. Subsequently, eigenimage analysis has been elaborated in a number of ways. Notable among these is canonical variate analysis (CVA) and multidimensional scaling (Friston et al 1996b, 1996c). Canonical variate analysis was introduced in the context of ManCova (multiple analysis of covariance) and uses the generalised eigenvector solution to maximise the variance that can be explained by some explanatory variables relative to error. CVA can be thought of as an extension of eigenimage analysis that refers explicitly to some explanatory variables and allows for statistical inference.

In fMRI, eigenimage analysis (*e.g.* Sychra *et al* 1994) is generally used as an exploratory device to characterise coherent brain activity. These variance components may, or may not be, related to experimental design. For example, endogenous coherent dynamics have been observed in the motor system at very low frequencies (Biswal *et al* 1995). Despite its exploratory power, eigenimage analysis is fundamentally limited for two reasons. Firstly, it offers only a linear decomposition of any set of neurophysiological measurements and second, the particular set of eigenimages or spatial modes obtained is uniquely determined by constraints that are biologically implausible. These aspects of PCA confer inherent limitations on the interpretability and usefulness of eigenimage analysis of biological time-series and have motivated the exploration of nonlinear PCA and neural network approaches.

Two other important approaches deserve mention here. The first is independent component analysis (ICA). ICA uses entropy maximisation to find, using iterative schemes, spatial modes or their dynamics that are approximately *independent*. This is a stronger requirement than *orthogonality* in PCA and involves removing high order correlations among the modes (or dynamics). It was first used to analyse EEG signals (for a review see Makeig *et al* 2004) and has proved very useful in disambiguating patterns of activation on the scalp and, in particular, in identifying artefacts (*e.g.* eye movements, ballisto-cardiogram, *etc.*). It was introduced, initially, to fMRI as *spatial* ICA (McKeown *et al* 1998) in which the independence constraint was applied to the modes (with no constraints on their temporal expression). More recent approaches in fMRI use, by analogy with magneto- and electrophysiological time-series analysis, *temporal* ICA where the dynamics are enforced to be independent. This requires an initial dimension reduction (usually using conventional eigenimage analysis). Finally, there has been an interest in cluster analysis (Baumgartner et al 1997). Conceptually, this can be related to eigenimage analysis through multidimensional scaling and principal co-ordinate analysis.

All these approaches are interesting, but tell one nothing about how the brain works or allow one to ask specific questions. Simply demonstrating statistical dependencies among regional brain responses (*i.e.* demonstrating functional connectivity) does not address how these responses were caused. To address this one needs explicit models of integration or more precisely, effective connectivity.

III.3. Structural Equation Modelling

Established methods for estimating effective connectivity from neurophysiological time-series include structural equation modelling and models based on multivariate auto-regressive processes (McIntosh and Gonzalez-Lima 1994; Büchel and Friston 1997; Harrison *et al* 2003). In these models, which are often linear, there is no designed perturbation and the inputs are treated as unknown and stochastic. Furthermore, the inputs are usually assumed to express themselves instantaneously such that, at the point of observation, the change in states will be zero. From Eq(4), assuming a linear model and that the states are directly observed, we have

$$
\begin{aligned}
\dot{x}(t) &= f(x,u) \\
&= Ax + Cu \\
&= 0 \quad . \\
x &= -A^{-1}Cu \\
y &= x
\end{aligned}
\tag{7}
$$

This is the regression equation used in SEM where $A = A' - I$ and A' contains the off-diagonal connections among regions. The key point here is that A is estimated by assuming u is some random innovation with known covariance. This is not really tenable for designed experiments when u represents carefully structured experimental inputs. Although SEM and related autoregressive techniques are useful for establishing dependence among regional responses, they are not surrogates for informed causal models based on the underlying dynamics of these responses.

III.4. Dynamic Causal Modelling

The central idea, behind dynamic causal modelling (DCM), is to treat the brain as a deterministic nonlinear dynamic system that is subject to inputs and produces outputs. Effective connectivity is parameterised in terms of coupling among unobserved brain states (*e.g.* neuronal activity in different regions). A key aspect of DCM is that interactions are modelled among neuronal populations, at a cortical level, using neuroimaging time series (EEG or fMRI). The aim of these dynamic causal models (DCMs) is to estimate, and make inferences about, the coupling among brain areas and how that coupling is influenced by changes in experimental context (*e.g.* time or cognitive set). The basic idea is to construct a reasonably realistic neuronal model of interacting cortical regions or nodes. This model is then supplemented with a forward model of how neuronal or synaptic activity translates into a measured response. This enables the parameters of the neuronal model (*i.e.* effective connectivity) to be estimated from observed data.

Intuitively, the DCM approach regards an experiment as a designed perturbation of neuronal dynamics that are promulgated and distributed throughout a system of coupled anatomical nodes to change region-specific neuronal activity. These changes engender, through a measurement-specific forward model, responses that are used to identify the architecture and time constants of the system at a neuronal level. This represents a departure from conventional approaches (*e.g.* structural equation modelling and autoregression models), in which one assumes the observed responses are driven by endogenous or intrinsic noise (*i.e.* innovations). In contradistinction, dynamic causal models assume the responses are driven by designed changes in inputs. An important conceptual aspect of dynamic causal models pertains to how the experimental inputs enter the model and cause neuronal responses. Experimental variables can elicit responses in one of two ways. First, through direct influences on specific anatomical nodes; this would be appropriate, for example, in modelling sensory evoked responses in early visual cortices. The second class of input exerts its effect vicariously, through a modulation of the coupling among nodes. These sorts of experimental variables would normally be more enduring, for example attention to a particular attribute or the maintenance of some perceptual set.

III.4.1 Dynamic Causal Modelling with Bilinear Models

The distinction between different sorts of input is seen most clearly in relation to particular forms of causal models used for estimation, for example the bilinear approximation

$$\dot{x} = f(x,u,\theta) \\ = Ax + uBx + Cu \\ y = g(x) + \varepsilon$$

$$A = \frac{\partial f}{\partial x} \quad B = \frac{\partial^2 f}{\partial x \partial u} \quad C = \frac{\partial f}{\partial u} \tag{8}$$

This is an approximation to any model of how changes in neuronal activity in one region x_i are caused by activity in the other regions. This is a particularly useful model for fMRI where one does not have enough information to model neuronal processes in great detail. Here the output function $g(x)$ embodies a hemodynamic model, linking neuronal activity to BOLD, for each region (*e.g.* that in Figure 6). The matrix A represents the connectivity among the regions in the absence of input u. Effective connectivity is the influence that one neuronal system exerts over another in terms of inducing a response $\partial\dot{x}/\partial x$. This latent connectivity can be thought of as the coupling in the absence of experimental perturbations. The matrix B is effectively the change in latent coupling, induced by the input. It encodes the input-sensitive changes in A or, equivalently, the modulation of effective connectivity by experimental manipulations. Because B is a second-order derivative it is referred to as *bilinear*. Finally, the matrix C embodies the extrinsic influences of inputs on neuronal activity. The parameters $\theta = \{A, B, C\}$ are the connectivity or coupling matrices that we wish to identify and define the functional architecture and interactions among brain regions at a neuronal level. Because Eq(8) has exactly the same form as Eq(4) we can express it as a GLM and estimate the parameters using EM in the usual way (see Friston *et al* 2003). Generally estimation in the context of highly parameterised models like DCMs requires constraints in the form of priors. These priors enable conditional inference about the connectivity estimates. The sorts of questions that can be addressed with DCMs for fMRI are now illustrated by looking at how attentional modulation might be mediated in sensory processing hierarchies in the brain.

III.4.2. DCM and Attentional Modulation as Measured with fMRI

It has been established that the superior posterior parietal cortex (SPC) exerts a modulatory role on V5 responses using Volterra-based regression models (Friston and Büchel 2000) and that the inferior frontal gyrus (IFG) exerts a similar influence on SPC using structural equation modelling (Büchel and Friston 1997). The example here shows that DCM leads to the same conclusions but starting from a completely different construct. The experimental paradigm and data acquisition parameters are described in the legend to Figure 8. This Figure also shows the location of the regions that entered into the DCM. These regions were based on maxima from conventional SPMs testing for the effects of photic stimulation, motion and attention. Regional time courses were taken as the first eigenvariate

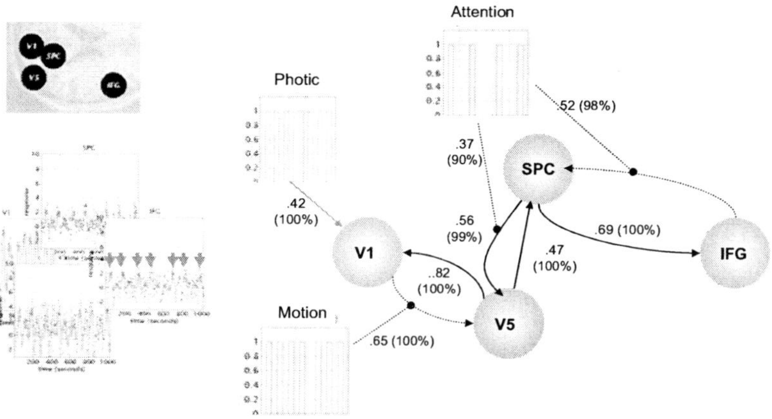

Figure 8.Results of an fMRI DCM analysis of attention to visual motion. Right panel: Functional architecture based upon the conditional estimates shown alongside their connections, with the percent confidence that they exceeded threshold in brackets. The most interesting aspects of this architecture involve the role of motion and attention in exerting bilinear effects. Critically, the influence of motion is to enable connections from V1 to the motion-sensitive area V5. The influence of attention is to enable backward connections from the inferior frontal gyrus (IFG) to the superior parietal cortex (SPC). Furthermore, attention increases the influence of SPC on V5. Dotted arrows connecting regions represent significant bilinear effects in the absence of a significant intrinsic coupling. Left Panel: Fitted responses based upon the conditional estimates and the adjusted data are shown for each region in the DCM. The insert (upper left) shows the location of the regions. Subjects were studied with fMRI under identical stimulus conditions (visual motion subtended by radially moving dots) whilst manipulating the attentional component of the task (detection of velocity changes). The data were acquired from a normal subject at 2 Tesla using a Magnetom VISION (Siemens, Erlangen) whole body MRI system, equipped with a head volume coil. Contiguous multi-slice T2*-weighted fMRI images were obtained with a gradient echo-planar sequence (TE = 40ms, TR = 3.22 seconds, matrix size = 64x64x32, voxel size 3x3x3mm). Each subject had 4 consecutive 100-scan sessions comprising a series of 10-scan blocks under 5 different conditions D F A F N F A F N S. The first condition (D) was a dummy condition to allow for magnetic saturation effects. F (Fixation) corresponds to a low-level baseline where the subjects viewed a fixation point at the centre of a screen. In condition A (Attention) subjects viewed 250 dots moving radially from the centre at 4.7 degrees per second and were asked to detect changes in radial velocity. In condition N (No attention) the subjects were asked simply to view the moving dots. In condition S (Stationary) subjects viewed stationary dots. The order of A and N was swapped for the last two sessions. In all conditions, subjects fixated the centre of the screen. During scanning there were no speed changes. No overt response was required in any condition.

of 8mm spherical volumes of interest centred on the maxima shown in the figure. The inputs, in this example, comprise one sensory perturbation and two contextual inputs. The sensory input was simply the presence of photic stimulation and the first contextual one was presence of motion in the visual field. The second contextual input, encoding attentional set, was unity during attention to speed changes and zero otherwise. The outputs corresponded to the four regional eigenvariates in (Figure 8, left panel). The intrinsic connections were constrained to conform to a hierarchical pattern in which each area was reciprocally connected to its supraordinate area. Photic stimulation entered at, and only at, V1. The effect of motion in the visual field was modelled as a bilinear modulation of the V1 to V5 connectivity and attention was allowed to modulate the backward connections from IFG and SPC.

The results of the DCM are shown in Figure 8 (right panel). Of primary interest here is the modulatory effect of attention that is expressed in terms of the bilinear coupling parameters for this input. As expected, we can be highly confident that attention modulates the backward connections from IFG to SPC and from SPC to V5. Indeed, the influences of IFG on SPC are negligible in the absence of attention (dotted connection). It is important to note that the only way that attention can affect brain responses was through this bilinear effect. Attention-related responses are seen throughout the system (attention epochs are marked with arrows in the plot of IFG responses in Figure 8).

This attentional modulation is accounted for, sufficiently, by changing just two connections. This change is, presumably, instantiated by instructional set at the beginning of each epoch.

The second thing, this analysis illustrates, is how functional segregation is modelled in DCM. Here one can regard V1 as 'segregating' motion from other visual information and distributing it to the motion-sensitive area V5. This segregation is modelled as a bilinear 'enabling' of V1 to V5 connections when, and only when, motion is present. Note that in the absence of motion the intrinsic V1 to V5 connection was trivially small (in fact the estimate was -0.04). The key advantage of entering motion through a bilinear effect, as opposed to a direct effect on V5, is that we can finesse the inference that V5 shows motion-selective responses with the assertion that these responses are mediated by afferents from V1. The two bilinear effects above represent two important aspects of functional integration that DCM is able to characterise.

III.4.3. Dynamic Causal Modelling with Neural Mass Models and EEG

In the previous section the bilinear approximation to any DCM was illustrated through its use with fMRI to study attentional modulation. The parameters of bilinear DCMs include first-order effective connectivity A and its experimentally induced changes B. Although the bilinear approximation is useful it is not possible to model nonlinear interactions among neuronal subpopulations explicitly. We conclude this review with a DCM that embraces a number of neurobiological facts and takes us much closer to a mechanistic understanding of how brain responses are generated. This example concerns responses measured with ERPs. ERPs have been used for decades as electrophysiological correlates of perceptual and cognitive operations. However, the exact neurobiological mechanisms underlying their generation are largely unknown. In this section we use, as far as possible, neuronally plausible models to understand event-related responses. These models show that changes in connectivity are sufficient to explain certain ERP components.

Specifically we will look at the mismatch negativity (MMN) (Näätänen 2003): The MMN is a negative component of the ERP to any discriminative change in some repetitive aspect of auditory stimulation. It is thought that the genesis of the MMN is based on the presence of a memory trace, formed by preceding stimuli, which lasts about 10 seconds. The generators of the MMN are usually found bilaterally, in the auditory and frontal cortex. If the unexpected nature of rare stimuli depends on the perceptual learning of frequent stimuli, then the MMN may be due to plastic changes in connectivity that mediate this learning. In particular, we will show that the MMN can be explained by a learning-related difference in top-down connections between frontal and primary auditory cortices. This final example shows that recent advances in the modelling of evoked responses now afford measures of connectivity among cortical sources that can be used to revisit classical phenomena in a more mechanistic way.

III.4.4. Hierarchical Neural Mass Models

The minimal DCM for ERPs, we have developed (David *et al*, in revision), uses the connectivity rules described in Felleman and Van Essen (1991) to assemble a network of coupled sources. These rules are based on a partitioning of the cortical sheet into supra-, infra-granular layers and granular layer (layer 4). Bottom-up or forward connections originate in agranular layers and terminate in layer 4. Top-down or backward connections target agranular layers. Lateral connections originate in agranular layers and target all layers. These long-range or extrinsic cortico-cortical connections are excitatory and arise from pyramidal cells.

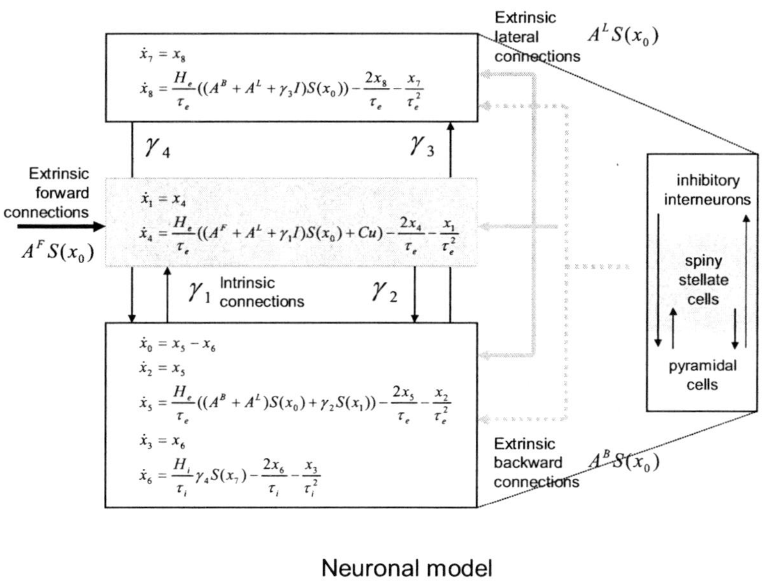

Figure 9. Schematic of the DCM used to model electrical responses. This schematic shows the state equation describing the dynamics of sources or regions. Each source is modelled with three subpopulations (pyramidal, spiny stellate and inhibitory interneurons) as described in Jansen and Rit (1995) and David and Friston (2003). These have been assigned to granular and agranular cortical layers and receive forward, backward and lateral connections according to specific laminar connectivity patterns.

Each region or source is modelled using a neural mass model described in Jansen and Rit (1995). This model emulates the activity of a cortical area using three neuronal subpopulations, assigned to granular and agranular layers. A population of excitatory pyramidal (output) cells receives inputs from inhibitory and excitatory populations of interneurons, via intrinsic connections (intrinsic connections are confined to the cortical sheet). Within this model, excitatory interneurons can be regarded as spiny stellate cells found predominantly in layer 4 and in receipt of forward connections. Excitatory pyramidal cells and inhibitory interneurons will be considered to occupy agranular layers and receive backward and lateral inputs (Figure 9).

To model event-related responses, the network receives inputs via input connections. These connections are exactly the same as forward connections and deliver inputs u to the spiny stellate cells in layer 4. In the present context, inputs u model subcortical auditory inputs. The vector C controls the influence of the input on each source. The lower, upper and leading diagonal matrices A^F, A^B, A^L encode forward, backward and lateral connections respectively. The DCM here is specified in terms of the state equations shown in Figure 9 and a linear output equation

$$
\begin{aligned}
\dot{x} &= f(x,u,\theta) \\
y &= Lx_0 + \varepsilon
\end{aligned}
\tag{9}
$$

where x_0 represents the transmembrane potential of pyramidal cells and L is a lead field matrix coupling electrical sources to the EEG channels. This should be compared to the DCM above for hemodynamics. Here the equations governing the evolution of neuronal states are much more complicated and realistic, as opposed to the bilinear approximation in Eq(8). Conversely, the output equation is a simple linearity, as opposed to the nonlinear observer used for fMRI. As an example, the state equation for the inhibitory subpopulation is[3]

$$
\begin{aligned}
\dot{x}_7 &= x_8 \\
\dot{x}_8 &= \frac{H_e}{\tau_e}((A^B + A^L + \gamma_3 I)S(x_0)) - \frac{2x_8}{\tau_e} - \frac{x_7}{\tau_e^2}.
\end{aligned}
\tag{10}
$$

Within each subpopulation, the evolution of neuronal states rests on two operators (Figure 5). The first transforms the average density of pre-synaptic inputs into the average postsynaptic membrane potential. This is modelled by a linear transformation with excitatory (e) and inhibitory (i) kernels parameterised by $H_{e,i}$ and $\tau_{e,i}$. $H_{e,i}$ control the maximum post-synaptic potential and $\tau_{e,i}$ represent a lumped rate constant. The second operator S transforms the average potential of each subpopulation into an average firing rate. This is assumed to be instantaneous and is a sigmoid function. Interactions, among the subpopulations, depend on constants $\gamma_{1,2,3,4}$, which control the strength of intrinsic connections and reflect the total number of synapses expressed by each subpopulation. In Eq(10), the top line expresses the rate of change of voltage as a function of current. The

[3] Propagation delays on the extrinsic connections have been omitted for clarity here and in Figure 9.

second line specifies how current changes as a function of voltage, current and pre-synaptic input from extrinsic and intrinsic sources. Having specified the DCM one can estimate the coupling parameters from empirical data using EM as described above.

III.4.5. DCM and Perceptual Learning

The example shown in Figure 10 is an attempt to model the MMN in terms of changes in backward connections among cortical sources representing the primary auditory and orbitofrontal cortex. In this example, a preliminary classical source localisation was performed to contain, anatomically, the DCM. Cortical sources were localized symmetrically along the medial part of the upper bank of the Sylvian fissure, in the right middle temporal gyrus, left medial and posterior cingulate, and bilateral orbitofrontal cortex (Figure 10). These locations are in good agreement with the literature: Sources along the upper bank of the Sylvian fissure can be regarded as early auditory cortices, although they are generally located in the lower bank of the Sylvian fissure (Heschl's gyrus). Primary auditory cortices have major inter-hemispheric connections through the corpus callosum. In addition, these areas project to temporal and frontal lobes following different streams (Kaas and Hackett 2000; Romanski et al 1999). Finally, cingulate activations are often found in relation to oddball tasks, either auditory or visual (Linden et al 1999). Using prior knowledge about the connectivity and functional organization of the auditory system, we designed the following DCM (Figure 10): an extrinsic (thalamic) input entered bilaterally to primary auditory areas (A1), which were connected to ipsilateral orbitofrontal cortex (OFC). In the right hemisphere, an indirect forward pathway was also specified from A1 to OFC through the superior temporal gyrus (STG). All these connections were reciprocal. At the highest level in the hierarchy, OFC and left posterior cingulate cortex (PCC) were laterally and reciprocally connected.

To illustrate the potential of the DCM approach, we test here a functional hypothesis within the context of the above network. If we posit that modulation of the ERP (comparing frequent and rare events) is due to learning-related changes in connectivity, we have to specify the connections that can change. The characteristics of the MMN suggest that it could arise from increases (or decreases) in backward connections from OFC to A1. We allowed these connections to differ between rare and frequent ERPs. The results are shown in Figure 10 and reveal that such connectivity changes are indeed sufficient to generate a MMN (here in the PCC). If this model is a sufficient approximation to the real sources, these changes are a non-invasive measure of plasticity, mediating perceptual learning, in the human brain. Finally, note that several functional hypotheses can be tested, for instance by allowing different patterns of connectivity changes. The ensuing models can be then compared to determine the most likely model, using Bayesian model comparison (Penny *et al* 2004).

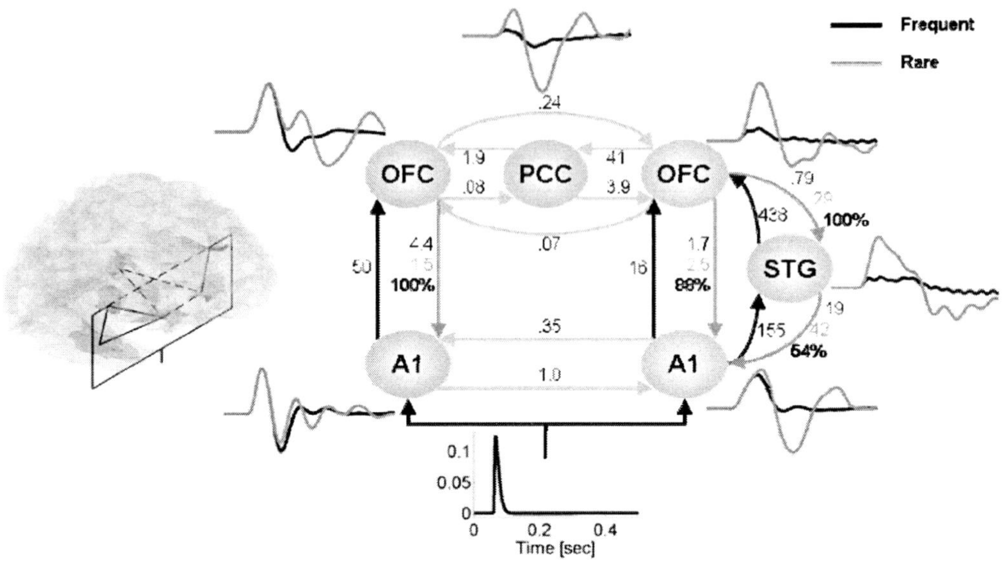

Figure 10. Summary of a DCM of ERPs, elicited during an auditory oddball paradigm, employing rare and frequent pure tones. Left: Transparent view of the cortical mesh from the top-right, showing the spatial configuration of the DCM: A bilateral extrinsic input acts on primary auditory cortices (A1) which are laterally interconnected through the corpus callosum (broken lines) and project to orbitofrontal regions (OFC) with reciprocal connections (solid line). In the right hemisphere, an indirect pathway was specified via a relay in the superior temporal gyrus (STS). At the highest level in the hierarchy, orbitofrontal and left posterior cingulate (PCC) cortices were assumed to be laterally and reciprocally connected. Right: Connectivity parameters and estimated time series after estimation of DCM parameters. This DCM tests for a modulation of backward connections between A1 and OFC by the sensory learning of frequent stimuli, relative to rare. The estimated coupling coefficients are shown by each connection. We also indicate the probability of connection strength change being greater than zero. These posterior inferences were based on the conditional variance of the contrast comparing the connections strengths directly. Predicted neuronal responses are shown alongside each region (black: frequent events, grey: rare events).
Auditory stimuli, 1000 or 2000 Hz tones with 5 ms rise and fall times and 80 ms duration, were presented binaurally. The tones were presented for 15 minutes, every 2 seconds in a pseudo-random sequence with 2000-Hz tones occurring 20% of the time and 1000-Hz tones occurring 80% of the time. The subject was instructed to keep a mental record of the number of 2000-Hz tones (non-frequent target tones). Data were acquired using 128 EEG electrodes with 1000 Hz sampling frequency. Before averaging, data were referenced to mean earlobe activity and band-pass filtered between 1 and 30 Hz. Trials showing ocular artefacts and bad channels were removed from further analysis.

IV. Conclusion

In this article we have reviewed some key models that underpin time-series analysis in neuroimaging and have touched briefly on ways of assessing specialisation and integration in the brain. These models can be regarded as a succession of modelling endeavours, drawing more and more on our understanding of how brain-imaging signals are generated, both in terms of biophysics and the underlying neuronal interactions. We have seen how hierarchical linear observation models encode the treatment effects elicited by experimental design.

General linear models based on convolution models imply an underlying dynamic input-state-output system. The form of these systems can be used to constrain convolution models and explore some of their simpler nonlinear properties. By creating observation models based on explicit forward models of neuronal interactions, one can start to model and assess interactions among distributed cortical areas and make inferences about coupling at the neuronal level. The next years will probably see an increasing realism in the dynamic causal models introduced above (see Horwitz *et al* 2001). There are already attempts to use plausible models of neuronal ensembles to estimate network parameters of evoked responses in EEG. These endeavours are likely to encompass fMRI signals in the near future enabling the conjoint modelling, or fusion, of different modalities and the marriage of computational neuroscience with the modelling of brain responses.

Acknowledgements

The Wellcome Trust funded this work.

References

Adler RJ. (1981). In "*The geometry of random fields*". Wiley New York

Aertsen A and Preißl H. (1991). Dynamics of activity and connectivity in physiological neuronal Networks. In *Non Linear Dynamics and Neuronal Networks*. Ed Schuster HG VCH publishers Inc. New York NY USA p281-302.

Ashburner J and Friston KJ. (2000). Voxel-based morphometry - the methods. *NeuroImage*. 11:805-21.

Bandettini PA, Jesmanowicz A, Wong EC and Hyde JS. (1993) Processing strategies for time course data sets in functional MRI of the human brain. *Mag. Res. Med.* 30:161-173.

Baumgartner R, Scarth G, Teichtmeister C, Somorjai R and Moser E. (1997). Fuzzy clustering of gradient-echo functional MRI in the human visual cortex Part 1: reproducibility. *J. Mag. Res. Imaging* 7:1094-1101.

Bendat JS. (1990). *Nonlinear System Analysis and Identification from Random Data*. John Wiley and Sons, New York USA

Berry DA and Hochberg Y. (1999). Bayesian perspectives on multiple comparisons. *J. Statistical Planning and Inference*. 82:215-227

Biswal B, Yetkin FZ, Haughton VM and Hyde JS. (1995). Functional connectivity in the motor cortex of resting human brain using echo-planar MRI. *Mag. Res. Med.* 34:537-541

Boynton GM, Engel SA, Glover GH and Heeger DJ. (1996). Linear systems analysis of functional magnetic resonance imaging in human V1. *J Neurosci.* 16:4207-4221.

Brookes MJ, Gibson AM, Hall SD, Furlong PL, Barnes GR, Hillebrand A, Singh KD, Holliday IE, Francis ST and Morris PG. (2004). A general linear model for MEG beamformer imaging. *Neuroimage*. 23(3):936-946.

Büchel C, Wise RJS, Mummery CJ, Poline J-B, and Friston KJ. (1996). Nonlinear regression in parametric activation studies. *NeuroImage* 4:60-66.

Büchel C and Friston KJ. (1997). Modulation of connectivity in visual pathways by attention: Cortical interactions evaluated with structural equation modelling and fMRI. *Cerebral Cortex* 7:768-778.

Buckner R, Bandettini P, O'Craven K, Savoy R, Petersen S, Raichle M and Rosen B. (1996). Detection of cortical activation during averaged single trials of a cognitive task using functional magnetic resonance imaging. *Proc. Natl. Acad. Sci. USA* 93:14878-14883.

Burock MA, Buckner RL, Woldorff MG, Rosen BR and Dale AM. (1998). Randomized Event-Related Experimental Designs Allow for Extremely Rapid Presentation Rates Using Functional MRI. *NeuroReport* 9:3735-3739.

Buxton RB and Frank LR. (1997). A model for the coupling between cerebral blood flow and oxygen metabolism during neural stimulation. *J. Cereb. Blood. Flow Metab.* 17:64-72.

Dale A and Buckner R. (1997). Selective averaging of rapidly presented individual trials using fMRI. *Hum. Brain Mapp.* 5:329-340.

David O, Friston KJ. (2003) A neural mass model for MEG/EEG: coupling and neuronal dynamics. *NeuroImage* 20:1743-55.

David O, Cosmelli D, Friston KJ. (2004a) Evaluation of different measures of functional connectivity using a neural mass model. *NeuroImage* 21(2):659-673.

David O, Harrison L, Kilner J, Penny W, and Friston KJ. (2004b) Studying effective connectivity with a neural mass model of evoked MEG/EEG responses. *Proceedings of the 14th international conference on biomagnetism BIOMAG 2004,* p. 135-138. Eds: Halgren E, Ahlfors S, Hämäläinen M and Cohen D. Boston, Ma., USA.

David O, Harisson L, and Friston KJ (in revision). Modelling event-related responses in the brain. NeuroImage.

Dempster AP, Laird NM and Rubin DR (1977). Maximum likelihood from incomplete data via the EM algorithm. *J. Roy. Stat. Soc. Series B* 39:1-38.

Durka PJ (2003). From wavelets to adaptive approximations: time-frequency parametrization of EEG. *Biomed Eng Online.* 2(1):1.

Fliess M, Lamnabhi M and Lamnabhi-Lagarrigue F (1983). An algebraic approach to nonlinear functional expansions. *IEEE Trans. Circuits Syst.* 30:554-570.

Felleman DJ, Van Essen DC. (1992). Distributed hierarchical processing in the primate cerebral cortex. *Cereb. Cortex* 1:1-47.

Freeman WJ. (1978). Models of the dynamics of neural populations. *Electroencephalogr. Clin. Neurophysiol. [Suppl]* 34: 9-18.

Friston KJ, Frith CD, Liddle PF and Frackowiak RSJ. (1991). Comparing functional (PET) images: the assessment of significant change. *J. Cereb. Blood Flow Metab.* 11:690-699.

Friston KJ, Frith CD, Passingham RE, Liddle PF and Frackowiak RSJ. (1992). Motor practice and neurophysiological adaptation in the cerebellum: A positron tomography study. *Proc. Roy. Soc. Lon. Series B* 248:223-228.

Friston KJ, Frith CD, Liddle PF and Frackowiak RSJ. (1993). Functional Connectivity: The principal component analysis of large data sets. *J Cereb. Blood Flow Metab.* 13:5-14.

Friston KJ, Jezzard PJ and Turner R. (1994). Analysis of functional MRI time-*series Hum. Brain Mapp.* 1:153-171.

Friston KJ, Holmes AP, Worsley KJ, Poline JB, Frith CD and Frackowiak RSJ. (1995a). Statistical Parametric Maps in functional imaging: A general linear approach *Hum. Brain Mapp.* 2:189-210.

Friston KJ, Frith CD, Turner R and Frackowiak RSJ. (1995b). Characterising evoked hemodynamics with fMRI. *NeuroImage* 2:157-165.

Friston KJ, Price CJ, Fletcher P, Moore C, Frackowiak RSJ and Dolan RJ. (1996a). The trouble with cognitive subtraction. *NeuroImage* 4:97-104.

Friston KJ, Poline J-B, Holmes AP, Frith CD and Frackowiak RSJ. (1996b). A multivariate analysis of PET activation studies. *Hum. Brain Mapp.* 4:140-151.

Friston KJ, Frith CD, Fletcher P, Liddle PF and Frackowiak RSJ. (1996c). Functional topography: multidimensional scaling and functional connectivity in the brain. *Cerebral Cortex* 6:156-164.

Friston KJ, Mechelli A, Turner R, Price CJ. (2000). Nonlinear responses in fMRI: the Balloon model, Volterra kernels, and other hemodynamics. *NeuroImage.* 12:466-77.

Friston KJ and Büchel C. (2000). Attentional modulation of effective connectivity from V2 to V5/MT in humans. *Proc Natl Acad Sci U S A.* 97:7591-6.

Friston KJ, Harrison L, Penny W. (2003) Dynamic causal modelling. *NeuroImage* 19:1273-302.

Gerstein GL and Perkel DH. (1969). Simultaneously recorded trains of action potentials: Analysis and functional interpretation. *Science* 164:828-830.

Goltz F. (1881). In "*Transactions of the 7th international medical congress*" (W MacCormac Ed) Vol. I JW Kolkmann London. p218-228.

Grafton S, Mazziotta J, Presty S, Friston KJ, Frackowiak RSJ and Phelps M. (1992). Functional anatomy of human procedural learning determined with regional cerebral blood flow and PET. *J Neurosci.* 12:2542-2548.

Harrison LM, Penny W. and Friston KJ. (2003). Multivariate autoregressive modelling of fMRI time series. *NeuroImage.* 19:1477-91.

Hoge RD, Atkinson J, Gill B, Crelier GR, Marrett S and Pike GB. (1999). Linear coupling between cerebral blood flow and oxygen consumption in activated human cortex. *Proc. Natl. Acad. Sci.* 96:9403-9408.

Holmes A and Ford I. (1993). A Bayesian approach to significance testing for statistic images from PET. In Quantification of Brain function, Tracer kinetics and Image analysis in brain PET. Eds. K. Uemura, NA. Lassen, T. Jones and I. Kanno. *Excerpta Medica, Int. Cong.* Series No. 1030: 521-534.

Horwitz B, Friston KJ and Taylor JG. (2001). Neural modelling and functional brain imaging: an overview. *Neural Networks* 13:829-846.

Jansen BH, Rit VG. (1995). Electroencephalogram and visual evoked potential generation in a mathematical model of coupled cortical columns. *Biol. Cybern* 73:357-366.

Kaas JH and Hackett TA. (2000). Subdivisions of auditory cortex and processing streams in primates. Proc. Natl. Acad. Sci. USA 97:11793-11799.

Kiebel SJ, Friston KJ. (2004a). Statistical parametric mapping for event-related potentials (I): Generic considerations. *NeuroImage* 22:492-502.

Kiebel SJ, Friston KJ. (2004b). Statistical parametric mapping for event-related potentials (II): A hierarchical temporal model. *NeuroImage* 22:503-520.

Kilner JM, Kiebel SJ, Friston KJ. (in press). Applications of random field theory to electrophysiology. *Neuroscience letters.*

Lange N and Zeger SL. (1997). Non-linear Fourier time series analysis for human brain mapping by functional magnetic resonance imaging (with discussion) J *Roy. Stat. Soc. Ser. C.* 46:1-29.

Lopes da Silva FH, Hoeks A, Smits H, and Zetterberg LH. 1974. Model of brain rhythmic activity. The alpha-rhythm of the thalamus. *Kybernetik.* 15: 27-37.

Lueck CJ, Zeki S, Friston KJ, Deiber MP, Cope NO et al (1989). The colour centre in the cerebral cortex of man. *Nature* 340:386-389.

Makeig S (1993). Auditory event-related dynamics of the EEG spectrum and effects of exposure to tones. *Electroencephalogr Clin Neurophysiol.* 86(4):283-93.

Makeig S, Debener S, Onton J and Delorme A (2004). Mining event-related brain dynamics. *Trends Cog. Sci.* 8(5):204:210.

Mandeville JB, Marota JJ, Ayata C, Zararchuk G, Moskowitz MA, B Rosen B, and Weisskoff RM. (1999). Evidence of a cerebrovascular postarteriole Windkessel with delayed compliance. *J. Cereb. Blood Flow Metab.* 19:679-689.

McIntosh AR and Gonzalez-Lima F. (1994). Structural equation modelling and its application to network analysis in functional brain imaging. *Hum. Brain Mapp.* 2:2-22.

McKeown M, Jung T-P, Makeig S, Brown G, Kinderman S, Lee T-W and Sejnowski T. (1998). Spatially independent activity patterns in functional MRI data during the Stroop colour naming task. *Proc. Natl. Acad. Sci.* 95:803-810.

Näätänen R. (2003). Mismatch negativity: clinical research and possible applications. *Int. J. Psychophysiol.* 48:179:188.

Penny W, Stephan K, Mechelli A, and Friston K. (2004). Comparing dynamic causal models. *NeuroImage* 22(3):1157-1172.

Petersen SE, Fox PT, Posner MI, Mintun M and Raichle ME. (1989). Positron emission tomographic studies of the processing of single words. *J Cog. Neurosci.* 1:153-170.

Pikovsky,A., Rosenblum,M., and Kurths,J. (2001). *Synchronization. A universal concept in nonlinear sciences.* Cambridge University Press, Cambridge.

Price CJ, Wise RJS, Ramsay S, Friston KJ, Howard D, et al. (1992). Regional response differences within the human auditory cortex when listening to words. *Neurosci. Lett.* 146:179-182.

Price CJ and Friston KJ. (1997). Cognitive Conjunction: A new approach to brain activation experiments. *NeuroImage* 5:261-270.

Quian Quiroga R, Kraskov A, Kreuz T, and Grassberger P. (2002). Performance of different synchronization measures in real data: a case study on electroencephalographic signals. *Phys. Rev. E* 65: 041903.

Romanski LM, Tian B, Fritz J, Mishkin M, Goldman-Rakic PS, and Rauschecker JP (1999). Dual streams of auditory afferents target multiple domains in the primate prefrontal cortex. Nat Neurosci 2:1131-1136.

Rulkov NF, Sushchik MM, Tsimring LS, and Abarbanel HD. (1995). Generalized synchronization of chaos in directionally coupled chaotic systems. *Phys. Rev. E* 51: 980-994.

Schreiber T and Schmitz A. (2000). Surrogate time series. *Physica D* 142:346-382.

Sychra JJ, Bandettini PA, Bhattacharya N and Lin Q. (1994). Synthetic images by subspace transforms I Principal component images and related filters. *Med. Physics* 21:193-201.

Talairach P and Tournoux J. (1988). "*A Stereotactic coplanar atlas of the human brain*" Stuttgart Thieme.

Tallon-Baudry C, Bertrand O, Delpuech C and Pernier J. (1996). Stimulus specificity of phase-locked and non-phase-locked 40 Hz visual responses in human. *J Neurosci.* 16(13):4240-4249.

Tass P, Rosenblum M, Weule J, Kurths J, Pikovsky A, Volkmann J, Schnitzler A and Freund H-J. (1998). Detection of n:m phase locking from noisy data: Application to magnetoencephalography. *Phys Rev Lett.* 81:3291–3294.

Wilson HR, Cowan JD. (1972). Excitatory and inhibitory interactions in localized populations of model neurons. *Biophys.J.* 12:1-24.

Worsley KJ, Evans AC, Marrett S and Neelin P. (1992). A three-dimensional statistical analysis for rCBF activation studies in human brain. *J Cereb. Blood Flow Metab.* 12:900-918.

Worsley KJ, Marrett S, Neelin P, Vandal AC, Friston KJ and Evans AC. (1996). A unified statistical approach or determining significant signals in images of cerebral activation. *Hum. Brain Mapp.* 4:58-73.

In: Progress in Brain Mapping Research
Editor: F. J. Chen, pp. 159-175
ISBN 1-59454-580-4

Chapter 4

Positron Emission Tomography Studies in Parkinson's Disease: Recent Advances

Yen F. Tai and Paola Piccini*
MRC Clinical Sciences Centre and Division of Neuroscience, Faculty of Medicine, Imperial College London, Hammersmith Hospital, London, United Kingdom

Abstract

Positron emission tomography (PET) enables human brain functions to be investigated *in vivo*. The technique has greatly enhanced our understanding of central nervous system diseases by measuring changes in neurochemical levels, activation patterns and cerebral metabolism. The ability of PET for quantitative and dynamic assessments is particularly pertinent in the investigation of movement disorders such as Parkinson's disease, which are characterised by disturbances and fluctuations in the level of neurotransmitters in the basal ganglia neuronal circuits. The subjects may be examined in a resting state, whilst performing certain tasks, or after external interventions such as pharmacological challenges or electromagnetic stimulations. This chapter describes recent advances in the study of underlying biochemical abnormalities in Parkinson's disease using PET, and how these have enhanced our understanding of disease pathogenesis and progression.

Introduction

Idiopathic Parkinson's disease (PD) is a progressive neurodegenerative disorder characterised clinically by asymmetric tremor, rigidity and bradykinesia. One of the cardinal pathological features of PD is the loss of dopaminergic neurons in the pars compacta of

* Corresponding Author: Dr Paola Piccini, Cyclotron Building, Imperial College London. Hammersmith Hospital, Du Cane Road W12 0NN London U.K. Tel:+44 020 8383 3773 (direct); +44 020 8383 3162 (reception); Fax:+44 020 8383 2029; E-mail: paola.piccini@csc.mrc.ac.uk

substantia nigra [1]. The greatest loss occurs in the ventrolateral tier of pars compacta, with lesser involvement in the ventromedial and dorsal tiers. This unique pattern of cell loss in the substantia nigra results in a corresponding loss of its striatal terminals with caudal putamen being most affected, followed by rostral putamen and caudate nucleus. It was estimated that at the onset of symptoms, there is a greater than 50% loss of dopaminergic neurons in substantia nigra [2].

Current symptomatic treatments for PD are generally directed towards restoring dopaminergic transmission in the striatum. In early PD, the symptoms, particularly bradykinesia and rigidity, respond very well to treatments with dopamine replacement therapy (using levodopa) or dopamine agonists. However, this 'honeymoon' period usually lasts for only 3-5 years. With progression of disease, the therapeutic response becomes diminished or unpredictable. The patients can experience unpredictable fluctuations between a more mobile 'on' state and a more rigid 'off' state ('on-off' fluctuations). The duration of clinical benefit after each dose also becomes progressively shorter ('wearing off' fluctuations). Levodopa-induced dyskinesias (LIDs), a form of abnormal involuntary movements involving face, limbs and/or trunk, can also occur later on. Studies have shown that approximately 50% of PD patients develop motor fluctuations and LIDs after 5 to 6 years of levodopa therapy [3, 4]. These motor complications can be extremely resistant to pharmacological manipulations, and are a cause of significant morbidity in PD patients. In addition, there are other motor manifestations of PD such as tremor and non-motor manifestations such as depression which are not very responsive to dopaminergic therapy from the outset, as they are likely to be secondary to the involvement of non-dopaminergic systems in PD.

Animal models of PD are produced using dopaminergic neurotoxins such as 1-methyl-4-phenyl-1,2,3,6-tetrahydropyridine (MPTP) or 6-hydroxydopamine, or based on one of the several genetic models. However, these may not necessarily mimic the clinical course and progression, nor reflect the non-dopaminergic involvement, in human PD. Positron emission tomography (PET) offers an *in vivo* technique to investigate brain pathology. It is particularly useful in the study of pathogenesis and pathological progression in PD due to its ability to assess and quantify dynamic changes in neurochemical levels, neuroreceptors binding and cerebral metabolism in living humans. In this chapter, we will discuss recent advances in the understanding of the pathophysiology and progression of PD using PET, particularly looking at presynaptic dopaminergic terminal function, post-synaptic dopaminergic receptor status and contribution of non-dopaminergic neurochemicals.

Dopaminergic Dysfunction in PD

In normal individuals, the striatal dopamine levels are tightly regulated by several processes. Dopa is converted by aromatic amino acid decarboxylase (AADC) into dopamine in the cell bodies. The dopamine is then packaged into synaptic vesicles by type 2 vesicular monoamine transporters (VMAT2). Following a signal to release dopamine, depolarisation occurs and dopamine is released into the synaptic cleft, where it interacts with pre- and post-synaptic dopamine receptors. The concentration of this extracellular dopamine is regulated by presynaptic plasma membrane dopamine transporters, which reuptake synaptic dopamine into dopamine nerve terminals. The remaining dopamine in the synapse is broken down by catechol *O*-methyltransferase. The synaptic dopamine also binds to inhibitory presynaptic dopamine autoreceptors, and this provides a negative feedback to the terminals and cell bodies to reduce synthesis and release of dopamine.

Several PET ligands have been employed to study presynaptic dopaminergic function. One of the most commonly used ligands is ^{18}F-6-L-fluorodopa (^{18}F-Dopa). Once injected intravenously, ^{18}F-Dopa crosses blood brain barrier and is taken up by dopaminergic neurons, where it is converted by AADC into ^{18}F-Dopamine. This is stored in the vesicles and transported to presynaptic terminals before being released. The influx constants (Ki) of ^{18}F-dopa reflects dopa transport into the terminals, AADC activity and dopamine storage capacity [5]. ^{18}F-dopa PET can therefore provide an *in vivo* indicator of the function and integrity of pre-synaptic dopaminergic terminals. The ^{18}F-dopa uptake in the striatum also correlates well with nigral cell count [6]. Tracers that bind to presynaptic dopamine transporters such as ^{11}C-methylphenidate and ^{11}C-CFT, and dopamine terminal VMAT2 such as ^{11}C-dihydrotetrabenazine (^{11}C-DTBZ), have also been used as markers of presynaptic dopaminergic function. In PD, the loss of nigrostriatal dopaminergic projection is reflected by these PET markers as asymmetric loss of uptake or binding in the putamen, greatest in the side contralateral to the clinically more affected limbs [7, 8]. There is also a caudal-rostral gradient loss of uptake/binding, starting from caudal putamen, and eventually progressing to rostral putamen (see figure 1). The caudate nucleus is also affected in the later stages. The striatal dopaminergic function as measured by PET correlates inversely with the clinical severity of PD. The following sections discuss dopaminergic dysfunction in PD in the context of motor manifestations and cognitive impairment.

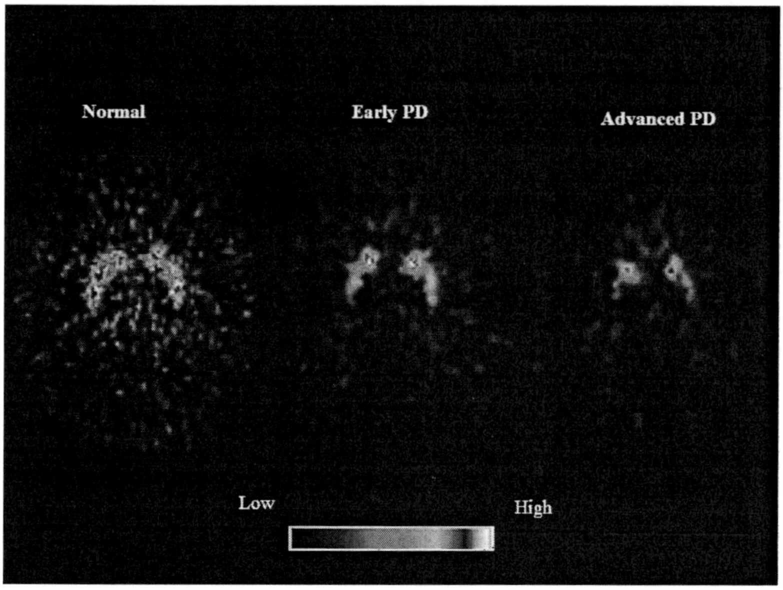

Figure 1. ^{18}F-Dopa PET parametric images showing progressive, asymmetric and caudal-rostral loss of striatal ^{18}F-Dopa uptake in PD, most marked in the caudal putamen contralateral to the clinically most affected limbs. (Images courtesy of Nicola Pavese)

Motor Manifestations

Presynaptic Dopamine Function

In normal individuals, there is a linear fallout of dopaminergic neurons in the pars compacta of substantia nigra at 4.7% per decade [2]. Age-related decline in striatal terminal dopaminergic function can be detected with ^{11}C-DTBZ PET (estimated to be about 6% per decade) [9], but not with ^{18}F-Dopa PET [10]. One possible explanation is that with age, the AADC enzyme is upregulated to increase dopamine production in the terminals to compensate for dopaminergic cell loss. An analogous phenomenon is also observed in early PD. It is widely believed that there is a significant loss of nigral dopaminergic cells before manifestation of parkinsonian signs. PET studies looking into presymptomatic carriers of mutations for familial PD, such as *parkin* [11] and *PINK1* [12], and monozygotic cotwins [13] have detected subclinical nigrostriatal dopaminergic dysfunction. A post-mortem study had predicted a 50% reduction in substantia nigra cell count before onset of symptoms in PD [2]. However, a ^{18}F-Dopa PET study estimated that at the onset of symptoms, there is only a 30% reduction in striatal ^{18}F-Dopa uptake [14]. This discrepancy is thought to be due to the upregulation of the AADC enzyme in the surviving dopaminergic terminals to increase dopamine turnover and to compensate for cell loss in early disease [5]. This was also demonstrated by Lee *et al* [15] who studied 35 PD patients using three presynaptic dopaminergic markers, ^{11}C-DTBZ, ^{18}F-Dopa and ^{11}C-methylphenidate, and compared the results with 16 healthy controls. They showed that in PD, the striatal terminal AADC activity appears to be relatively upregulated and dopamine transporter binding relatively downregulated compared with VMAT2 density. These are interpreted by the authors as compensatory mechanisms of the surviving dopaminergic terminals to enhance dopamine transmission in the denervated striatum. Such observations have also been noted in animal models of PD [16, 17].

In PD, the loss of nigrostriatal projection in the direct pathway results in the loss of inhibition of the internal segment of globus pallidus (GPi). The inhibitory GPi output to the thalamus thus becomes overactive, and reduces the excitatory thalamic output to the cortex. A ^{18}F-Dopa PET study showed that in early PD, the progressive decline in putamen ^{18}F-Dopa Ki is not accompanied by an appreciable decline in clinical scores [18]. During this period of relative clinical stability, there is a supranormal increase in the Ki of the GPi. It is thought that this represents an upregulation of inhibitory nigral projection to GPi to compensate for the loss of nigrostriatal projection (figure 2). In advanced PD with extensive nigral cell loss, this upregulation is lost and the GPi Ki is reduced to subnormal value. The nigropallidal neurons are localised in the dorsal tier of substantia nigra, which is relatively spared in early PD. With advancing disease, the pathology affects other parts of nigra, resulting in the loss of pallidal projection and the alteration of the firing pattern of the pallidum from steady tonic to burst firing. Therefore, the loss of GPi upregulation coincides with the onset of clinical progression and may contribute to the development of motor complications in PD. Interestingly, the authors also noted that in patients who individually exhibited motor fluctuations at the time of PET scans, their GPi also had the lowest ^{18}F-Dopa uptake.

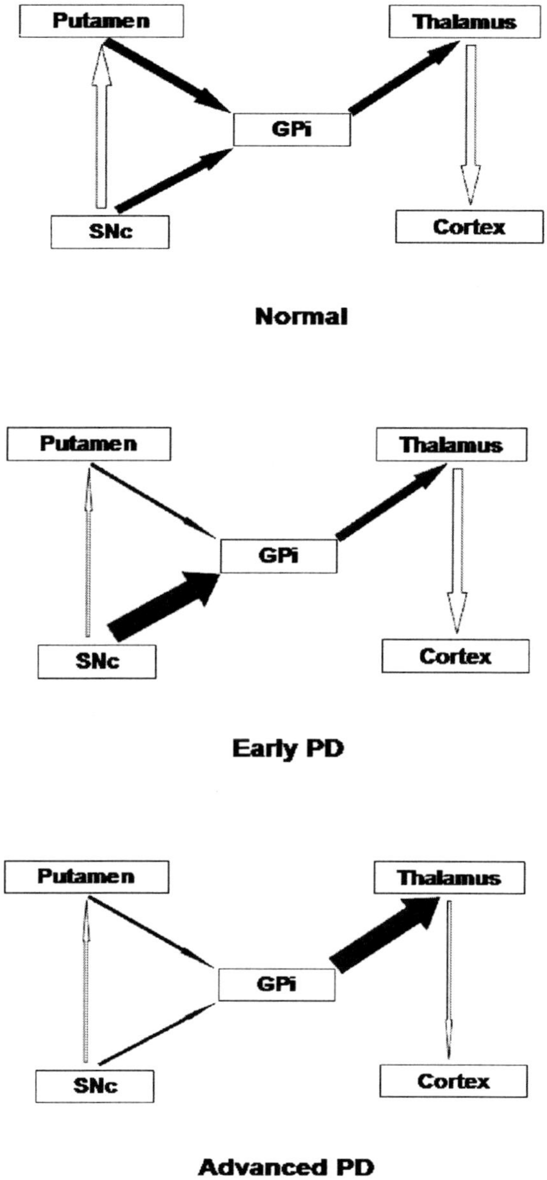

Figure 2. Simplified diagrams showing direct striatal output pathway in (i) normal where there is a balanced input to GPi from nigra and striatum. (ii) In early PD, the loss of excitatory nigrostriatal projection results in a reduction of inhibitory striatopallidal output. The GPi thus becomes overactive. This is compensated for by the upregulation of inhibitory nigropallidal projection and thus maintains the thalamic output to cortex. (iii) This upregulation is lost in advanced PD, resulting in excessive inhibitory GPi projection to thalamus and reduced thalamic output to cortex. Solid arrow = inhibitory projection; open arrow = excitatory projection; thick arrow = upregulation; thin arrow = downregulation. SNc = substantia nigra pars compacta; GPi = internal segment of globus pallidus. (Modified from Whone *et al* (18))

One of the first motor complications encountered in advanced PD is the 'wearing-off' fluctuations. Both pre- and post-synaptic mechanisms have been studied to elucidate the cause of this complication. In a ^{18}F-Dopa PET study, the 2-hour putamen ^{18}F-Dopa Ki values are lower for the 'wearing-off' fluctuators than stable responders [19]. However, there is significant overlap in the values between the two groups. The authors concluded that although the loss of nigro-striatal terminals predisposes PD patients towards the development of 'wearing-off' fluctuations, other factors may be implicated. Indeed, another study found that at 4-hour, the putamen ^{18}F-Dopa Ki values are much lower in the fluctuators than stable responders, suggesting greater fluctuation of synaptic dopamine level or faster dopamine turnover in the former group [7].

Using the principle of competition between endogenous neurotransmitters and administered tracers for the same neuroreceptors, it is possible to image acute fluctuations in the concentration of synaptic neurotransmitters using PET [20]. ^{11}C-raclopride competes with synaptic dopamine for post-synaptic dopamine D2 receptors. According to the classic occupancy model, when there is an increased synaptic release of dopamine after performing a task mediated by dopamine, or following pharmacological challenges with levodopa or a dopamine depleting agent such as methamphetamine, fewer dopamine D2 receptors will be available to ^{11}C-raclopride, and this is evidenced by a reduction in ^{11}C-raclopride binding. Data from microdialysis study performed on Rhesus monkeys suggest that after administering 0.2mg/kg of amphetamine, a 1% reduction in striatal ^{11}C-raclopride binding corresponds to at least an 8% increase in striatal extracellular dopamine levels [21].

Tedroff *et al* measured synaptic dopamine release in PD patients following levodopa challenge in a ^{11}C-raclopride PET study [22]. They found the greatest release of dopamine in the posterior putamen, followed by anterior putamen and caudate nucleus. The authors suggested that the fluctuation in levodopa-induced dopamine levels is related to the degree of striatal denervation. De la Fuente-Fernandez *et al* investigated 8 early PD patients with no motor complications using ^{11}C-raclopride PET at baseline and at 1 and 4 hours after administration of levodopa to measure dopamine turnover in these subjects. These subjects were then followed up to see if the pattern of dopamine release might relate to the risk of developing motor fluctuations in the future [23]. Of the 8 patients, half of them developed motor fluctuations after a mean interval of 1.75 years. There is no difference in putamen ^{11}C-raclopride binding between the fluctuators and stable responders at baseline. However, the fluctuators have three times greater reduction in putamen ^{11}C-raclopride binding 1 hour after levodopa administration compared to stable responders, indicating greater release of dopamine. After 4 hours, the ^{11}C-raclopride binding in the fluctuators group have returned to baseline level, whereas that in the stable responders group continues to decline. This is consistent with the clinical observation that with progression of PD, the onset of beneficial motor response to levodopa becomes more rapid, but the duration of this response also becomes shorter [24]. The authors employed the same PET methodology to compare striatal dopamine turnover in PD patients with and without peak-dose LIDs in another recent study. They found that dyskinetic patients had greater synaptic dopamine release 1-hour after levodopa administration than the stable responders, but the differences disappeared at 4-hour [25]. Taken together, the data indicate that a rapid turnover of dopamine may play a role in the development of 'wearing-off' fluctuations and LIDs.

The role of inhibitory presynaptic dopamine autoreceptors, which are important in the feedback control of dopamine synthesis and release in nigrostriatal terminals, in the development of complications in PD has also been studied. Torstenson *et al* investigated the effects of pharmacologically effective doses of bolus intravenous levodopa on striatal ^{11}C-Dopa uptake in PD [26]. The dorsal putamen ^{11}C-Dopa uptake was reduced by 23% in early PD patients but was increased by 40% in advanced patients with motor complications. The caudate uptake was unaffected in both groups of patients. In a follow-up study, the authors substituted levodopa with therapeutic doses of subcutaneous apomorphine, a dopamine D1- and D2-receptor agonist, and found that dorsal putamen ^{11}C-Dopa uptake was reduced by 28% in early PD patients but was unchanged in more advanced patients [27]. The authors concluded that in early PD, the presynaptic autoreceptors of remaining dopaminergic terminals in putamen are upregulated. When these upregulated autoreceptors are exposed to therapeutic doses levodopa or apomorphine, the negative feedback mechanisms result in marked downregulation of AADC in order to maintain a steady and physiological dopamine tone. In more advanced patients, further degeneration of dopaminergic terminals in putamen results in defective autoreceptors regulatory mechanisms. Levodopa, but not apomorphine, increases the activity of AADC via an uncertain mechanism, causing the synaptic dopamine level to swing abnormally high. This lends further support to the theory that rapidly fluctuating levels of dopamine in advanced PD is important for the pathogenesis of motor complications.

Post-Synaptic Dopamine Function

PET studies looking into post-synaptic dopaminergic receptors using ligands such as ^{11}C-raclopride or ^{11}C-methylspiperone, both dopamine D2 receptor ligands, showed normal caudate binding and either normal or slightly increased putamen binding in de novo drug-naïve PD patients. In more advanced patients, the striatal binding is either normal or slightly decreased [28, 29]. PET studies using dopamine D1 receptor antagonist ^{11}C-SCH23390 showed similar findings, with striatal binding preserved in de novo patients but slightly reduced in patients chronically treated with levodopa [30, 31].

It was postulated that deafferentation of striatal neurons in PD leads to supersensitivity of post-synaptic dopamine receptors. Subsequent exposure to high and pulsatile levels of levodopa results in the development of dyskinesias [32]. However, it was shown that high-dose levodopa can induce dyskinesias in primates even in the presence of intact nigrostriatal pathway [33]. A PET study has also revealed that there is no difference in striatal dopamine D1 and D2 receptors binding between stable responders and dyskinetic patients matched for disease duration [31]. Olanow *et al* suggested that changes in downstream neurons including dysregulation of genes and proteins, rather than the availability of striatal dopamine receptors per se, are responsible for the alterations in neuronal firing patterns and development of dyskinesias [34].

Cognitive Impairment/Dementia

Dementia is a common complication of PD with a prevalence of approximately 28% as reported by one community-based study [35]. Cognitive dysfunction in PD is characterised by a progressive decline in executive functions accompanied by attentional deficits and fluctuating cognition [36]. The underlying cause of dementia in PD is thought to be multi-factorial with dopaminergic deficiency in caudate nucleus and mesocortical areas, cholinergic deficiency in the basal nucleus of Meynert and cortical Lewy bodies all implicated [36]. A ^{18}F-Dopa PET study revealed a significant reduction in ^{18}F-Dopa uptake in the anterior cingulate, ventral striatum and right caudate nucleus of PD patients with dementia compared to those without, suggesting that dementia in PD is associated with impaired mesolimbic and caudate dopaminergic function [37]. The authors also detected a significant correlation between mini mental state examination (MMSE) scores and right caudate ^{18}F-Dopa uptake. Other PET studies have also reported significant correlations between caudate and frontal ^{18}F-Dopa uptake and cognitive functions in PD [38, 39]. Different parts of frontostriatal circuitry appear to mediate different aspects of cognitive functions. Higher-level executive functions such as planning and spatial recognition tasks depend on the integrity of the caudate-dorsolateral frontal dopamine pathway, whereas low-level control processes such as reversal learning and explicit retrieval of information are controlled by the ventrostriatal-ventrolateral frontal projections. In PD, the former pathway is more affected than the latter, and this is reflected by the pattern of executive functions impairment. Levodopa improves performances in tasks mediated by dorsolateral frontal cortex, but impairs performances in tasks mediated by the relatively intact ventrolateral frontal cortex, possibly due to dopamine 'overloading' in the pathway [40].

Using ^{11}C-raclopride PET, we have recently investigated the release of endogenous dopamine in a group of early non-demented PD patients and healthy volunteers whilst performing a visual search task as a test of executive functions. We showed that striatal dopamine release during the visual search task is significantly impaired in PD compared to controls, whereas the prefrontal dopamine release is relatively preserved [41]. Even in the more advanced stage of PD, the frontal release of dopamine appears to be well preserved compared to normal individuals as demonstrated in a ^{11}C-raclopride PET study after methamphetamine challenge [42]. These data suggest that the deficits of executive functions in PD are not due to intrinsic prefrontal dysfunction per se, but rather as a result of abnormal processing of striato-frontal input. Indeed, Carbon *et al* showed that in early PD, where the presynaptic dopaminergic function in caudate is only mildly impaired, there is a loss of the tight coupling between caudate dopaminergic input and thalamo-cortical activity during sequence learning as seen in normal individuals [43].

Non-Dopaminergic Dysfunction in PD

In PD, post-mortem studies have shown reduction in the levels of several non-dopaminergic neurotransmitters including noradrenaline, serotonin and acetylcholine. This is due to pathological involvement of areas such as locus coeruleus, raphe nuclei and basal nucleus of Meynert [44]. Clinical manifestations of these neurotransmitter deficiencies are usually poorly responsive to conventional treatments using levodopa or dopamine agonists. Lack of clinical improvements in several neurorestorative studies in PD despite evidence of restoration of some dopaminergic functions may be partially due to the persisting non-dopaminergic deficiencies [45]. A better understanding of the multi-system nature of neurodegeneration in PD is essential for the development of more effective therapies for PD in the future.

Serotonergic System

Parkinsonian tremor is characterised by a resting tremor of 3 to 5 Hz and postural tremor of 4 to 8 Hz. It is usually not as responsive to dopaminergic medications as other motor symptoms of PD such as bradykinesia and rigidity, suggesting involvement of non-dopaminergic system [46]. Several ^{18}F-Dopa PET studies had shown that decreases in striatal ^{18}F-Dopa uptake correlate with the degree of bradykinesia and rigidity, but not tremor, in PD [47, 48]. In addition, administration of MPTP in primates resulted in bradykinesia and rigidity but did not produce tremor reliably [49]. Using ^{11}C-WAY 100635 PET to examine cerebral 5-HT_{1A} receptors status in PD, Doder *et al* found a 27% reduction in the midbrain raphe 5-HT_{1A} binding in PD patients compared to healthy controls. The reduction reflects the known serotonergic neuronal loss in raphe nuclei in PD and/or 5-HT_{1A} receptors dysfunction. In addition, 5-HT_{1A} binding in the raphe correlates inversely with the severity of tremor, but not rigidity or bradykinesia [50], suggesting an important role of serotonergic neurons in the pathogenesis of tremor. However, the lack of efficacy of selective serotonin reuptake inhibitors (SSRIs) in the treatment of tremor in PD suggests other neurotransmitters are likely to be involved.

Noradrenergic System

In PD, the loss of noradrenergic neurons in the locus coeruleus is well documented [51]. Reduced levels of noradrenaline transporters in the locus coeruleus is also seen in major depression [52]. A post-mortem study revealed a greater loss of noradrenergic neurons in locus coeruleus in PD patients with depression compared to those without [53]. Using ^{11}C-RTI-32, which binds to dopamine and noradrenaline membrane transporters (DAT and NAT) with similar affinity, to study depressed and non-depressed PD patients matched for age and disease severity, the former group had lower ^{11}C-RTI-32 binding in the locus coeruleus and regions of the limbic system including the anterior cingulate cortex, thalamus, amygdala and ventral striatum [54]. ^{11}C-RTI-32 binding in these regions also correlated inversely with anxiety score. ^{11}C-RTI-32 binding does not distinguish between DAT or NAT, but based on known anatomical distribution of noradrenergic and dopaminergic neurons, low ^{11}C-RTI-32 binding in areas such as locus coeruleus is likely to reflect loss of noradrenergic neurons and their innervations, whereas that in the other regions is likely to be related to dopaminergic and/or noradrenergic dysfunction. Serotonergic dysfunction is implicated in the pathogenesis of primary depression. However, using ^{11}C-WAY 100635 PET, the same authors found reduction in raphe 5-HT_{1A} binding in both depressed and non-depressed PD patients but there is no significant difference between the two groups [55]. These results suggest that noradrenergic and dopaminergic, rather than serotonergic, dysfunction in the limbic system may be important for the pathogenesis of depression in PD. The clinical benefits of tricyclic antidepressants in depression in PD may be partially mediated through inhibition of noradrenaline uptake.

Cholinergic System

Pathological studies have revealed the loss of cholinergic basal forebrain neurons in Parkinson's disease with dementia, similar to that seen in Alzheimer's disease [56]. A recent study used ^{11}C-PMP PET to study cortical acetylcholinesterase (AChE) activity in patients with Parkinson's disease and mild Alzheimer's disease. The greatest reduction in cortical AChE was seen in Parkinson's disease with dementia, followed by Parkinson's disease without dementia. Patients with mild Alzheimer's disease, of whom the degree of dementia is similar to that of patients with Parkinson's disease dementia, had relatively preserved mean cortical AChE activity apart from the lateral temporal cortex which was selectively involved [57]. These, together with a recent therapeutic trial which showed moderate clinical improvements in patients who have dementia associated with Parkinson's disease taking cholinesterase inhibitor rivastigmine [58], indicate that cholinergic deficiency is an important cause of dementia in Parkinson's disease.

Opioid Binding

Opioid neuropeptides are important neurotransmitters in the basal ganglia and are normally present in high concentrations [59]. Endogenous opioids such as dynorphin and enkephalin are both co-transmitters of the inhibitory neurotransmitter GABA, acting via the direct and indirect basal ganglia pathways respectively. A post-mortem study which included 11 PD patients, 9 of which had LIDs, showed increased striatal opioid peptide gene expression compared to controls [60]. PD patients without dyskinesias had normal basal ganglia binding of ^{11}C-diprenorphine, a non-selective opioid PET tracer which binds to δ, μ, and κ subtype receptors with equal affinity [61]. However, in dyskinetic patients, the ^{11}C-diprenorphine binding is reduced in putamen, thalamus and cingulate [62]. There was also a significant correlation between the severity of dyskinesias and reduction in putamen opioid binding. The results suggest a greater occupancy of opioid receptors by endogenous opioids in dyskinetic PD. It is thought that enhanced level of enkephalin and dynorphin transmission results in underactive inhibitory output from the GPi to thalamus, and thereby causes dyskinesia [63]. However, clinical studies using non-selective opioid antagonists such as naloxone to treat LIDs in PD have yielded disappointing results thus far [64, 65]. The authors of one of the studies [64] surmised that using an opioid antagonist that is selective for δ and μ subtype receptors may be necessary to demonstrate the anti-dyskinetic property shown in a preclinical study [66].

Microglial Activation

^{11}C-(R)-PK11195 binds to peripheral benzodiazepine binding sites, which are selectively expressed in the central nervous system by activated microglia. Microglia are normally present in the central nervous system in a quiescent state but can become activated in response to various insults such as trauma, ischaemia, inflammation and neurodegeneration [67]. Microglia activation is linked to the activation of caspase cascades and release of pro-inflammatory cytokines, both of which lead to neuronal death [68]. Activated microglia have been detected in post-mortem PD brains [69] and inhibition of microglial activation in the MPTP-model of PD using minocycline is shown to be neuroprotective [70], suggesting the role of activated microglia in the pathogenesis and/or progression of PD. A ^{11}C-(R)-PK11195 PET study demonstrated increased microglial activation in midbrain of PD patients, and the degree of activation correlates positively with clinical disability but negatively with putamen binding of a dopamine transporter marker ^{11}C-CFT [71]. This suggests a close association between microglial activation and nigrostriatal dysfunction, but does not clarify if the link is causative or reactive. The authors of this study did not find activation in the striatum, which is in contradiction to another report which found increased ^{11}C-(R)-PK11195 binding in the striatum but not in the midbrain, and there was no correlation between ^{11}C-(R)-PK11195 binding and putamen ^{18}F-Dopa uptake [72]. The discrepancy between the two studies could be due to differences in methodological approach and subject inclusion as the former study included de novo drug-naïve PD patients only.

Blood-Brain Barrier

The discovery of MPTP as a cause of parkinsonism has led to the hypothesis that exposure to and impaired clearance of neurotoxins are implicated in the pathogenesis of idiopathic PD [73]. P-glycoprotein (P-gp) is a membrane transporter encoded by the MDR1 gene. It is present in the endothelial cells of blood-brain barrier and acts to extrude potentially toxic substances across the barrier. A specific polymorphism in the P-gp MDR1 gene is found more commonly in patients with parkinsonism related to pesticides exposure [74]. Kortekaas *et al* used ^{11}C-verapamil, which is a substrate for P-gp, and PET to investigate blood-brain barrier function in PD [75]. They demonstrated that compared to controls, PD patients had significantly increased ^{11}C-verapamil uptake in midbrain, an area where significant neuronal loss is found in PD. The authors interpreted the finding as showing localised impairment of P-gp function in PD, and suggested a link between impaired blood-brain barrier clearance of toxins and the pathogenesis of PD. However, it is not entirely clear why the blood-brain barrier function should be impaired in a region-specific manner and the results may require further confirmation [76].

Conclusion

PET is a powerful *in vivo* tool for investigation of brain pathology especially when complemented by other techniques such as molecular analyses and post-mortem studies. Its advantages over other imaging tools include the ability to image neurochemical fluctuations in addition to haemodynamic changes. Appreciation of the progressive and multi-system nature of neurodegeneration in PD will allow us to have a better understanding of its pathogenesis and pathophysiology, which will in turn enable scientists to develop better symptomatic and neuroprotective/restorative treatments in the future.

References

[1] Bernheimer H, Birkmayer W, Hornykiewicz O, Jellinger K, Seitelberger F. Brain dopamine and the syndromes of Parkinson and Huntington. Clinical, morphological and neurochemical correlations. *J Neurol Sci* 1973;20(4):415-55.

[2] Fearnley JM, Lees AJ. Ageing and Parkinson's disease: substantia nigra regional selectivity. *Brain* 1991;114(Pt 5):2283-301.

[3] Poewe WH, Lees AJ, Stern GM. Low-dose L-dopa therapy in Parkinson's disease: a 6-year follow-up study. *Neurology* 1986;36(11):1528-30.

[4] Hely MA, Morris JG, Reid WG, O'Sullivan DJ, Williamson PM, Rail D, et al. The Sydney Multicentre Study of Parkinson's disease: a randomised, prospective five year study comparing low dose bromocriptine with low dose levodopa-carbidopa. *J Neurol Neurosurg Psychiatry* 1994;57(8):903-10.

[5] Brooks DJ. Imaging end points for monitoring neuroprotection in Parkinson's disease. *Ann Neurol* 2003;53(Suppl 3):S110-8; discussion S118-9.

[6] Snow BJ, Tooyama I, McGeer EG, Yamada T, Calne DB, Takahashi H, et al. Human positron emission tomographic [18F]fluorodopa studies correlate with dopamine cell counts and levels. *Ann Neurol* 1993;34(3):324-30.

[7] Leenders KL, Palmer AJ, Quinn N, Clark JC, Firnau G, Garnett ES, et al. Brain dopamine metabolism in patients with Parkinson's disease measured with positron emission tomography. *J Neurol Neurosurg Psychiatry* 1986;49(8):853-60.

[8] Frey KA, Koeppe RA, Kilbourn MR, Vander Borght TM, Albin RL, Gilman S, et al. Presynaptic monoaminergic vesicles in Parkinson's disease and normal aging. *Ann Neurol* 1996;40(6):873-84.

[9] Taylor SF, Koeppe RA, Tandon R, Zubieta JK, Frey KA. In vivo measurement of the vesicular monoamine transporter in schizophrenia. *Neuropsychopharmacology* 2000;23(6):667-75.

[10] Sawle GV, Colebatch JG, Shah A, Brooks DJ, Marsden CD, Frackowiak RS. Striatal function in normal aging: implications for Parkinson's disease. *Ann Neurol* 1990;28(6):799-804.

[11] Khan NL, Scherfler C, Graham E, Bhatia KP, Quinn N, Lees AJ, et al. Dopaminergic dysfunction in unrelated, asymptomatic carriers of a single parkin mutation. *Neurology* 2005;64(1):134-6.

[12] Khan NL, Valente EM, Bentivoglio AR, Wood NW, Albanese A, Brooks DJ, et al. Clinical and subclinical dopaminergic dysfunction in PARK6-linked parkinsonism: an 18F-dopa PET study. *Ann Neurol* 2002;52(6):849-53.

[13] Piccini P, Burn DJ, Ceravolo R, Maraganore D, Brooks DJ. The role of inheritance in sporadic Parkinson's disease: evidence from a longitudinal study of dopaminergic function in twins. *Ann Neurol* 1999;45(5):577-82.

[14] Morrish PK, Rakshi JS, Bailey DL, Sawle GV, Brooks DJ. Measuring the rate of progression and estimating the preclinical period of Parkinson's disease with [18F]dopa PET. *J Neurol Neurosurg Psychiatry* 1998;64(3):314-9.

[15] Lee CS, Samii A, Sossi V, Ruth TJ, Schulzer M, Holden JE, et al. In vivo positron emission tomographic evidence for compensatory changes in presynaptic dopaminergic nerve terminals in Parkinson's disease. *Ann Neurol* 2000;47(4):493-503.

[16] Zigmond MJ, Abercrombie ED, Berger TW, Grace AA, Stricker EM. Compensations after lesions of central dopaminergic neurons: some clinical and basic implications. *Trends Neurosci* 1990;13(7):290-6.

[17] Stachowiak MK, Keller RW, Jr., Stricker EM, Zigmond MJ. Increased dopamine efflux from striatal slices during development and after nigrostriatal bundle damage. *J Neurosci* 1987;7(6):1648-54.

[18] Whone AL, Moore RY, Piccini PP, Brooks DJ. Plasticity of the nigropallidal pathway in Parkinson's disease. *Ann Neurol* 2003;53(2):206-13.

[19] de la Fuente-Fernandez R, Pal PK, Vingerhoets FJ, Kishore A, Schulzer M, Mak EK, et al. Evidence for impaired presynaptic dopamine function in parkinsonian patients with motor fluctuations. *J Neural Transm* 2000;107(1):49-57.

[20] Laruelle M. Imaging synaptic neurotransmission with in vivo binding competition techniques: a critical review. *J Cereb Blood Flow Metab* 2000;20(3):423-51.

[21] Breier A, Su TP, Saunders R, Carson RE, Kolachana BS, de Bartolomeis A, et al. Schizophrenia is associated with elevated amphetamine-induced synaptic dopamine concentrations: evidence from a novel positron emission tomography method. *Proc Natl Acad Sci U S A* 1997;94(6):2569-74.

[22] Tedroff J, Pedersen M, Aquilonius SM, Hartvig P, Jacobsson G, Langstrom B. Levodopa-induced changes in synaptic dopamine in patients with Parkinson's disease as measured by [11C]raclopride displacement and PET. *Neurology* 1996;46(5):1430-6.

[23] de la Fuente-Fernandez R, Lu JQ, Sossi V, Jivan S, Schulzer M, Holden JE, et al. Biochemical variations in the synaptic level of dopamine precede motor fluctuations in Parkinson's disease: PET evidence of increased dopamine turnover. *Ann Neurol* 2001;49(3):298-303.

[24] Nutt JG, Holford NH. The response to levodopa in Parkinson's disease: imposing pharmacological law and order. *Ann Neurol* 1996;39(5):561-73.

[25] de la Fuente-Fernandez R, Sossi V, Huang Z, Furtado S, Lu JQ, Calne DB, et al. Levodopa-induced changes in synaptic dopamine levels increase with progression of Parkinson's disease: implications for dyskinesias. *Brain* 2004;127(Pt 12):2747-54. Epub 2004 Aug 25.

[26] Torstenson R, Hartvig P, Langstrom B, Westerberg G, Tedroff J. Differential effects of levodopa on dopaminergic function in early and advanced Parkinson's disease. *Ann Neurol* 1997;41(3):334-40.

[27] Ekesbo A, Rydin E, Torstenson R, Sydow O, Laengstrom B, Tedroff J. Dopamine autoreceptor function is lost in advanced Parkinson's disease. *Neurology* 1999;52(1):120-5.

[28] Brooks DJ, Ibanez V, Sawle GV, Playford ED, Quinn N, Mathias CJ, et al. Striatal D2 receptor status in patients with Parkinson's disease, striatonigral degeneration, and progressive supranuclear palsy, measured with 11C-raclopride and positron emission tomography. *Ann Neurol* 1992;31(2):184-92.

[29] Dentresangle C, Veyre L, Le Bars D, Pierre C, Lavenne F, Pollak P, et al. Striatal D2 dopamine receptor status in Parkinson's disease: an [18F]dopa and [11C]raclopride PET study. *Mov Disord* 1999;14(6):1025-30.

[30] Rinne JO, Laihinen A, Nagren K, Bergman J, Solin O, Haaparanta M, et al. PET demonstrates different behaviour of striatal dopamine D-1 and D-2 receptors in early Parkinson's disease. *J Neurosci Res* 1990;27(4):494-9.

[31] Turjanski N, Lees AJ, Brooks DJ. In vivo studies on striatal dopamine D1 and D2 site binding in L-dopa-treated Parkinson's disease patients with and without dyskinesias. *Neurology* 1997;49(3):717-23.

[32] Mouradian MM, Heuser IJ, Baronti F, Fabbrini G, Juncos JL, Chase TN. Pathogenesis of dyskinesias in Parkinson's disease. *Ann Neurol* 1989;25(5):523-6.

[33] Zeng BY, Pearce RK, MacKenzie GM, Jenner P. Alterations in preproenkephalin and adenosine-2a receptor mRNA, but not preprotachykinin mRNA correlate with occurrence of dyskinesia in normal monkeys chronically treated with L-DOPA. *Eur J Neurosci* 2000;12(3):1096-104.

[34] Olanow W, Schapira AH, Rascol O. Continuous dopamine-receptor stimulation in early Parkinson's disease. *Trends Neurosci* 2000;23(10 Suppl):S117-26.

[35] Aarsland D, Tandberg E, Larsen JP, Cummings JL. Frequency of dementia in Parkinson disease. *Arch Neurol* 1996;53(6):538-42.

[36] Bosboom JL, Stoffers D, Wolters E. Cognitive dysfunction and dementia in Parkinson's disease. *J Neural Transm* 2004;111(10-11):1303-15. Epub 2004 Jun 30.

[37] Ito K, Nagano-Saito A, Kato T, Arahata Y, Nakamura A, Kawasumi Y, et al. Striatal and extrastriatal dysfunction in Parkinson's disease with dementia: a 6-[18F]fluoro-L-dopa PET study. *Brain* 2002;125(Pt 6):1358-65.

[38] Holthoff-Detto VA, Kessler J, Herholz K, Bonner H, Pietrzyk U, Wurker M, et al. Functional effects of striatal dysfunction in Parkinson disease. *Arch Neurol* 1997;54(2):145-50.

[39] Rinne JO, Portin R, Ruottinen H, Nurmi E, Bergman J, Haaparanta M, et al. Cognitive impairment and the brain dopaminergic system in Parkinson disease: [18F]fluorodopa positron emission tomographic study. *Arch Neurol* 2000;57(4):470-5.

[40] Owen AM. Cognitive dysfunction in Parkinson's disease: the role of frontostriatal circuitry. *Neuroscientist* 2004;10(6):525-37.

[41] Sawamoto N, Hotton GR, Pavese N, Piccini P, Brooks DJ. Frontal endogenous dopamine release detected with 11C-Raclopride during a visual search task in healthy subjects and Parkinson's disease patients. *Neurology* 2005;64(Suppl 1):A274.

[42] Piccini P, Pavese N, Brooks DJ. Endogenous dopamine release after pharmacological challenges in Parkinson's disease. *Ann Neurol* 2003;53(5):647-53.

[43] Carbon M, Ma Y, Barnes A, Dhawan V, Chaly T, Ghilardi MF, et al. Caudate nucleus: influence of dopaminergic input on sequence learning and brain activation in Parkinsonism. *Neuroimage* 2004;21(4):1497-507.

[44] Hornykiewicz O. Biochemical aspects of Parkinson's disease. *Neurology* 1998;51(2 Suppl 2):S2-9.

[45] Lang AE, Obeso JA. Challenges in Parkinson's disease: restoration of the nigrostriatal dopamine system is not enough. *Lancet Neurol* 2004;3(5):309-16.

[46] Lang AE, Lozano AM. Parkinson's disease. Second of two parts. *N Engl J Med* 1998;339(16):1130-43.

[47] Otsuka M, Ichiya Y, Kuwabara Y, Hosokawa S, Sasaki M, Yoshida T, et al. Differences in the reduced 18F-Dopa uptakes of the caudate and the putamen in Parkinson's disease: correlations with the three main symptoms. *J Neurol Sci* 1996;136(1-2):169-73.

[48] Vingerhoets FJ, Schulzer M, Calne DB, Snow BJ. Which clinical sign of Parkinson's disease best reflects the nigrostriatal lesion? *Ann Neurol* 1997;41(1):58-64.

[49] Wilms H, Sievers J, Deuschl G. Animal models of tremor. *Mov Disord* 1999;14(4):557-71.

[50] Doder M, Rabiner EA, Turjanski N, Lees AJ, Brooks DJ. Tremor in Parkinson's disease and serotonergic dysfunction: an 11C-WAY 100635 PET study. *Neurology* 2003;60(4):601-5.

[51] Paulus W, Jellinger K. The neuropathologic basis of different clinical subgroups of Parkinson's disease. *J Neuropathol Exp Neurol* 1991;50(6):743-55.

[52] Klimek V, Stockmeier C, Overholser J, Meltzer HY, Kalka S, Dilley G, et al. Reduced levels of norepinephrine transporters in the locus coeruleus in major depression. *J Neurosci* 1997;17(21):8451-8.

[53] Chan-Palay V, Asan E. Alterations in catecholamine neurons of the locus coeruleus in senile dementia of the Alzheimer type and in Parkinson's disease with and without dementia and depression. *J Comp Neurol* 1989;287(3):373-92.

[54] Remy P, Doder M, Lees A, Turjanski N, Brooks D. Depression in Parkinson's disease: loss of dopamine and noradrenaline innervation in the limbic system. *Brain* 2005;16:16.

[55] Doder M, Rabiner EA, Turjanski N, Lees AJ, Brooks DJ. Brain serotonin 1A receptors in Parkinson's disease with and without depression measured by positron emission tomography with 11C-WAY 100635. *Mov Disord* 2000;15(Suppl 3):213(abstract).

[56] Whitehouse PJ, Hedreen JC, White CL, 3rd, Price DL. Basal forebrain neurons in the dementia of Parkinson disease. *Ann Neurol* 1983;13(3):243-8.

[57] Bohnen NI, Kaufer DI, Ivanco LS, Lopresti B, Koeppe RA, Davis JG, et al. Cortical cholinergic function is more severely affected in parkinsonian dementia than in

Alzheimer disease: an in vivo positron emission tomographic study. *Arch Neurol* 2003;60(12):1745-8.

[58] Emre M, Aarsland D, Albanese A, Byrne EJ, Deuschl G, De Deyn PP, et al. Rivastigmine for dementia associated with Parkinson's disease. *N Engl J Med* 2004;351(24):2509-18.

[59] Haber SN, Watson SJ. The comparative distribution of enkephalin, dynorphin and substance P in the human globus pallidus and basal forebrain. *Neuroscience* 1985;14(4):1011-24.

[60] Nisbet AP, Foster OJ, Kingsbury A, Eve DJ, Daniel SE, Marsden CD, et al. Preproenkephalin and preprotachykinin messenger RNA expression in normal human basal ganglia and in Parkinson's disease. *Neuroscience* 1995;66(2):361-76.

[61] Burn DJ, Rinne JO, Quinn NP, Lees AJ, Marsden CD, Brooks DJ. Striatal opioid receptor binding in Parkinson's disease, striatonigral degeneration and Steele-Richardson-Olszewski syndrome, A [11C]diprenorphine PET study. *Brain* 1995;118(Pt 4):951-8.

[62] Piccini P, Weeks RA, Brooks DJ. Alterations in opioid receptor binding in Parkinson's disease patients with levodopa-induced dyskinesias. *Ann Neurol* 1997;42(5):720-6.

[63] Henry B, Brotchie JM. Potential of opioid antagonists in the treatment of levodopa-induced dyskinesias in Parkinson's disease. *Drugs Aging* 1996;9(3):149-58.

[64] Fox S, Silverdale M, Kellett M, Davies R, Steiger M, Fletcher N, et al. Non-subtype-selective opioid receptor antagonism in treatment of levodopa-induced motor complications in Parkinson's disease. *Mov Disord* 2004;19(5):554-60.

[65] Rascol O, Fabre N, Blin O, Poulik J, Sabatini U, Senard JM, et al. Naltrexone, an opiate antagonist, fails to modify motor symptoms in patients with Parkinson's disease. *Mov Disord* 1994;9(4):437-40.

[66] Henry B, Fox SH, Crossman AR, Brotchie JM. Mu- and delta-opioid receptor antagonists reduce levodopa-induced dyskinesia in the MPTP-lesioned primate model of Parkinson's disease. *Exp Neurol* 2001;171(1):139-46.

[67] Kreutzberg GW. Microglia: a sensor for pathological events in the CNS. *Trends Neurosci* 1996;19(8):312-8.

[68] Tatton WG, Chalmers-Redman R, Brown D, Tatton N. Apoptosis in Parkinson's disease: signals for neuronal degradation. Ann Neurol 2003;53(Suppl 3):S61-70; discussion S70-2.

[69] McGeer PL, Itagaki S, Boyes BE, McGeer EG. Reactive microglia are positive for HLA-DR in the substantia nigra of Parkinson's and Alzheimer's disease brains. *Neurology* 1988;38(8):1285-91.

[70] Wu DC, Jackson-Lewis V, Vila M, Tieu K, Teismann P, Vadseth C, et al. Blockade of microglial activation is neuroprotective in the 1-methyl-4-phenyl-1,2,3,6-tetrahydropyridine mouse model of Parkinson disease. *J Neurosci* 2002;22(5):1763-71.

[71] Ouchi Y, Yoshikawa E, Sekine Y, Futatsubashi M, Kanno T, Ogusu T, et al. Microglial activation and dopamine terminal loss in early Parkinson's disease. *Ann Neurol* 2005;57(2):168-75.

[72] Gerhard A, Pavese N, Hotton GR, Es M, Turkheimer F, Oertel W, et al. Microglial activation in Parkinson's disease - Its Longitudinal Course and Correrlation with

Clinical Parameters: An 11C(R)-PK11195 PET study. *Neurology* 2004;62(Suppl5):A432.

[73] Calne DB, Langston JW. Aetiology of Parkinson's disease. *Lance*t 1983;2(8365-66):1457-9.

[74] Drozdzik M, Bialecka M, Mysliwiec K, Honczarenko K, Stankiewicz J, Sych Z. Polymorphism in the P-glycoprotein drug transporter MDR1 gene: a possible link between environmental and genetic factors in Parkinson's disease. *Pharmacogenetics* 2003;13(5):259-63.

[75] Kortekaas R, Leenders KL, van Oostrom JC, Vaalburg W, Bart J, Willemsen AT, et al. Blood-brain barrier dysfunction in parkinsonian midbrain in vivo. *Ann Neurol* 2005;57(2):176-9.

[76] Stoessl AJ, McGeer PL. Hot spots: can positron emission tomography offer insights into the pathogenesis of PD? *Ann Neurol* 2005;57(2):161-2.

In: Progress in Brain Mapping Research
Editor: F. J. Chen, pp. 177-204
ISBN 1-59454-580-4

Chapter 5

An Application of Eigensystem and Frequency Analysis in Brain Functional Mapping

***Mercedes Cabrerizo*[1], *Malek Adjouadi*[2] *and Melvin Ayala*[3]**
Department of Electrical and Computer Engineering,
Florida International University

Abstract

The objective of this study was to evaluate the feasibility of using an eigensystem-based study in EEG data in order to validate brain functional mappings associated with the characterization effects of an Auditory/Comprehension paradigm. The study associates key parameters, which relate the correlation between electrodes and the EEG activity and also analyzes key frequency bands (Alpha, Beta, Delta, and Theta) in order to corroborate findings that associate brain activity with specific auditory/comprehension tasks. The theoretical perspective for this research is established to set course for the elaboration of topographical analysis in order to distinguish the areas of the brain displaying prominent activities while specific events are taking place. The new visualization methods are established to assess and appreciate brain activity that characterizes such events. A mathematical framework is thus created in order to support both the algorithm designed to extract such activity, and the visualization methods of EEG activity. This study primarily explored the human brain mechanisms/patterns responsible for auditory language comprehension and response phases in a non-invasive manner. Conceivably, as the EEG and subjective effects of these tasks become better understood, their use as a helpful tool in mapping the different functions of the brain will become more effective. Such a representation can thus provide new insight on how

[1] Department of Electrical and Computer Engineering, Florida International University 10555 W. Flagler Street, Miami FL 33174, Tel: (30 5) 348-3019, Email: mercedes.cabrerizo@fiu.edu
[2] E-mail: adjouadi@fiu.edu
[3] E-mail: ayalam@fiu.edu

different subjects react during auditory and response tasks. The algorithm as developed in this study could be extended in its application to other brain functional mapping tasks given its simple but effective mathematical foundation.

Keywords: EEG data, Auditory/Comprehension paradigm, brain functional mappings, eigensystem study.

1. Introduction

The objective of this research endeavor is to interpret EEG signals during auditory and comprehension activities in order to assess and model induced EEG behavioral patterns. The localization of major brain activity during auditory and comprehension tasks is of clinical relevance in order to ascertain task-related brain functional mappings. Among the four lobes of the brain, which are frontal, parietal, temporal and occipital, the software algorithm developed in this study will assess the amount of relative involvement of each of the four lobes during an auditory/compression process. The brain functional mapping will thus be assessed using intra and inter subject comparisons. The acquisition of the data is carried out during a standard test of comprehension provided by the Department of Neuroscience at Miami Children's Hospital.

The brain is by far the most complex and least understood component of the human machinery. In adults, auditory problems may manifest through difficulty in retaining auditory information, inattentiveness, sound sensitivity, or speech/language and other voice concerns. Preliminary research findings of this study expand on earlier findings suggesting involvement of the Broca's and Wernicke's areas in language functions. This particular research endeavor may thus prove useful when valid behavioral patterns or profiles as determined are found to serve as a basis for analysis to determine if the patient has a learning problem due to auditory processing.

2. Method

2.1. Data Acquisition

The EEG data was recorded from fifteen normal subjects (age 23-42) with 12 males and 3 females during the Auditory/Comprehension test from 41 scalp sites. The electrodes were placed according to the Modified Combinatorial Nomenclature (MCN) (Greenstein et al. 2000). The EEG data collection was performed in continuous mode using a 500 Hz sampling frequency for all subjects.

The EEG recording time for each subject was limited to 10 minutes. The subjects that took part in the experiment had standard requirements placed on them prior to the test. Each subject was laid down in a bed and a brief explanation about the test was given to them before starting with the procedure. The test administered to the subject is a standard auditory test used in psychological assessments, in which the subject has to supply the missing word in 34 sentences. The test administered was test number 15 from Woodcock-Johnson III (Woodcock et al. 2001, p. 16). This is an oral comprehension test that measures the ability of a subject to comprehend a short audio-recorded passage and then supply the missing word. The test begins with simple analogies and associations and progresses to more complex passages. This test is known to have a median reliability of 0.89 in the adult range. At the time of the test, it was required from the subject to have his/her eyes closed and to maintain maximum possible relaxation in order to reduce the effect of artifacts in the EEG signal. Thirty to forty seconds of background brain activity of the relaxed subject were recorded with the eyes closed in order to have a baseline data for comparative purposes.

2.2. Recording Apparatus

EEG +data was recorded using an Electrical Source Imaging system with 256 electrodes, the ESI-256 recording system as illustrated in Figure 1, under standard clinical settings. The main modules of the system consist of 8 SynAmps (synchronous amplifiers). Software support consists of the Acquire program. The host computer executing this program controls the data acquisition of the SynAmp. This program performs all of the acquisition process, including the display and storage of data. The ESI-256 interface was used to exploit in an optimal fashion the existing online preprocessing and visualization tools.

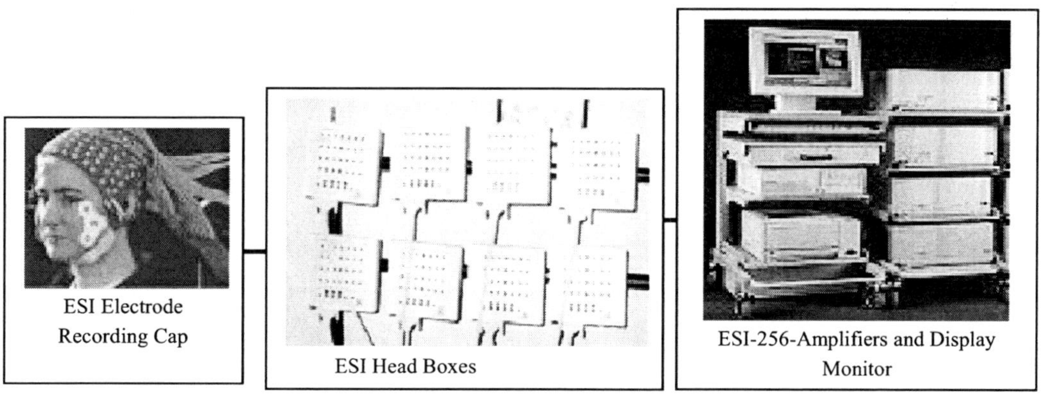

Figure 1. The ESI-256 EEG Recording System

2.3. Mathematical Foundation and Implementation of the EEG-Based Eigensystem Study

EEG data recorded from all the channels was initially preprocessed through the ESI-256 in order to eliminate common EEG artifacts together with the background noise. The algorithm is designed to contend with 7 files per subject, consisting of the baseline file and 6 auditory/response files. The program reads the files and creates a matrix with 41 columns, where each column represents a temporal digitized data record from a single electrode. The vertical axis thus represents all electrodes used in the experiment, and the horizontal axis displays the EEG data recorded at 500 Hz sampling frequency.

The algorithm integrated the following processing steps that led to the desired results:

- Removing the DC offset from the EEG signals by subtracting the average behavior for each electrode;
- Filtering unwanted noise of the EEG signals by applying Daubechies family of wavelet functions (Misiti et al. 1996; Vetterli et al. 1995);
- Averaging 6 epochs of EEG, during auditory and response phases in time domain;
- Subtracting the baseline of a subject from the averaged EEG signal of the auditory and answering blocks in time domain;
- Computing the mean voltage for each electrode in time domain as derived in Equation 1

$$\overline{V} = \frac{1}{N}\sum_{w=i}^{w=j} X_w \text{ , with } i = f_{c1}\,\frac{N}{2}\cdot 2\cdot f_s \text{ and } j = f_{c2}\,\frac{N}{2}\cdot 2\cdot f_s \tag{1}$$

N being the total number of samples; f_{c1} and f_{c2} are the cut off frequencies, f_s is the sampling frequency and X_w is the vector containing the EEG data values;

- Computing the empirical standard deviation $\sigma_X(p)$ of the voltages and calculating two thresholds T_1 and T_2 such that $T_1 = \sigma_X(p)$ and $T_2 = 2\ \sigma_X(p)$. These thresholds are applied (in the positive as well as in the negative direction) with respect to the absolute mean voltage μ of the signal in order to consider only those values within the following demarcated ranges: $[\mu+T_1, \mu+T_2]$, $[\mu+T_2, \infty)$, $[\mu-T_2, \mu-T_1]$, and $(-\infty, \mu-T_2]$.
- Establishing topographical representations using a gray-color-coding scheme in order to visualize in the brain those regions that reflect increasing and decreasing changes with respect to the mean voltage of each specific channel.

The visual graph proposed as presented in Figures 5 to 10 represents the shape of a human head with its 41 electrodes positioned in the same MCN order. In order to have an understanding of the behavior of the brain, two thresholds were established. The darkest gray colors are the ones that belong to the positive threshold of 2 and 1 standard deviations. The same reasoning was followed using the two lightest gray colors for the negative threshold of 2 and 1 standard deviation in the negative direction. This visualization approach provides a temporal depiction of the dynamic neural processes underlying the allocation of attention during the performance of auditory and response phases.

- Applying the Eigensystem study-based algorithm to each of the delineated regions of the brain: frontal left (FL), frontal right (FR), temporal left (TL), temporal right (TR), parietal left (PL), parietal right (PR), occipital left (OL), and occipital right (OR).

Eigensystem techniques have been sufficiently applied to EEG analysis for important applications such as source localization (Soong et al. 1995; Zhukov et al. 2000) and in many other traditional image and signal processing applications (Duda et al. 2001). This new algorithm applies the eigensystem analysis in an innovative way to explore and compare brain region activations based on standard deviation measurements. For this purpose, nine groups of electrodes were considered in the eigensystem analysis, whose names are very explicit in terms of their localization over the scalp. The groups of electrodes were established as defined in Table 1.

Table 1. Standard region definitions and corresponding electrodes

Group Number (r)	Group Name	Electrodes within the Group
1.	Frontal Left (FL)	FP_1, AF_7, F_7, FT_7, AF_3, F_3, FC_3
2.	Frontal Right (FR)	FP_2, AF_8, F_8, FT_8, AF_4, F_4, FC_4
3.	Temporal Left (TL)	FT_7, T_7, TP_7
4.	Temporal Right (TR)	FT_8, T_8, TP_8
5.	Parietal Left (PL)	TP_7, P_7, PO_7, CP_3, P_3, PO_3
6.	Parietal Right (PR)	TP_8, P_8, PO_8, CP_4, P_4, PO_4
7.	Occipital Left (OL)	PO_7, PO_3, O_1
8.	Occipital Right (OR)	PO_8, PO_4, O_2
9.	Central (C)	FC_3, C_3, CP_3, FC_Z, C_Z, CP_Z, FC_4, C_4, CP_4

Figure 2 illustrates the electrode nomenclature used to represent the nine preset regions. The frontal left and frontal right regions contain seven electrodes each. The temporal left, temporal right, occipital left and occipital right regions contain three electrodes each. The parietal left and right regions have six electrodes each. The central region contains nine electrodes.

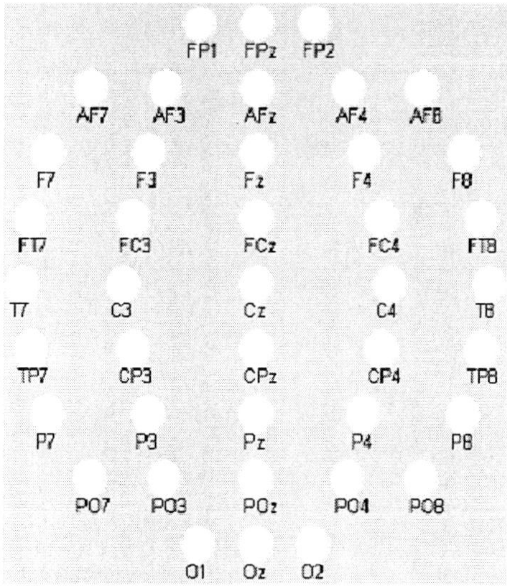

Figure 2. Nomenclature for electrode localization

The eigensystem-based algorithm was applied to each one of these groups. The first step was to calculate the covariance matrix, whose size varies from one group to another depending on the number of electrodes residing in each group. For a specific brain area with M electrodes, the particular input matrix X contained as many rows as there are samples in the signal (i.e., N) and as many columns as electrodes that are present in the area (i.e., M).

$$X = \begin{bmatrix} x_{11} & x_{12} & \cdots & x_{1M} \\ x_{21} & x_{22} & \cdots & x_{2M} \\ \vdots & \vdots & \cdots & \vdots \\ x_{N1} & x_{N2} & \cdots & x_{NM} \end{bmatrix}$$

The covariance matrix C of the input matrix X whose elements denoted as c_{pq} is derived as follows:

$$c_{pq} = \frac{1}{N-1} \sum_{i=1}^{N} (X_{ip} - \overline{X}_p)(X_{iq} - \overline{X}_q)^T \tag{2}$$

where X_{ip} and X_{iq} are the elements of vectors X_p and X_q which contain the N data samples recorded by electrodes p and q, respectively. Similarly, $\overline{X}_p$ and $\overline{X}_q$ represent the averages of the signals representing electrodes p and q, respectively.

The covariance matrix C is established in the following form:

$$C = \begin{bmatrix} c_{11} & c_{12} & \cdots & c_{1M} \\ c_{21} & c_{22} & \cdots & c_{2M} \\ \vdots & \vdots & \vdots & \vdots \\ c_{M1} & c_{M2} & \cdots & c_{MM} \end{bmatrix}$$

The covariance matrix C is symmetric (where $c_{pq} = c_{qp}$ for p,q = 1,2,…,M) which makes it opportune for fast eigensystem implementation (Gonzalez and Woods, 2002).

The matrix decomposition of the covariance matrix C into the so-called eigenvectors and eigenvalues was performed next. This procedure generated eigenvalues $\lambda_1, \lambda_2, \ldots, \lambda_M$ and their corresponding linearly independent eigenvectors $v_1, v_2, \ldots, v_M$. For further consideration, the matrices composed by the corresponding eigenvectors (V) and eigenvalues (D) are constructed:

$$V \equiv [v_1 \quad v_2 \quad \cdots \quad v_M] = \begin{bmatrix} v_{11} & v_{21} & \cdots & v_{M1} \\ v_{12} & v_{22} & \cdots & v_{M2} \\ \vdots & \vdots & \ddots & \vdots \\ v_{1M} & v_{2M} & \cdots & v_{MM} \end{bmatrix}$$

$$D \equiv \begin{bmatrix} \lambda_1 & 0 & \cdots & 0 \\ 0 & \lambda_2 & \cdots & 0 \\ \vdots & \vdots & \ddots & \vdots \\ 0 & 0 & \cdots & \lambda_M \end{bmatrix}$$

The elements of the main diagonal of D are also represented by vector $E = [\lambda_1\ \lambda_2\ ...\ \lambda_M]$.

This eigensystem analysis was applied to 9 different areas of the brain. Each area had a specific number of electrodes in accordance with the MCN nomenclature. For this purpose, 9 different sub matrixes $X_{sub}(r)$ were created, where r = 1, 2,..., 9 (see Table 1). The comparison of the eigensystem values among these areas is assessed while taking into consideration the topographic variations in the different areas.

Due to the different number of electrodes considered in each area, comparing the vectors of eigenvalues of these areas could lead to a misconception. That is why a new criterion was needed in order to compare all these areas regardless of the number of electrodes that are present them. To clarify this assertion, suppose that two regions 1 and 2 represented by $X_{sub}(1)$ and $X_{sub}(2)$ have to be compared, with three and two electrodes, respectively. Suppose also that the normalized eigenvalue vector is $E_{X_{sub}(1)}$ = [0.7 0.2 0.1] for region 1 and $E_{X_{sub}(2)}$ = [0.5 0.5] for region 2. Both systems are illustrated in Figure 3:

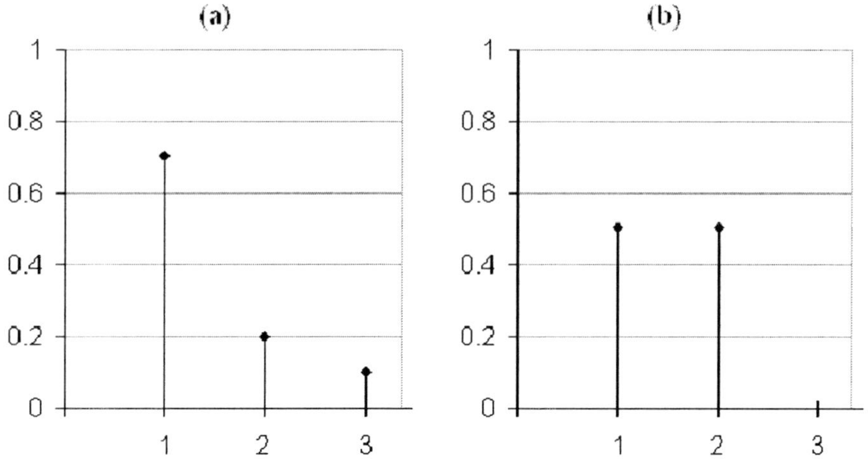

Figure 3. Example of the plot of the eigenvalues of two systems: (a) Eigenvalues for system $X_{sub}(1)$ with 3 dimensions, and (b) Eigenvalues for system $X_{sub}(2)$ with 2 dimensions

An optimized way to contrast such regions is in defining a criterion that selects a region with the highest correlation. It is known by fact, that the largest eigenvalue is the one that takes the direction of maximum variance; therefore, if it is determined that a certain region has the highest standard deviation with respect to others, then it can be concluded that that region is the one with the highest correlation. In direct application to EEG data, the area of the brain, which has the highest standard deviation of the eigenvalues, is assumed to be the area whose electrodes are more correlated. Therefore, to allow comparing such regions irrespective of the number of electrodes within them, a new evaluation criterion had to be established.

Eigenvalues are not correlation amplitudes. But through their analysis, one can conclude how well a multidimensional system is correlated among its dimensions. In a multidimensional system with a perfect one to one correlation between all dimensions, the vector of eigenvalues would be [N, 0, 0, …, 0] where N is the number of dimensions. That is, only one eigenvalue will be different from zero. In the case of an uncorrelated multidimensional system, at least 2 eigenvalues will be different from zero, and the more uncorrelated across the dimensions the system the more nonzero eigenvalues will be. When expressed statistically, this means that when the correlation between the dimensions decreases, the standard deviation (or variance) of the eigenvalues increases. Intuitively, it can be thus concluded that the standard deviation of the eigenvalues of a system belonging to a brain region relates to the degree of correlation in the EEG activity for this specific region.

Since the brain was subdivided into nine areas, the goal was to find a specific area whose electrodes are more correlated. The correlation of the electrode signals belonging to one specific region relates to the level of EEG activity inside that specific region. Equation 3 returns the optimum index $Index_{opt}$ of the stipulated area $X_{sub}(r)$, which has the greatest standard deviation of its eigenvalues. The optimal index is thus defined as:

$$Index_{opt} = \arg(\max_{r} \sigma_E(r)) \tag{3}$$

where $\sigma_E(r)$ is the standard deviation of the eigenvalues for region r and is calculated as:

$$\sigma_E(r) = \sqrt{\frac{\sum_{i=1}^{M(r)} (E_{X_{sub}(r),\, i} - \overline{E}_{X_{sub}(r)})^2}{M(r)-1}} \tag{4}$$

where, $\overline{E}$ is the mean of vector E which represents the eigenvalues of the specific sub matrix $X_{sub}(r)$, and *M(r)* is the number of electrodes present in region r.

Applying equation 3 to the example shown in Figure 3, yields $Index_{opt} = 1$, since $X_{sub}(1)$ is the one with the highest standard deviation of the eigenvalues. From this it can be concluded, that the electrode signals are more correlated in region 1.

In retrospect, for each of these 9 groups, the eigenvalues were calculated and the standard deviation of this set of eigenvalues was considered for ascertaining the standard deviations among these different groups. The original EEG signals were divided into the auditory/comprehension phase of the test and the response phase of the test, in order to carry-out comparative studies between them.

It should be noted that analysis of EEG activities relied on the accepted belief that the surface and scalp-recorded electrical activity results from extracellular current flow associated with summated EPSPs (excitatory post synaptic potential) and IPSPs (inhibitory post synaptic potential). The EEG thus reflects summated PSPs (Daly and Pedley, page 110). The recorded potential, when recorded in monopolar fashion to a distant reference point (like our recording in the study), is proportional to the solid angle subtended by a dipole layer at the position of the recording electrode. The magnitude of the recorded potential at any point around the dipole layer is determined by the dipole layer and the solid angle subtended at the recording electrode position. Therefore, it is not an unreasonable assumption too assume that all the neural generator dipoles are oriented perpendicular to the cortical surface. Especially since the belief here is that each recording electrode reflects the dipole underneath it.

2.4. Eigensystem Analysis

The main contribution of this study is in associating key parameters of the eigensystem to brain activities during auditory comprehension and response phases. The standard deviation values of the set of eigenvalues resultant of the different regions are represented in Tables 2 and 3. Note that all of the highest standard deviations are located in the frontal region.

During the auditory phase, the highest standard deviation of the eigenvalues was found to be in the left frontal area of the brain for 5 subjects and in the right frontal area for the remaining 4 subjects. In the response phase, the highest standard deviation of the eigenvalues was found to be in the left frontal area for 5 subjects and in the right frontal area for the remaining 4 subjects.

Table 2. Standard deviation of the set of eigenvalues of the different groups of electrodes during the auditory phase for the nine subjects

Subject	FL	FR	TL	TR	PL	PR	OL	OR	C
Subject 1	593	527	146	222	308	472	362	492	530
Subject 2	364	721	46	149	85	116	88	115	174
Subject 3	920	385	81	95	94	163	107	151	294
Subject 4	184	800	27	48	171	180	213	173	146
Subject 5	397	429	52	43	77	55	52	40	155
Subject 6	406	200	105	63	152	109	121	124	175
Subject 7	2300	1200	198	147	75	85	50	59	184
Subject 8	2100	2000	131	200	140	268	115	240	349
Subject 9	332	718	88	142	253	220	232	199	298

Since EEG changes are taken into consideration in both the positive and negative direction with respect to the mean of the signal, the highest positive and the lowest negative voltage values with respect to a baseline are considered important. In Tables 4 and 5, all the predefined regions of the brain are ordered starting from the region with the highest relative positive activity down to the smallest relative negative activity (i.e. activity with respect to the mean). Therefore, the first and last regions represented for each subject in tables 4 and 5 have equal importance in our analysis because they are the regions which present higher activation with respect to the EEG baseline. Consequently, these regions are considered to be the most active during the auditory and response phases.

Table 3. Standard deviation of the set of eigenvalues of the different groups of electrodes during the response phase for the nine subjects

Subject	FL	FR	TL	TR	PL	PR	OL	OR	C
Subject	2700	2300	487	648	543	756	511	603	1200
Subject2	619	1200	116	223	188	253	170	240	341
Subjet 3	1500	1100	113	158	134	223	121	172	472
Subject 4	1200	3100	91	178	270	247	296	193	283
Subject 5	1100	944	119	296	137	300	95	177	333
Subject 6	570	349	174	224	161	145	126	157	207
Subject 7	14000	9100	1900	1400	319	307	155	131	614
Subject 8	2400	2900	221	373	228	422	178	338	475
Subject 9	1700	3200	213	223	287	195	236	174	495

Table 4. Descending order of activity with respect to the baseline during listening phase

Subject	Regions from Highest to Lowest
Subject 1	FL,C, FR, OR, PR, OL, PL, TR, TL
Subject 2	FR, FL, C, TR, PR, OR, OL, PL, TL
Subject 3	FL, FR, C, PR, OR, OL, TR, PL, TL
Subject 4	FR, OL, FL, PR, OR, PL, C, TR, TL
Subject 5	FL, C, FR, OR, PR, OL, PL, TR, TL
Subject 6	FL, FR, C, PL, OR, OL, PR, TL, TR
Subject 7	FL, FR, TL, C, TR, PR, PL, OR, OL
Subject 8	FL, FR, C, PR, OR, TR, PL, TL, OL
Subject 9	FR, FR, C, PL, OL, PR, OR, TR, TL

Table 5. Descending order of the activity with respect to the baseline during response phase

Subject	Regions from Highest to Lowest
Subject 1	FL, FR, C, PR, TR, OR, PL, OL, TL
Subject 2	FR, FR, C, PR, OR, TR, PL, OL, TL
Subject 3	FL,,FR, C, PR, OR, TR, PL, OL,TL
Subject 4	FR, FL, OL, C, PL, PR, OR, TR, TL
Subject 5	FL, FR, C, PR, TR, OR, PL, TL, OL
Subject 6	FL, FR, TR, C, TL, PL, OR, PR, OL
Subject 7	FR, TL, TR, FL, C, PL, PR, OL, OR
Subject 8	FR, FL, C, PR, TR, OR, OL, TL, OL
Subject 9	FR, FL, C, PL, OL, TR, TL, PR, OR

2.5. Frequency Domain: Implementation Steps and Computational Analysis

After processing the acquired information, an additional frequency analysis for the same data was conducted for comparative purposes with the intent to reinforce the conclusions drawn from the eigensystem-based analysis as means for initial validation. In this second part of the study, the following steps were performed:

STEP 1: The relative mean power and absolute mean voltage were computed for each electrode in time domain and frequency domain for Delta (1-4Hz), Theta (4-8Hz), Alpha (8-13 Hz), Beta 1 (13-20Hz), and Beta 2 (20-30Hz), as derived in Equations 5 and 6.

$$\overline{P_r} = \frac{\frac{1}{N}\sum_{i=1}^{N}[x(i)]^2}{\frac{1}{N}\sum_{i=1}^{N}[y(i)]^2} \tag{5}$$

$$\overline{V} = \frac{1}{N}\sum_{w=i}^{w=j} X_w \tag{6}$$

where, i and j are defined as: $i = f_{c1}\frac{N}{2}\cdot 2\cdot f_s$ and $j = f_{c2}\frac{N}{2}\cdot 2\cdot f_s$, N being the total number of samples, with x representing the voltage values for a specific band, y representing the voltage values for all the bands, f_{c1} and f_{c2} are the cut off frequencies, f_s is the sampling frequency, and X_w is the vector containing the real values of the Fourier Transform (Proakis et al. 1996).

STEP 2: Computing the empirical standard deviation $\sigma_X(p)$ for the signal and frequency spectrum of each electrode p and calculating two thresholds T_1 and T_2 such that $T_1 = \sigma_X(p)$ and $T_2 = 2\sigma_X(p)$. These thresholds are applied both in the positive and in the negative directions with respect to the absolute mean voltage μ of the signal, in order to consider only those values within the following demarcated ranges: $[\mu+T_1, \mu+T_2]$, $[\mu+T_2, \infty)$, $[\mu-T_2, \mu-T_1]$, and $(-\infty, \mu-T_2]$.

STEP 3: Creating specific data arrays that contain the number of active electrodes in each hemisphere. This is performed for each frequency band and for all subjects.

STEP 5: Establishing topographical representations using a gray-color-coding scheme in order to visualize those regions in the brain that reflect increasing and decreasing changes with respect to the mean voltage of each specific channel. The gray color used in accordance to step 2 of section 2.5 are from darkest to lighest gray (descending gray scale), beginning in the range $[\mu+T_2, \infty)$, follow by $[\mu+T_1, \mu+T_2]$, and $[\mu-T_2, \mu-T_1]$, and ending in the range $(-\infty, \mu-T_2]$. The visual graph proposed represents the shape of a human head with 41 electrodes positioned in the same MCN order.

During the frequency analysis, the fluctuations in the spectra are displayed for both tasks (auditory phase and response phase). The spectral arrays are thus viewed as gray color topographic maps illustrating the resulting brain activities in order to establish relationships between brain waves at different cortex locations. This visualization approach provides a temporal depiction of the dynamic neural processes underlying the allocation of attention during the performance of auditory and response phases.

2.6. Hemispheric Lateralization Analysis

According to prior findings about right and left handed people, in about 98 percent of right-handers, the left hemisphere accomplishes most language processing functions. In those people who are non-right handers, which include left-handed and ambidextrous people, language functions are far more likely to involve the right hemisphere. In this study, it was found that the left hemisphere accomplishes most language processing functions in 56% of the subjects (5 out of 9 subjects) during the listening phase, and in 44% of the subjects (4 out of 9 subjects) during the response phase. At this stage of the study however, and given the small sample of subjects used (9), such an assessment calls for more clinical studies before such statistics are deemed appropriate. Table 6 provides the initial results based on this left- vs. right-handed analysis.

Table 6. Area of the brain with major activity for each of the nine subjects during auditory and response phases

Subjects	Auditory Phase	Response Phase
Subject #1→ Right-Handed	Frontal Left	Frontal Left
Subject #2→ Right-Handed	Frontal Right	Frontal Right
Subject #3→ Right-Handed	Frontal Left	Frontal Left
Subject #4→ Left-Handed	Frontal Right	Frontal Right
Subject #5→ Right-Handed	Frontal Right	Frontal Left and Right
Subject #6→ Right-Handed	Frontal Left and Right	Frontal Right
Subject #7→ Right-Handed	Frontal Left	Frontal Left and Right
Subject #8→ Right-Handed	Frontal Left and Right	Frontal Right
Subject #9→ Right-Handed	Frontal Left and Right	Frontal Right

The results however yielded 100% of the main voltage activity to be located in the frontal lobe of the brain. This agrees with the knowledge that the lobe of the brain that is related to such activities as reasoning, planning, parts of speech and movement (motor cortex), emotions, and problem solving is the frontal lobe (Lokhorst et al. 1996). As for the activity in the left and right hemispheres of the brain, the numbers are equilibrated, 50% of the subjects showed major activity on the left side and 50% on the right side.

2.7. Energy Distribution

Another technique used to analyze the data was through the energy distribution. The procedure consisted of calculating the percentage of energy for each electrode. Figures 4 and 5 establish the energy contribution of each electrode with respect to the different groups created using the different standard deviations. For example, from electrode #5 in Figure 4, can be seen that more than 95% of the data had the amplitude of the voltage in the range [μ-T_1, μ+T_1] from the mean of the data under analysis (white color according to the legend), the rest had the voltage in the interval [μ-T_2, μ-T_1] (lightest gray color).

The electrodes that show more energy are #1, #2, #3, #26 and #27. The numbers given for the forty-one electrodes is as indicated earlier; electrode #1 corresponds to FP_1, Electrodes #2 to AF_7, Electrodes #3 was assigned to F_7, Electrodes#26 to FP_2, and Electrode #27 matches with AF_8. By the letter F in all the names of the electrodes, signifies that all of them belong to the frontal lobe.

In this case it is relevant to mention that in the auditory task, in addition to electrodes #1, #2, #26, #27 like, electrode #17 corresponding to FP_Z and located in the frontal lobe was also involved.

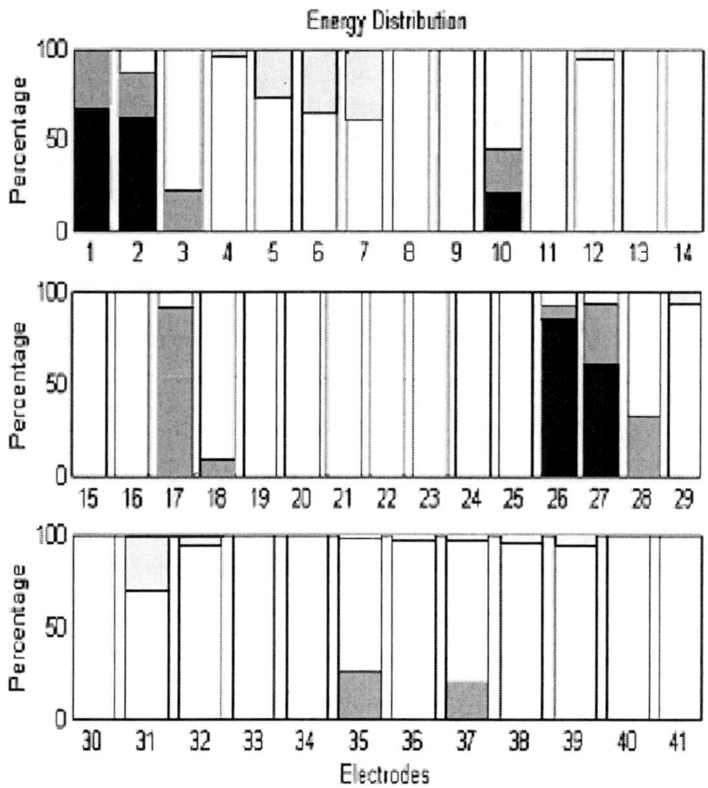

Figure 4. Energy distribution of the average of the listening

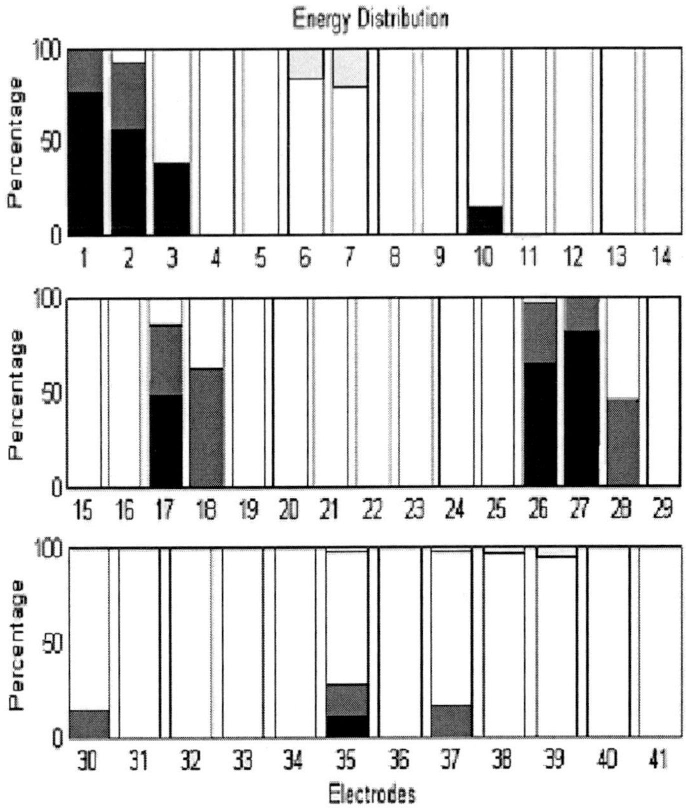

Figure 5. Energy distribution of the average of the answering

3. Results

3.1. Tabulated Results of the Analysis

Tables were constructed illustrating the percentage of voltage activity present in the different lobes of the brain during the auditory and response phases. Some weighted decisions had to be made about those electrodes whose assumed positions in between lobes. For instance, if an electrode is on the boundary between the frontal and the temporal lobes, this electrode is assumed to contribute a weight of 0.5 to the frontal cortex and 0.5 to the temporal cortex. Obviously, those electrodes that are within the boundaries of a given lobe are assigned a weight of 1 in contribution to that lobe. The tables presented below contain percentages of the groups of electrodes in the different lobes of the brain, as represented by the color assigned to them. Also, the tables show the percentage that these groups represent on the left and right sides of the brain. Tables 7-9 show the different values corresponding to the auditory phase, and tables 10-12 show the different values for the response phase.

Table 7. Percentage of the range between +1s and +2s (darkest gray colors) on the different lobes of the brain during auditory task for subjects 1 through 9

$[\mu+T_1, \infty)$	Frontal	Temporal	Parietal	Central	Occipital	Left	Right
Subject 1	9.76	0	0	0	0	6.25	3.12
Subject 2	15.75	0	0	1.22	0	6.25	12.50
Subject 3	7.32	0	0	0	0	9.38	0
Subject 4	14.63	0	0	0	0	3.12	12.50
Subject 5	14.63	0	0	0	0	6.25	9.38
Subject 6	19.51	0	0	0	0	9.38	9.38
Subject 7	17.07	0	0	0	0	12.50	6.25
Subject 8	12.20	0	0	0	0	6.25	6.25
Subject 9	12.20	0	0	0	0	6.25	6.25

Table 8. Percentage of the range between +1s and -1s (white color) on the different lobes of the brain during auditory task for subjects 1 through 9

White	Frontal	Temporal	Parietal	Central	Occipital	Left	Right
Subject 1	25.61	6.10	20.73	14.63	13.41	34.38	43.75
Subject 2	21.95	6.10	20.73	13.41	13.41	34.38	37.50
Subject 3	30.49	9.76	21.95	14.63	13.41	37.50	50
Subject 4	20.738	4.88	23.18	13.42	13.42	37.51	34.38
Subject 5	23.17	9.76	21.95	14.63	13.41	43.75	37.51
Subject 6	10.98	7.32	21.95	9.76	13.41	40.62	18.75
Subject 7	20.73	9.76	24.39	14.63	13.41	37.50	43.75
Subject 8	25.61	9.76	24.39	14.63	13.41	43.75	43.75
Subject 9	25.61	9.76	24.39	14.63	13.41	43.75	43.75

Table 9. Percentage of the range between -1s and +1s (lightest gray colors) on the different lobes of the brain during auditory task for subjects 1 through 9

$[\mu-T_1, -\infty)$	Frontal	Temporal	Parietal	Central	Occipital	Left	Right
Subject 1	2.44	3.6585	3.66	0	0	9.38	3.12
Subject 2	0	3.66	3.66	0	0	9.38	0
Subject 3	0	0	2.44	0	0	3.12	0
Subject 4	2.44	4.88	1.22	1.22	0	9.38	3.12
Subject 5	0	0	2.44	0	0	0	3.12
Subject 6	7.32	2.44	2.44	4.88	0	0	21.88
Subject 7	0	0	0	0	0	0	0
Subject 8	0	0	0	0	0	0	0
Subject 9	0	0	0	0	0	0	0

Table 10. Percentage of the range between +1s and +2s (darkest gray colors) on the different lobes of the brain during answering task for subjects 1 through 9

$[\mu+T_1, \infty)$	Frontal	Temporal	Parietal	Central	Occipital	Left	Right
Subject 1	12.20	0	0	0	0	6.25	3.12
Subject 2	15.85	0	0	1.22	0	6.25	12.50
Subject 3	17.07	0	0	0	0	9.38	6.25
Subject 4	17.07	0	0	0	0	6.25	9.38
Subject 5	14.63	0	0	0	0	6.25	6.25
Subject 6	14.63	2.44	0	0	0	6.25	12.50
Subject 7	14.63	0	0	0	0	9.38	9.37
Subject 8	14.63	0	0	0	0	6.25	9.37
Subject 9	12.20	0	0	0	0	3.12	6.25

Table 11. Percentage of the range between +1s and -1s (white color) on the different lobes of the brain during answering task for subjects 1 through 9

White	Frontal	Temporal	Parietal	Central	Occipital	Left	Right
Subject 1	23.17	9.76	21.95	14.63	13.41	40.62	43.75
Subject 2	21.95	8.54	20.73	13.41	13.41	37.50	37.50
Subject 3	20.73	9.76	24.39	14.63	13.41	40.62	43.75
Subject 4	20.73	9.76	24.39	14.63	13.41	43.75	40.62
Subject 5	23.17	9.76	24.39	14.63	13.41	43.75	43.75
Subject 6	19.51	6.10	21.95	9.76	13.41	40.62	25
Subject 7	23.17	9.76	24.39	14.63	13.41	40.62	40.62
Subject 8	25.61	9.76	24.39	14.63	13.41	43.75	43.75
Subject 9	25.61	9.76	24.39	14.63	13.41	46.88	43.75

Table 12. Percentage of the range between -1s and +1s (lightest gray colors) on the different lobes of the brain during answering task for subjects 1 through 9

$[\mu-T_1, -\infty)$	Frontal	Temporal	Parietal	Central	Occipital	Left	Right
Subject 1	2.44	0	2.44	0	0	3.124	3.124
Subject 2	0	1.22	3.66	0	0	6.25	0
Subject 3	0	0	0	0	0	0	0
Subject 4	0	0	0	0	0	0	0
Subject 5	0	0	0	0	0	0	0
Subject6	3.66	1.22	2.44	4.88	0	3.12	12.5
Subjec 7	0	0	0	0	0	0	0
Subjet 8	0	0	0	0	0	0	0
Subject 9	0	0	0	0	0	0	0

Table 13. Percentage of the three ranges of activities on the different lobes of the brain for the average of the voltage activity during listening task

	Frontal	Temporal	Parietal	Central	Occipital	Left	Right
$[\mu+T_1, \infty)$	14.63	0	0	0	0	9.38	6.25
White	23.17	8.54	20.73	14.63	13.41	34.38	43.75
$[\mu-T_1, -\infty)$	0	1.22	3.66	0	0	6.25	0

Table 14. Percentage of the three ranges of activities on the different lobes of the brain for the average of the voltage activity during answering task

	Frontal	Temporal	Parietal	Central	Occipital	Left	Right
$[\mu+T_1, \infty)$	14.63	0	0	0	0	6.25	9.38
White	23.17	9.76	24.39	14.63	13.41	43.75	40.62
$[\mu-T_1, -\infty)$	0	0	0	0	0	0	0

The results for the auditory phase yielded 100% of the main voltage activity to be located in the frontal lobe of the brain. This agrees with the knowledge that the lobe of the brain that is related to such activities as reasoning, planning, parts of speech and movement (motor cortex), emotions, and problem solving is the frontal lobe. As for the activity in the left and right sides of the brain, the numbers are equilibrated, 50% of the subjects showed major activity on the left side and 50% on the right side. For the results obtained during the answering phase, the main activity is located in the right frontal lobe of the brain.

3.2. Frequency Analysis

A detailed analysis of different frequency bands was additionally performed in order to identify those frequencies in the EEG signals that best characterize brain activity associated with an auditory/comprehension test. The objectives were to:

- Analyze the differences that exist between auditory/receptive phase vs. response/expressive phase;
- Visualize through gray-color-coded maps the different activities of the cerebral hemispheres (right vs. left); and
- Allow for comparisons to assess similar/dissimilar behaviors between EEG signals of any new subject and EEG signals of other subjects already in the database.

The results obtained reveal the following relevant findings: (a) Greater activation of the left hemisphere was evident during the receptive phase; (b) Greater activation of the frontal and temporal lobes during the auditory and response phases, recalling that Broca's area is located in the frontal lobe and that Wernicke's area is located where the parietal lobe meets the temporal lobe.

Tables 15 and 16 present the regions that show activity of the different frequency bands with respect to the mean of the signal during the auditory and response phases. In general, note that the more active regions of the brain are the frontal and temporal regions.

Table 15. Frequency analysis for the auditory phase

Auditory Phase	Positive	Negative
Alpha	Right frontal	Temporal and parietal Left and Right (more to the Left)
Beta 1	Right frontal and occipital	Temporal and parietal and some frontal to the Right and Left hemispheres
Beta 2	Occipital left and right, partially parietal	Temporal Left
Delta	Bilateral frontal (more oriented to left hemisphere)	Not much activity. Some rare activity in the temporal Right lobes
Theta	Bilateral frontal (Left and Right hemisphere)	Temporal and parietal Left

Table 16. Frequency analysis for the response phase

Response Phase	Positive	Negative
Alpha	Right frontal	Temporal and parietal on both hemispheres (greater on the Left)
Beta 1	Right frontal	Temporal and parietal in both hemispheres (more to the Left)
Beta 2	Occipital and parietal Left	Parietal Left
Delta	Bilateral frontal (more oriented to right hemisphere)	Not much activity. Some rare activity in the central right lobes
Theta	Bilateral frontal	Almost no activity

Brain functional maps based on the frequency domain as obtained in this clinical study during auditory and response phases are shown in Figures 6-11. Only the results of 3 subjects are shown for illustrative purposes for both listening and response phases. Other subjects showed similar type of functional mappings. The circular dots represent the positions of the electrodes used in this study and the gray color bar on the right side represents the different ranges based on the two thresholds of 1 and 2 standard deviation(s) with respect to the mean (T_1 and T_2), following the demarcated ranges: $[\infty, \mu+T_2)$, $[\mu+T_1, \mu+T_2]$, $[\mu-T_2, \mu-T_1]$, and $[\mu-T_2, -\infty)$. Note that the deeper colors represent stronger deviations from the baseline in the positive direction of these subjects, and the lighter colors represent stronger deviations from the baseline in the negative direction as indicated in step 5 of section 2.5.

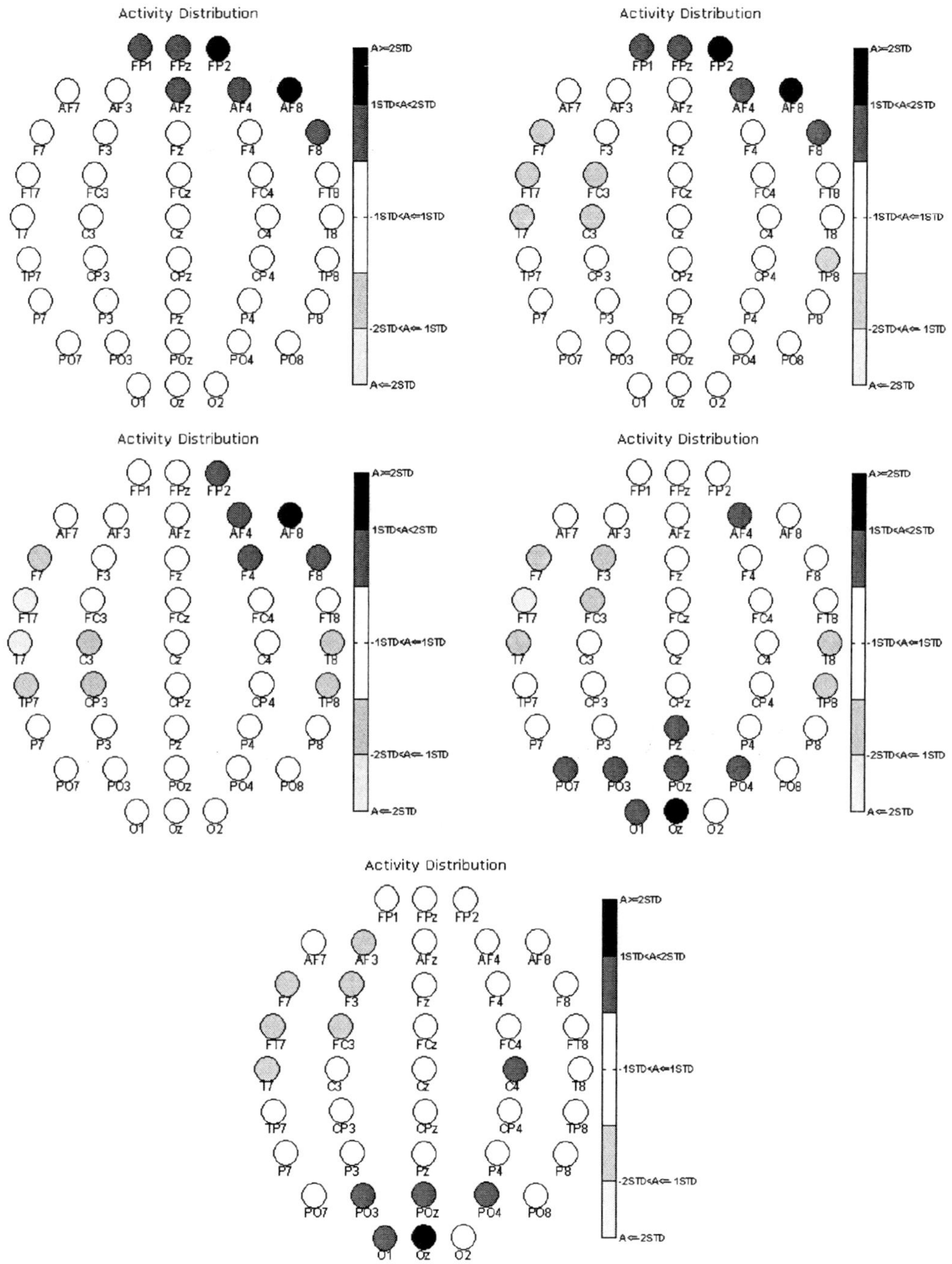

Figure 6. Illustrative frequency activities (Delta, Theta, Alpha, Beta 1, and Beat2) during auditory phase for subject 1

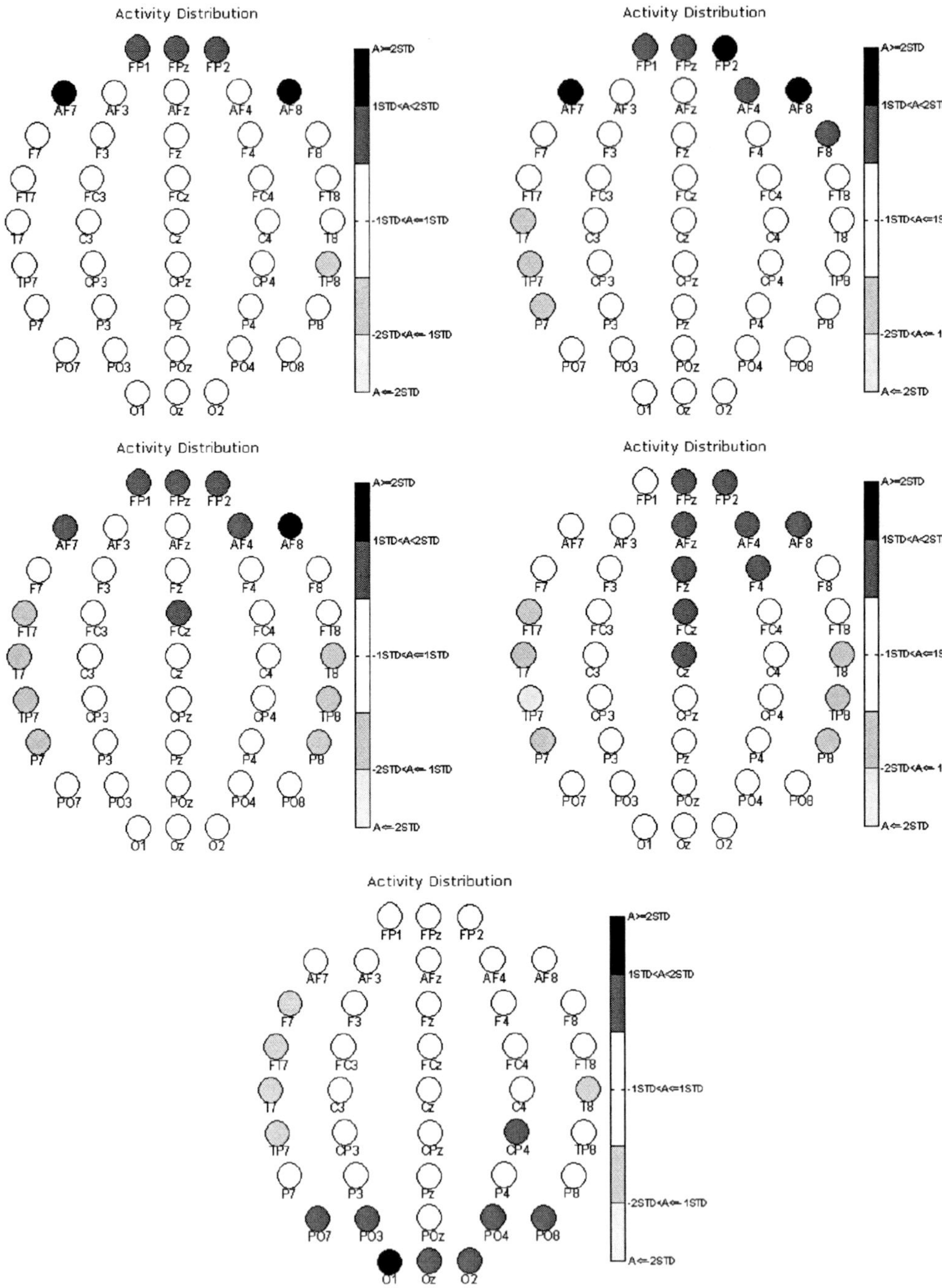

Figure 7. Illustrative frequency activities (Delta, Theta, Alpha, Beta 1, and Beat2) during auditory phase for subject 2

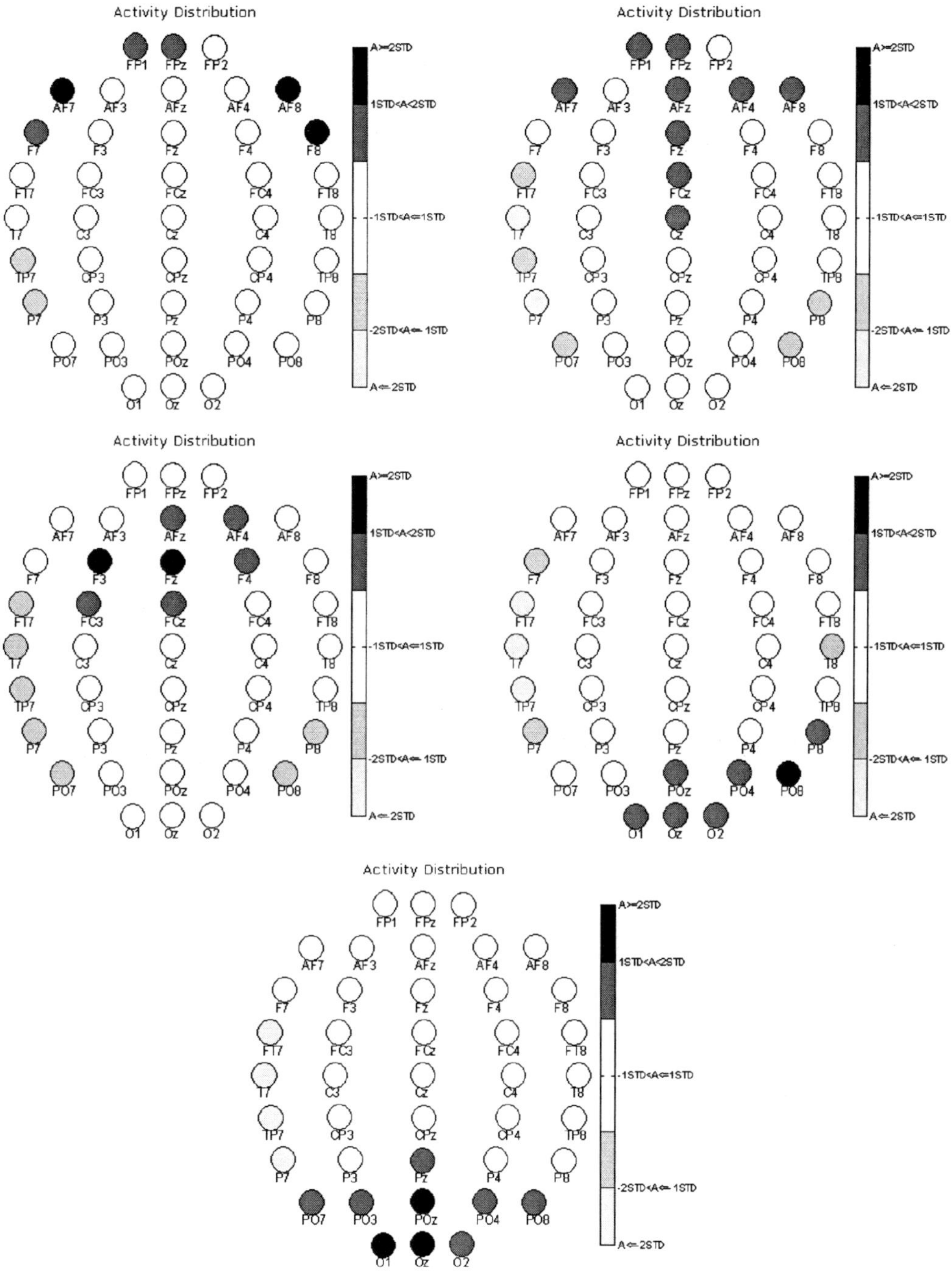

Figure 8. Illustrative frequency activities (Delta, Theta, Alpha, Beta 1, and Beat2) during auditory phase for subject 3

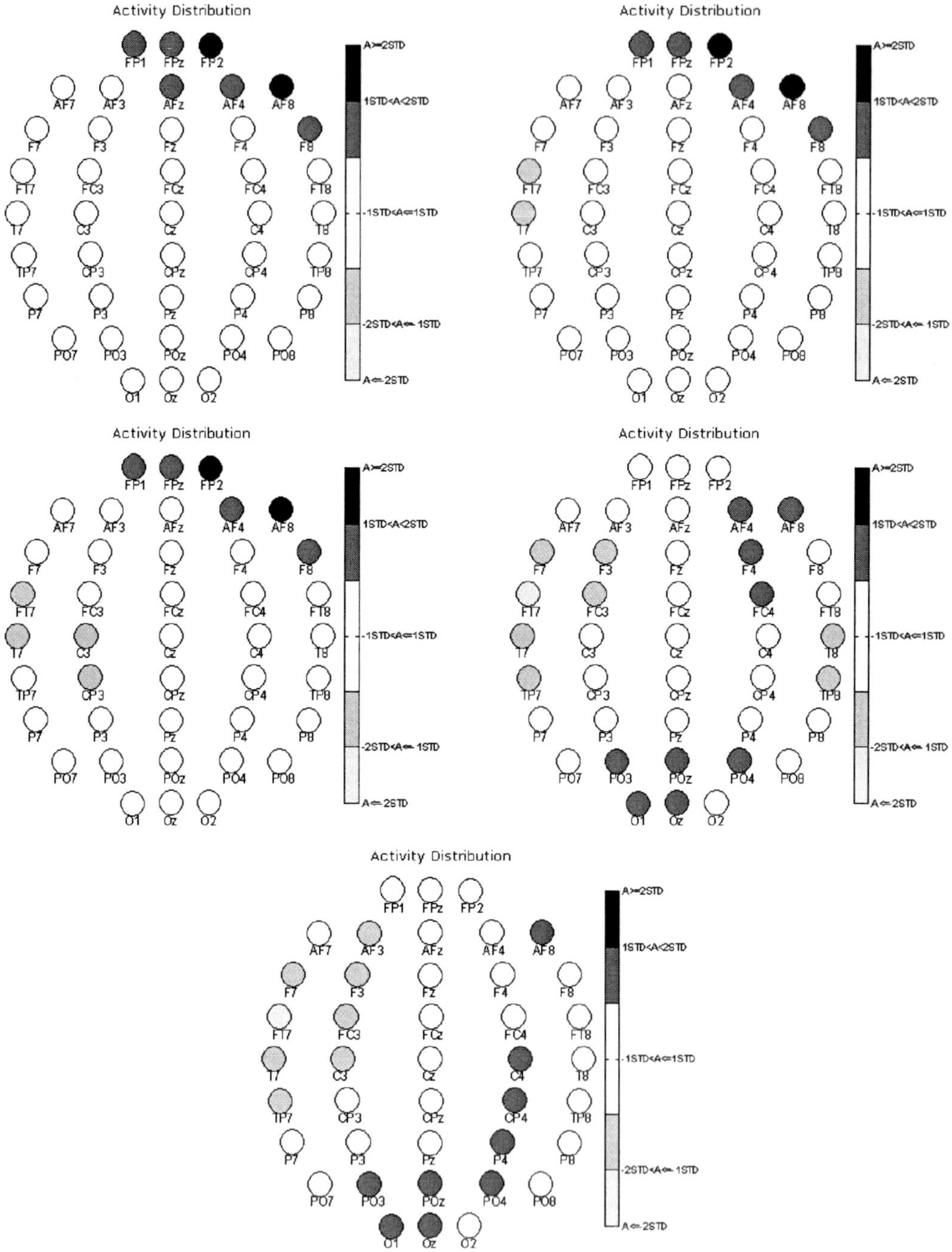

Figure 9. Illustrative frequency activities (Delta, Theta, Alpha, Beta 1, and Beat2) during the response phase for subject 1

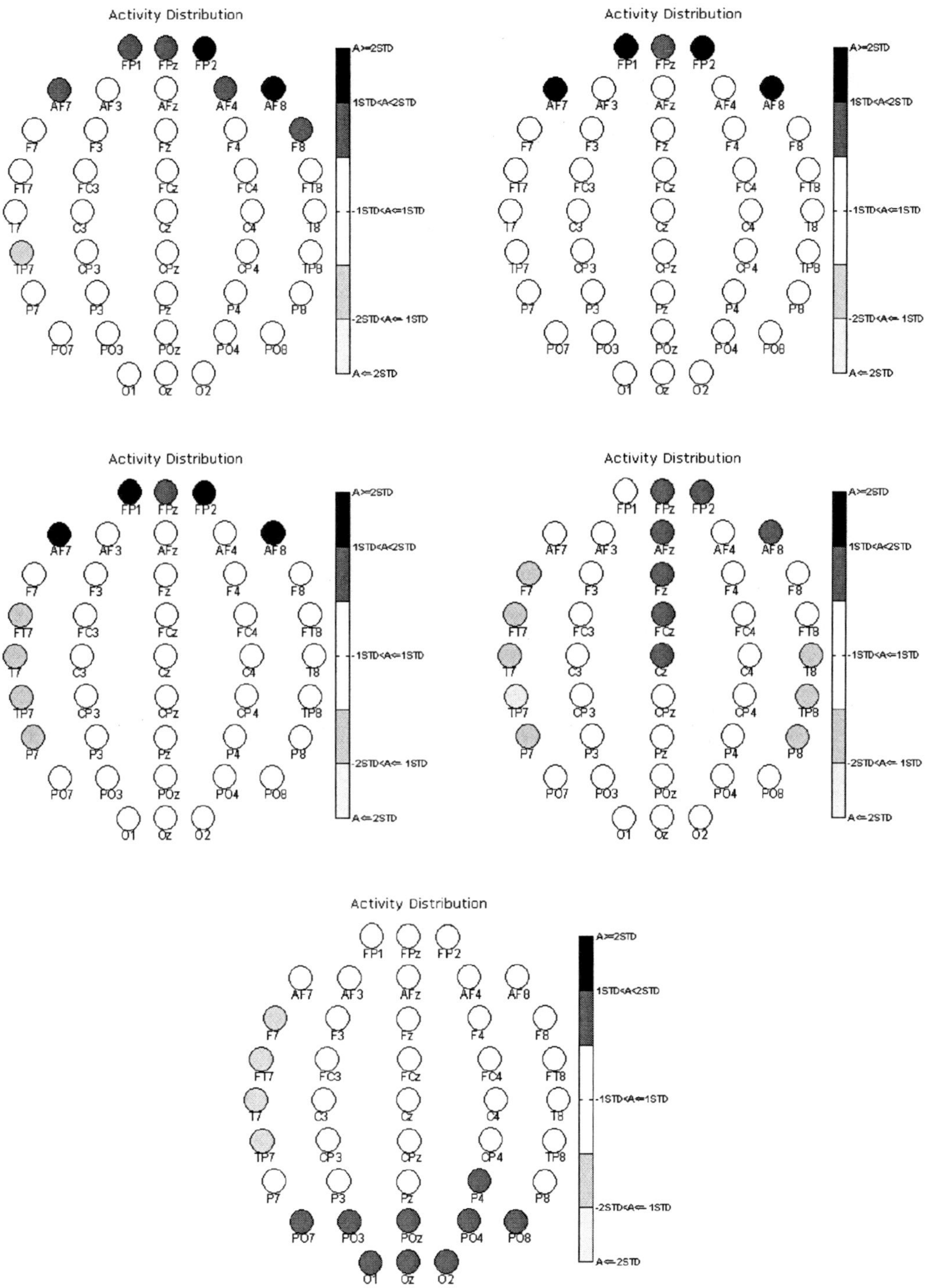

Figure 10. Illustrative frequency activities (Delta, Theta, Alpha, Beta 1, and Beat2) during the response phase for subject 2

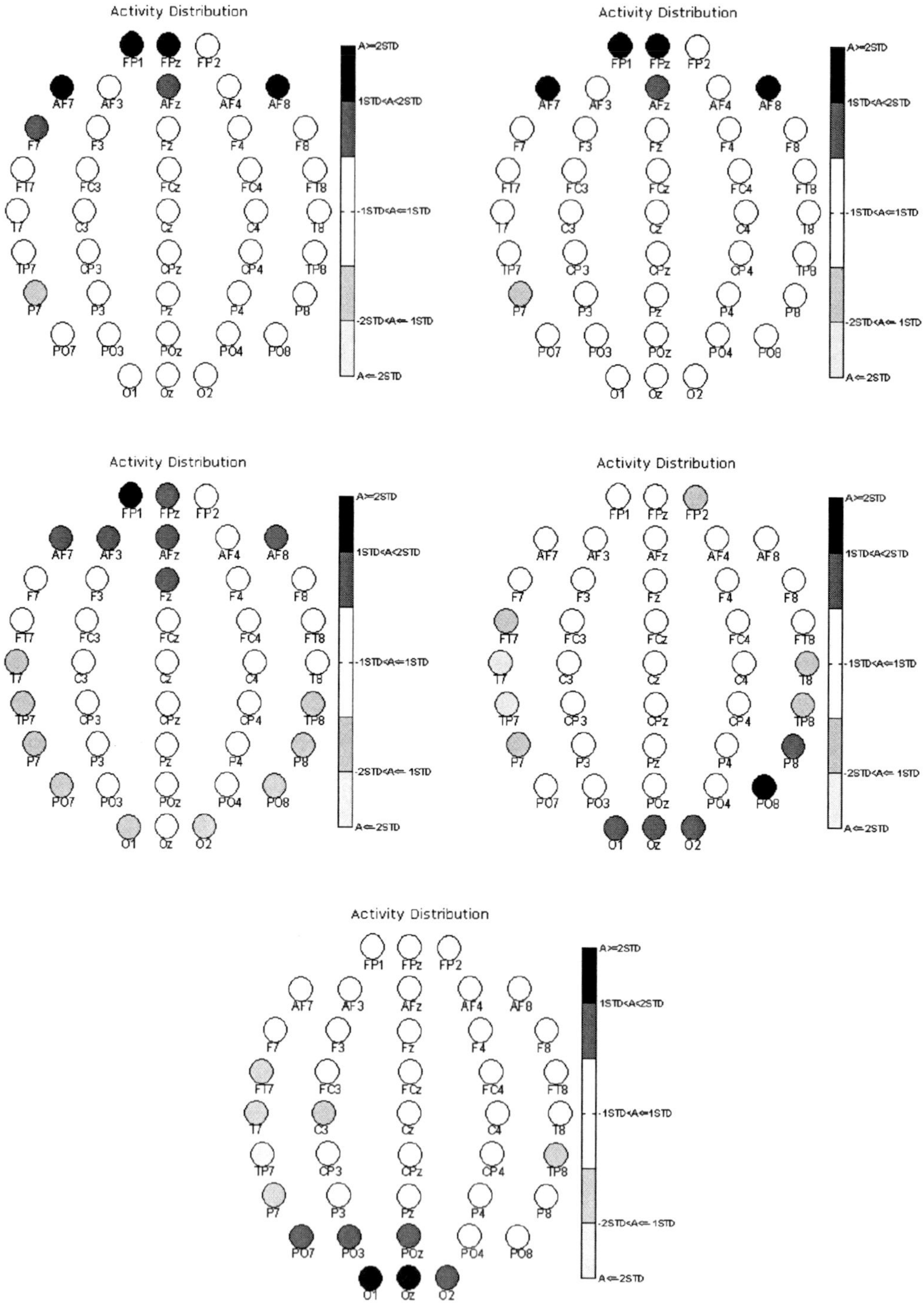

Figure 11. Illustrative frequency activities (Delta, Theta, Alpha, Beta 1, and Beat2) during the response phase for subject 3

3.3. Asymmetry Analysis

The results reveal that there were substantial but characterizing differences in hemispheric activation at the frontal, temporal, parietal, and occipital sites. Equation (7) was used to calculate the asymmetry ratio, which relates left hemisphere activation to the right hemisphere activation.

$$K = \frac{(R - L)}{(R + L)} \tag{7}$$

with K denoting the asymmetry ratio, and where R and L representing the number of electrodes active in the right and left hemisphere, respectively. The active electrodes are considered to be the ones that present activation values greater than one standard deviation or better, as aforementioned. Thus, if the ratio is negative, that means that the left hemisphere was more active than the right and vice versa if the ratio is positive.

As an illustration of the results based on this asymmetry ratio, Figure 12 consolidates the results of the 9 subjects considered out of the 15 tested by computing the centroids of activity. A decision to exclude 6 subjects was made in view of the artifacts, such as body movements or eye blinks present in the EEG. Nevertheless, further analysis would have required preprocessing to identify or remove these artifacts (Adjouadi et al., 2004 and 2005) on those excluded subjects.

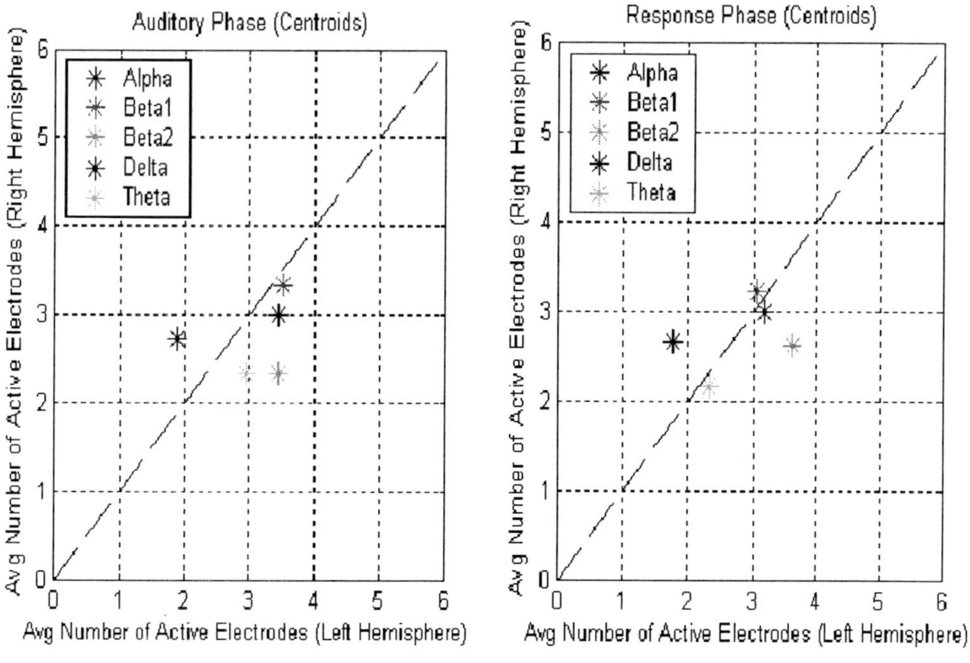

Figure 12. Centroids of activity of the right and left hemispheres for all subjects in terms of auditory (left) vs. response (right) phases

The centroids are defined in terms of the x and y axes for each one of the frequency bands analyzed, which correspond to the average number of electrodes found to be active in the left and right hemisphere, respectively. Note that during the auditory phase, there was more activation in the left hemisphere; nevertheless during the response phase, there was also some activation in the right hemisphere.

4. Conclusion

A thorough examination of EEG recordings through the eigensystem reveals that eigenvectors associated with the largest eigenvalues produce an activity pattern located in the frontal area of the brain directly attributable to those characteristic behaviors found in the Alpha, Beta, Delta, and Theta frequency bands. The corresponding eigenvalues and eigenvectors reveal that during the auditory phase, the majority of the subjects have the highest standard deviation of the eigenvalues located in the frontal left area of the brain. Nevertheless, the majority of the subjects analyzed during the response phase have the highest value of the standard deviation in the right frontal part of the brain. These results using the standard deviation come in support of the results supported earlier. The integration of the two studies (time and frequency domain) constitutes a unified method for assessing EEG activity during an auditory/response session. The regions of activity found in this study conform to earlier findings suggesting involvement of the Broca's and Wernicke's areas.

During the auditory/comprehension phase, changes in the beta frequency, which is involved with mental activity, are more predominant in the left hemisphere. This corroborates the premise that the left hemisphere is associated with more logical thought patterns and analytical approaches to problem solving (Happe et al. 2002; Kholosi et al. 1999). Changes in the delta band, the slowest frequency that is associated with less concentration, are predominant in the right hemisphere (McEvoy et al. 2001). The right hemisphere dominance is associated more with relatively less skill in logical thoughts. Theta frequency activity is evidently increased in the frontal region of the brain during the auditory-comprehension phase. This concurred with previous research that claims that theta activity is increased during internal focus (Gevins et al. 2000). Evident changes of alpha activity are observed in the parietal and frontal regions of the brain. These results are in agreement with previous studies that claim that EEG alpha rhythm in response to manipulations of task practice shows activity in the frontal and parietal regions (Mizuki 1987; Matsuoka 1990). During the response phase, it is revealed that the frontal region is the one that is more active. Since Broca's area is located in the frontal lobe and it is associated with the production of language, the positive changes of most of the frequency bands are concentrated in the frontal cortex (Martini 2001). With respect to the decreasing changes, the alpha band seems to localize its activity in the temporal and parietal lobes of both hemispheres, even though the activity is more oriented to the left hemisphere than to the right.

The main contribution of this study was is in validating brain functional mappings associated with the characterization effects of an auditory/comprehension task. When compared to existing methods, the contribution of the proposed algorithm is that it determines which areas in the brain are more active during these specific tasks by performing a unique eigensystem analysis. There is also the added value in relating in a unique way the standard deviation of the eigenvalues together with an optimum index (independent of region size) to the different brain activities. Through the development of this automated algorithm, clinical practitioners will be able to obtain detailed topographical brain maps and visualize them in order to learn which cortical lobes of the brain are active during an auditory comprehension test. Also, since the development of the algorithm is base on a non-invasive technique EEG-based technique, the method proposed can be easily implemented in a clinical environment.

Acknowledgments

This research was supported by the National Science Foundation Grants EIA-9906600, HRD- 0317692, CNS 042615, and the Office of Naval Research Grant N00014-99-1-0952, as well as the NSF Graduate Research Fellowship in support of Ms. Mercedes Cabrerizo. The support of Miami Children's Hospital is greatly appreciated.

References

Adjouadi, M., Sanchez, D., Cabrerizo, M., Ayala, M., Jayakar, P., Yaylali, I., and Barreto A., Interictal Spike Detection Using the Walsh Transform. *IEEE Transactions on Biomedical Engineering,* 51 (5), 2004: 868-873.

Adjouadi, M., Cabrerizo, M., Ayala, M., Sanchez, D., Jayakar, P., Yaylali, I., and Barreto, A., A New Approach to the Analysis of Epileptogenic Data Using Statistically Independent Operators, *Journal of Clinical Neurophysiology*, Vol 22(1), pp. 53-64, January/February 2005.

Duda, R. O., Hart, P.E., and Stork, D.G, *Pattern Classification*, John Wiley and Sons, 2001, New York.

Gevins, A.S. and Remond, A., Methods of analysis of brain electrical and magnetic signals, Handbook of Electroencephalography and Clinical Neurophysiology, Vol. 1: *Methods of Analysis of Brain Electrical and Magnetic Signals*, Elsevier: Amsterdam, 1987.

Gevins, A., and Smith, M. E., Neurophysiological measures of working memory and individual differences in cognitive ability and cognitive style, Cerebral Cortex, 2000, 10: 829-839.

Gonzalez, R. C. and Woods, R. E., *Digital Image Processing*, Prentice Hall, New Jersey; 2nd edition, 2002.

Greenstein, B. and Greenstein, A., Color atlas of neuroscience, *Neuroanatomy and Neurophysiology,* Thieme Stuttgart New York, 2000.

Happe, S., Anderer, P., Gruber G., Klösch, G., Saletu, B., and Zeitlhofer J., Scalp topography of the spontaneous k-complex and of delta-waves in human sleep, *Brain Topogra*phy, 2002, 15(1): 29-36.

Kholosi, M., McIntosh, A., Heath, B., Lithgow, B., and Cosic I., An analysis of brain waves by a 'thought comparator' to facilitate responsive functioning of electrical devices, *Proc.*

of the Inaugural Conference of the Victorian Chapter of the IEEE Engineering in Medicine and Biology Society, Caulfield, Vic, 22-23 Feb 99, 80 - 83, 1999.

Lokhorst, G. J. C., The first theory about hemispheric specialization: Fresh light on an old codex, *Journal of the History of Medicine and Allied Sciences*, 1996, 51(3): 293-312.

Martini, F. H., *Fundamentals of anatomy and physiology*, fifth edition, Prentice Hall, New Jersey, 2001.

Matsuoka, S., Theta rhythms: states of consciousness, Brain Topography, 1990, 3(1): 203-207.

McEvoy, L. K., Pellouchoud, E., Smith, M. E., and Gev*ins, A., Neurophysiological signals of working memory in normal aging,* Cognitive Brain Research, 2001, 11: 363-376.

Misiti, M., Misiti Y., Oppenhein, G., and Poggi, J., *Wavelet toolbox user's guide*, MathWorks Inc, 1996.

Mizuki, Y., Frontal Lobe: Mental function and EEG, *Am. J. EEG Technol*, 1987 (27):91-101.

Proakis, J. G. and Dimitris, G. M., *Digital signal processing - principles, algorithms and applications*, Prentice Hall, Third Edition, 1996.

Soong, A. C. K. and Koles, Z. J., Principal-Component localization of the sources of the background EEG. *Biomedical Engineering*, IEEE Transactions on, 1995, 42(1): 59-67.

Vetterli, M. and Kovacevic, J., Wavelets and subband coding, Prentice Hall, NJ, 1995.

Woodcock, R., McGrew, K., and Mather, N., *Woodcock-Johnson III*, Riverside Publishing Company, 2001.

Zhukov, L., Weinstein, D., and Johnson, C., Independent component analysis for EEG source localization, *IEEE Engineering in Medicine and Biology Magazine*, 2000, 19(3):87-96.

In: Progress in Brain Mapping Research
Editor: F. J. Chen, pp. 205-229
ISBN 1-59454-580-4

Chapter 6

New Dimension of Cognitive Neuroscience Research with Near-Infrared Spectroscopy: Free-Motion Neuroimaging Studies

Yoko Hoshi[7], and Shing-Jen Chen[2]
[1]Department of Integrated Neuroscience, Tokyo Institute of Psychiatry
[2]Research and Clinical Center for Child Development,
Graduate School of Education, Hokkaido University

Abstract

Near-infrared spectroscopy (NIRS) is a completely non-invasive neuroimaging technique, which does not require strict motion restriction and can be used in a daily life environment. Especially, a portable NIRS instrument combined with a wireless telemetry system (the wearable NIRS system) allows subjects to move during measurements like with portable ECG and EEG instruments. Thus, NIRS enables neuroimaging studies on children, the elderly, and patients with psychoneurological problems, who have not been fully examined until now. Yet several challenges that the NIRS field has spent more than 25 years attempting to overcome remain unsolved. These limiting factors in advancement of NIRS are addressed here: (1) light propagation in the human head remains unexplained, (2) detecting signals that resulted from the cerebral hemodynamic changes, poses a substantial challenge, (3) achieving data quantification requires a considerable amount of research. Nevertheless, its advantages of complete noninvasiveness and ease in operation are expected to provide new directions of neuroimaging studies that other neuroimaging techniques are unable to offer. This chapter focuses on free-motion neuroimaging studies, a novel neuroimaging study, with the wearable NIRS system. We also describe the basic theory, techniques, problems, and future prospects of NIRS.

---

[7] Corresponding address: Yoko Hoshi. Department of Integrated Neuroscience, Tokyo Institute of Psychiatry 2-1-8 Kamikitazawa, Setagaya-ku, Tokyo 156-8585 Japan. Tel: +81-3-3304-5701; Fax: +81-3-3329-8035 ; e-mail: yhoshi@prit.go.jp

Introduction

Near-infrared spectroscopy (NIRS), a noninvasive optical technique, can measure changes in hemoglobin (Hb) concentrations in the brain tissue. In 1977, Jöbsis first described the in vivo application of NIRS (Jöbsis, 1977), and the application of NIRS is gaining ground in clinically monitoring tissue oxygenation (Brazy et al., 1985; Rea et al., 1985; Wyatt et al., 1986). Furthermore, NIRS is also being employed in human brain mapping, referred to as functional near-infrared spectroscopy (fNIRS), as our team, as well as others, demonstrated NIRS had the potential to perform neuroimaging studies in 1993 (Hoshi et al., 1993a; Kato et al., 1993; Villringer et al., 1993). Current advancement in NIRS technologies enabled several types of NIRS instruments to be commercially available. Among them, instruments for continuous wave (CW) measurements based on the modified Beer-Lambert law (CW-type instruments), which include the earliest NIRS instruments, are readily available commercially. Instruments of this type allow us to observe dynamic changes in regional cerebral blood flow (rCBF) in real time by measuring concentration changes in cerebral Hb. Using NIRS, several types of brain activities, such as motor and cognitive activities have been assessed (Colier et al., 1999; Heekeren et al., 1997; Sato et al., 1999; Shimada et al., 2004; Tanosaki et al., 2001). NIRS is completely non-invasive, does not require strict motion restriction and can be used in a daily life environment, it enables neuroimaging studies on children, the elderly, and patients with psychoneurological problems who have not been fully examined until now because of difficulty in measuring by other neuroimaging techniques, such as PET (positron emission tomography) and fMRI (functional magnetic resonance imaging). Furthermore, a portable NIRS instrument combined with a wireless telemetry system (the wearable NIRS system) allows subjects to move during measurements i.e., portable ECG and EEG instruments. Thus, it is also expected that NIRS provides new directions for cognitive neuroscience research, such as assessments of the brain activity during dynamic movements.

At the same time, the accuracy and reliability of NIRS have not yet been widely accepted. This is mainly attributable to incomplete knowledge of which region in the brain is sampled by near-infrared (NIR) light, difficulty in selective detection of NIRS signals arising from the cerebral tissue, and the problem of quantification. Despite a number of theoretical and experimental investigations, NIR light propagation in the human head remains to be fully understood. It has been the major problem with NIRS that concentration changes in Hb cannot be quantified with CW-type instruments, which has hindered NIRS from being widely employed in clinical medicine and research. Over the past 25 years, work in the field of NIRS has concentrated on solving this problem. Many different approaches to quantification have been tried, and the quantitative accuracy of time-resolved spectroscopy (TRS) and phase-resolved spectroscopy (PRS) have been established. However, the difficulty of quantification has not yet been completely overcome (see PROBLEMS OF NIRS). Because of the problem of quantification, amplitude of NIRS signals cannot be compared between subjects and/or regions within a given subject. However, such comparisons have actually been made on an invalid assumption in a large number of published studies. Recently, cross-talk between oxygenated (oxy-Hb) and deoxygenated hemoglobin (deoxy-Hb) estimated by NIRS has also been argued as a potential source of error (Strangman et al., 2003; Uludağ et al., 2004).

Although there remain many problems to be solved, the potential benefits of NIRS are considerable. NIRS allows new neuroimaging studies that are different from those with PET and fMRI. It is thus expected that NIRS will open new dimensions in brain research and clinical applications. In this chapter, we will first outline the basic principles of NIRS, which will aid in understanding the potential and limitations of the technique. Then, we will give an example of a novel application of NIRS, a free-motion neuroimaging study with the wearable NIRS system, and also clarify the problems and identify the limitations of NIRS measurements. Finally, its future prospects will be described.

Near-Infrared Spectroscopy

Near-infrared (NIR) light, especially between 700 and 900 nm, easily passes through biological tissue because the light in this region is less scattered and absorbed by only a few biological chromophores such as hemoglobin (Hb), myoglobin (Mb), and cytochrome oxidase (CytOx) in mitochondria. The spectra of Hb and Mb in the NIR region vary with their oxygenation states. The spectrum of CytOx also varies with its oxidation state. Thus, by measuring the transmitted light through the tissue we can obtain information about the oxygenation-deoxygenation states of Hb and Mb and the oxidation-reduction state (the redox state) of CytOx. Many different types of NIRS measurements, which are associated with each type of instrumentation, have been developed. In the following sections, three main categories of NIRS measurements are described: continuous wave (CW), time-domain (TRS), and frequency-domain (PRS) measurements.

1. Continuous Wave Measurement (CW Measurement)

In CW-type instruments, the light sources (laser diodes, LDs or light emitting diodes, LEDs) emit light continuously at constant amplitude and the light intensity detected at a position a few centimeters away from the incident point is measured (Fig. 1A). Instruments of this type calculate relative concentration changes in chromophores according to the modified Beer-Lambert law (Eq. 1) (Delpy et al., 1988),

$$A = -\log I/I_0 = \varepsilon CL + S \qquad \text{(Eq. 1)}$$

where I and I_0 are the intensities of detected and incident light, respectively, ε is the molar absorption coefficient, C is concentration, and L is the length that light travels through the tissue (optical pathlength), and S denotes optical attenuation mainly due to scattering.

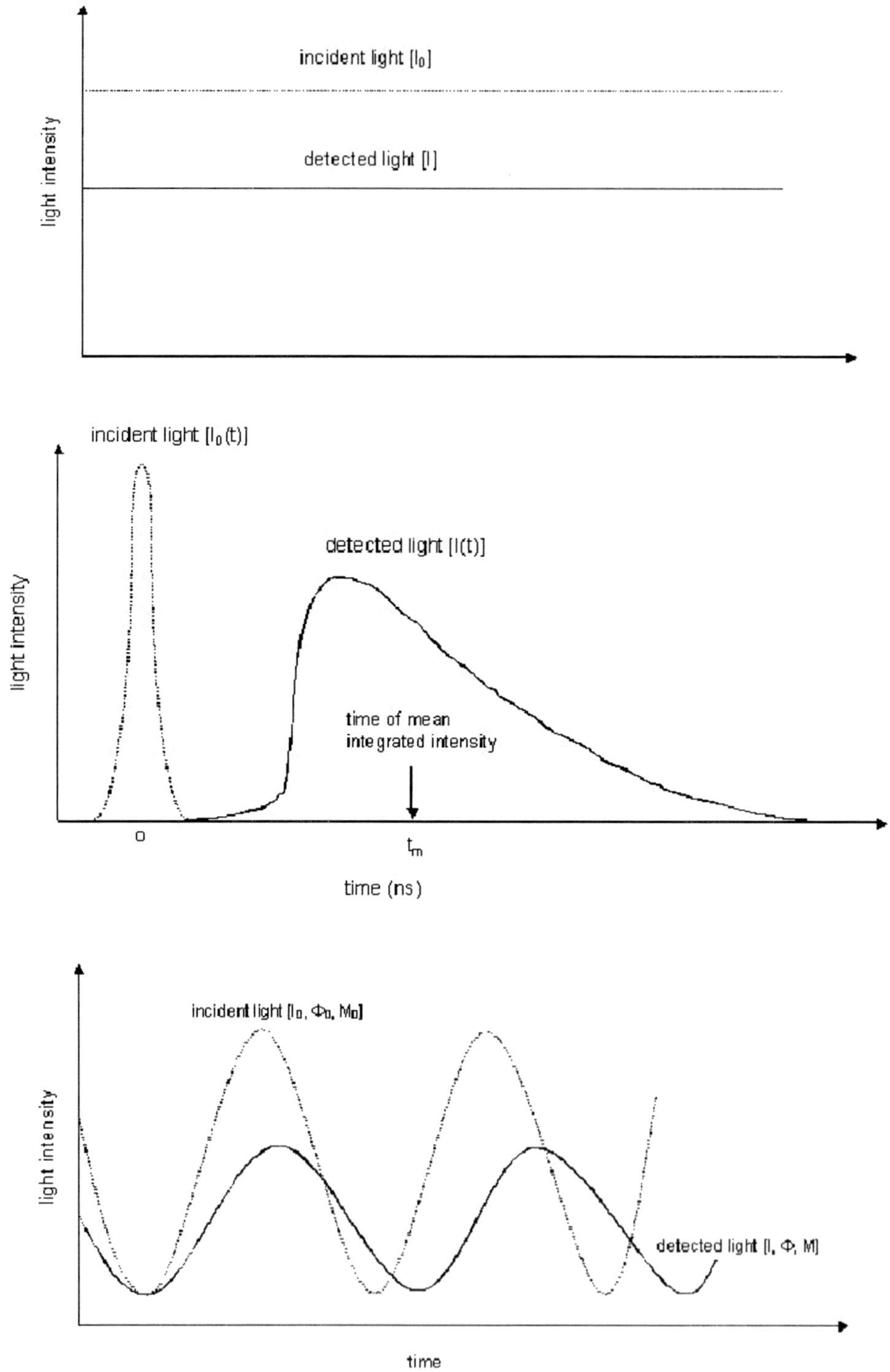

Figure 1. Schematic illustration of the three main types of NIRS measurements. A, continuous wave measurement; B, time-domain measurement; C, frequency-domain measurement; I, intensity; Φ, phase shift; M, modulation depth

When the scalp is illuminated by light of a certain wavelength (λ_1), absorbance ($A_{\lambda 1}$) is written as

$$A_{\lambda 1} = \varepsilon_{\lambda 1}[\text{oxy-Hb}]L_{\lambda 1} + \varepsilon'_{\lambda 1}[\text{deoxy-Hb}]L_{\lambda 1} + \varepsilon''_{\lambda 1}[\text{oxidizedCytOx}]L_{\lambda 1} + S_{\lambda 1}, \quad \text{(Eq. 2)}$$

where [oxy-Hb], [deoxy-Hb], [oxidized CytOx] are concentrations of oxygenated hemoglobin, deoxygenated hemoglobin, and oxidized CytOx, respectively. To minimize the effect of $S_{\lambda 1}$, a dual-wavelength method is often used, in which absorbance differences between measurement and reference wavelengths ($A_{\lambda 1} - A_{\lambda r} = A_{\lambda 1-r}$) are calculated. When the condition changes from one to another, $S_{\square 1-r}$ can be considered a constant. In the case that concentration changes in each chromophore are global within the head, the change in the absorbance difference ($\Delta A_{\lambda 1-r}$) is expressed as

$$\Delta A_{\lambda 1-r} = \varepsilon_{\lambda 1-r}\,\Delta\,[\text{oxy-Hb}]L_{\lambda 1-r} + \varepsilon'_{\lambda 1-r}\,\Delta\,[\text{deoxy-Hb}]\,L_{\lambda 1-r} + \varepsilon''_{\lambda 1-r}\,\Delta\,[\text{oxidized CytOx}]\,L_{\lambda 1-r} \quad \text{(Eq. 3)}$$

For measurements of living tissue, such as brain tissue, multiple wavelengths are used and Eq. 3 stands for each pair of wavelengths. By solving the simultaneous equations on the assumption that $L_{\lambda n-r}$ is the same for all pairs of measurement and reference wavelengths, and constant during the measurement period, concentration changes in oxy-Hb, deoxy-Hb, and oxidized CytOx are calculated. Summation of changes in oxy-Hb and deoxy-Hb provides the changes in total hemoglobin (t-Hb). The optical pathlength (total pathlength, t-PL) is longer than the distance between the source and detector because of the scattering effects. When the change in concentrations is not global, for example, regional brain activation, the optical pathlength in Eq. 3 is replaced by a partial pathlength (p-PL) through a region of uniform absorption change (Fig. 2).

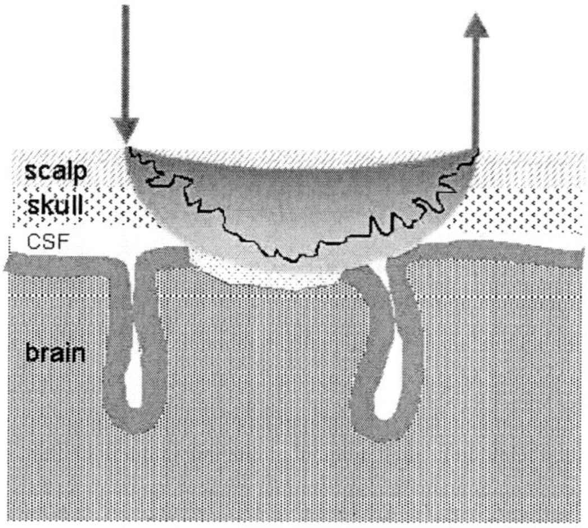

Figure 2. Schematic representation of NIR light traveling through the head. The pink dotted area denotes cortical activation. Determination of the pathlength through this region (p-PL) is required for quantification of cerebral Hb concentration changes

Since CW-type instruments cannot measure either t-PL or p-PL, instruments of this type do not provide absolute values of concentration changes but rather relative ones with an arbitrary unit (a. u.). However, the temporal resolution of CW-type instruments is high (in general, faster than 500 msec) and they allow continuous measurement for a prolonged time.

The redox state of CytOx is very useful for monitoring tissue oxygenation. Because changes in the redox state of CytOx, however, occur only under severely hypoxic conditions (Hoshi et al., 1997a), CytOx is not measured in neuroimaging studies with NIRS.

2. Time-Domain Measurement (Time-Resolved Spectroscopy, TRS)

In time-resolved spectroscopy (TRS), ultrashort (picosecond order) laser pulses are applied to the tissue, and the emerging intensity is detected as a function of time (the temporal point spread function, TPSF) with picosecond resolution (Fig. 1B) (Chance et al., 1988; Deply et al., 1988). Because time-resolved instruments have been developed as laboratory-based devices, they are difficult to use in the clinical environment. However, recent advances in technology have made possible the development of a compact 64-channel time-resolved optical imaging system (Eda et al., 1999). A single-channel TRS instrument that will expand clinical applications of NIRS has also been developed and is commercially available (Oda et al., 1999).

A temporal profile of the intensity of the detected light has information about optical properties of the head, that is, grand absorption (μ_a) and reduced scattering (μ_s') coefficients of the scalp, skull, CSF (cerebrospinal fluid), and brain. Propagation of photons in the living tissue, which is assumed to be a homogeneous medium, can be described by the diffusion approximation (Eq. 4) (Ishimaru, 1978),

$$-\frac{1}{c}\frac{\partial\varphi(\mathbf{r},t)}{\partial t} = \nabla[D(\mathbf{r})\nabla\varphi(\mathbf{r},t)] - \mu_a(\mathbf{r})\varphi(\mathbf{r},t) + S(\mathbf{r},t) \qquad \text{(Eq. 4)}$$

where $\varphi(\mathbf{r}, t)$ is the diffuse photon fluence rate at position $\boldsymbol{r}$ and the time t, c is the speed of light in the tissue, $D = 1/3\ \mu_s'\ (\boldsymbol{r})$ is the optical diffusion coefficient, μ_a is the absorption coefficient, μ_s' is the reduced scattering coefficient and $S(r, t)$ is the photon source. For a semi-infinite half-space geometry, the solution of Eq. 4 for the impulse input is expressed by Eq. 5 (Patterson et al., 1989),

$$R(l, t) = \frac{z_0\exp(-\mu_a ct)}{(4\pi Dct)^{3/2}\, t}\exp\left[-\frac{l^2 + z_0^2}{4Dct}\right] \qquad \text{(Eq. 5)}$$

where R (l, t) is the intensity of the reflected light, l and t are the distance and time from the impulse input, respectively, and $z_0 = 1/\mu_s$'. By fitting Eq. 5 to the observed temporal profiles,

μ_a and μ_s' are determined. As with CW measurements, using multiple wavelengths and determining μ_a for each wavelength, absolute values of Hb concentrations in the head are estimated.

The mean transit time of scattered photons is calculated from TPSF (t_m in Fig. 1B). The mean total optical pathlength (t-PL) is determined by multiplying light speed in the media by the mean transit time of scattered photons. It should be noted, however, that the mean t-PL determined by TRS measurements of the head is a summation of partial optical pathlengths (p-PLs) within the cerebral and extracerebral tissues.

3. Frequency-Domain Measurement (Phase-Resolved Spectroscopy, PRS)

The information contained in the temporal profile of the emerging light intensity through TRS can also be obtained by phase-resolved spectroscopy (PRS), the relation between the time and frequency information being the Fourier transform (Duncan et al., 1993; Sevic et al., 1991). In frequency-domain instruments, the light source is intensity-modulated at radio frequencies, and measurements are made not only of the detected light intensity (I), but also of its phase shift (Φ) and modulation depth (M) with respect to the incident light (Fig. 1C) (Lackowiz et al., 1990). It has been demonstrated that for typical tissues, and at frequencies below 200 MHz, the phase shift is linearly related to the mean optical pathlength (Arridge et al., 1992). Frequency-domain methods are a low-cost alternative to pulse-based methods for time-resolved methods. Several multichannel frequency-domain instruments are now in common use (Toronov et al., 2001)

NIR Light Propagation in the Head

Knowledge about which regions in the brain are sampled by NIRS light is still incomplete, although a number of theoretical and experimental investigations on NIR light propagation in the human head have been performed (Boas et al., 2002; Firbank et al., 1998; Fukui et al., 2003; Gratton et al., 1994). Recent models for the theoretical analysis of light propagation in the head are based on an inhomogeneous structure. These models consist of multiple layers, such as the scalp, skull, CSF, and the brain, which can be divided into the gray and white matters (Okada et al., 1997). Theoretical analyses of models consisting of three- or four-layered slabs, the latter incorporating a clear CSF layer, have demonstrated that light propagation in the adult head is highly affected by the presence of a low-scattering CSF layer (Okada et al., 1997). This indicated that the light penetration in the adult brain might be limited to the outer cortical gray matter, which has been confirmed by their later study, in which light propagation in head models generated from an MRI scan was predicted by Monte Carlo simulation (Firbank et al., 1998). A more recent study has reported that a large source-detector spacing only broadens the sampling region on the brain surface and affects the penetration depth in the adult head to a lesser degree, whereas the intensely sensitive region in the neonatal head is confined in the gray matter; however, the deeper region of the white matter is sampled with a large source-detector spacing (Fukui et al., 2003). In theoretical analysis, optical properties in each layer of the head are critical for prediction of the light propagation, though μ_a and μ_s' in each layer used for analysis are different from study to study. This is attributable to the fact that in situ measurements of the optical properties are not feasible. Thus, further investigation is required to confirm the validity of the theoretically predicted light propagation.

Interpretation of NIRS Signals

1. NIRS Signals in Activated Areas

Regional brain activation is accompanied by increases in rCBF and the regional cerebral oxygen metabolic rate ($rCMRO_2$). It is widely accepted that the degree of the increase in rCBF exceeds that of the increase in $rCMRO_2$ (Fox et al., 1986), which results in a decrease in deoxy-Hb in venous blood. Thus, increases in t-Hb and oxy-Hb with a decrease in deoxy-Hb are expected to be observed in activated areas in NIRS measurements (Fig. 3). However, deoxy-Hb and t-Hb do not necessarily show these changes: no change in t-Hb with an increase in oxy-Hb and a reciprocal decrease in deoxy-Hb, and an increase or no change in deoxy-Hb accompanying increases in t-Hb and oxy-Hb were observed (Hoshi et al., 1993b; Kato et al., 1993; Kleinschmidt et al., 1996).

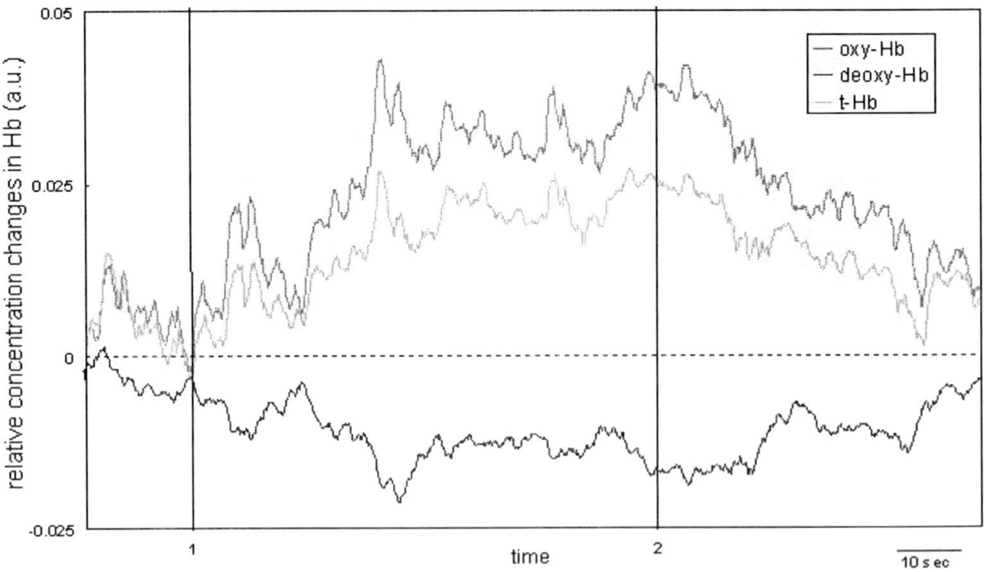

Figure 3. Changes in oxy-Hb, deoxy-Hb, and t-Hb in the left frontal region during the performance of a mental task (random number generation task). The task was performed between 1 and 2. Baselines were selected from the resting state, and these values are taken as zero for each signal. Changes from baseline are represented as a relative amount with an arbitrary unit. Upward (plus) and downward (minus) trends show increases and decreases in values, respectively

Comparing cerebral hemodynamic signals obtained simultaneously by NIRS and fMRI, some labs have reported that deoxy-Hb measured optically does not necessarily decrease in BOLD-fMRI signal increased areas (Hess et al., 2000; Kleinschmidt et al., 1996), while others have observed simultaneous reduction of deoxy-Hb in activation areas detected by fMRI (Tronov et al., 2001). Hess et al., (2000) have hypothesized that the hemodynamic basis of BOLD-fMRI signals is not necessarily a washout of deoxy-Hb, as is generally assumed. Instead, a positive BOLD signal can also be caused by a local increase of blood volume, even if deoxy-Hb levels are persistently elevated. Using a newly developed perfused rat brain model, we recently examined direct effects of each change in CBF and $CMRO_2$ on cerebral hemoglobin oxygenation to interpret NIRS signals (Hoshi et al., 2001). We confirmed that directions of changes in oxy-Hb are always the same as those of rCBF, whereas the direction of changes in deoxy-Hb is determined by changes in venous blood oxygenation and volume. It has also been confirmed that small changes in CBF are not accompanied by those in t-Hb. Thus, oxy-Hb is the most sensitive indicator of changes in rCBF in NIRS measurements.

2. Fluctuations in NIRS Signals at Rest

CW measurements have revealed that even under resting conditions, the Hb oxygenation state fluctuates (Hoshi et al., 1997b; Toronov et al., 2000). These fluctuations are divided into two types. One is fluctuations whose general patterns are systemic and that are related to such physiological activities as the systemic arterial pulse oscillations (~1 Hz) and respiration (0.2-0.3 Hz). The other is slower hemoglobin waves (frequency < 0.05 Hz), of which the temporal pattern varies with each brain region. It is well known that the cerebral blood flow velocity (CBFV) measured by transcranial Doppler ultrasound shows slow oscillation, which is thought to be attributed to small pial artery oscillations (Auer et al., 1983; Lindegaard et al., 1987). The frequency and characteristics of fluctuations in the hemoglobin oxygenation state are similar to those of the CBFV oscillations. It is thus likely that the fluctuations in the hemoglobin oxygenation state also originate from small artery oscillations. Our simultaneous measurements with NIRS and EEG have suggested the possibility that these oscillations are a result of vasomotor responses to spontaneous neuronal activity (Hoshi et al., 1998). Both the faster and slower fluctuations of the hemoglobin oxygenation state sometimes have amplitudes comparable with those of the signals evoked by functional activity. Thus, taking into account these fluctuations is critical for interpretation of NIRS signals.

Free-Motion Neuroimaging Studies with the Wearable NIRS System

NIRS has been used in a wide variety of studies on brain function (Colier et al., 1999; Heekeren et al., 1997; Horovitz et al., 2004; Sato et al, 1999; Schroeter et al., 2002; Shimada et al., 2004; Tanosaki et al., 2001). In earlier studies, which were performed with single- or two-channel instruments, the validity and accuracy of NIRS were confirmed by comparing with results obtained from other neuroimaging modalities, whereas recent studies, which include measurements using multichannel NIRS instruments, have revealed new information about brain functions.

Measurements with less motion restriction in daily life environment open new dimensions in neuroimaging studies. Using a 30-channel CW-type instrument, Miyai et al. (2001) succeed in visualizing cortical activation patterns associated with human gait. Mere alternating foot movements activated regions similar to those associated with walking but the regions were less broad, while actual gait imagery increased activities of different regions. From these findings, they proposed the use of NIRS for evaluating cerebral activation patterns during pathological gait and rehabilitative intervention. To expand such free-motion neuroimaging studies, we have recently developed a single-channel wearable near-infrared (NIR) monitoring system, which allows subjects to move around during measurements and examiners to see hemodynamic changes in real time (Fig. 4). Here, we will report a preliminary study with this system, in which we examined the role of the frontopolar cortex in motor control in children.

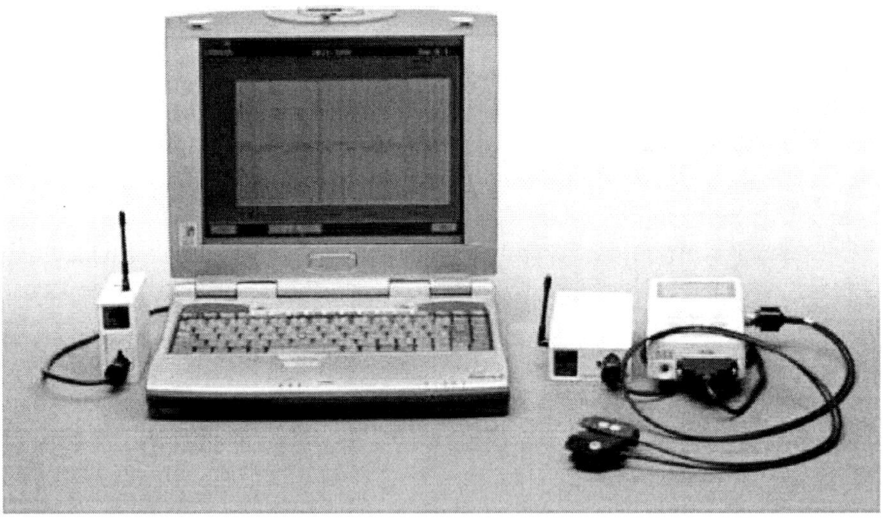

Figure 4. The wearable NIRS system.

1. The Objective

Several electrophysiological studies have indicated that the prefrontal cortex is at least partly related to a motor programming for various voluntary movements, which includes motor preparation, execution, judgment, motivation, and learning (Gemba, 2002). This is supported by the fact that motor behavior is often affected in individuals with prefrontal lesions, who do not even suffer from motor paralysis. Some interlimb coordination is inherent and present at birth (Fagard, 1994; Hirschfeld and Forssberg, 1994), whereas children's development of upper extremity control requires a rather extended learning process. It is, thus, supposed that the functional development of the prefrontal cortex is related to motor development in children. However, we remain largely in the dark regarding how the prefrontal cortex, especially the frontopolar cortex, which is thought to be essential for complex cognitive processing, contributes to motor control. In part, it is due to methodological limitations. PET, fMRI, and even multichannel NIRS are not appropriate to assess the brain activity during dynamic movements. In contrast, the wearable NIRS system is expected to be suitable for this aim. We, therefore, applied this system to examine brain activity-associated hemodynamic changes during voluntary movements in the frontopolar cortex of preschool and school children.

2. The Wearable NIRS System (Fig. 4)

The details of the portable NIRS instrument used here (HEO 200, Omron Ltd. Inc., Japan) have been reported elsewhere (Shiga et al., 1997). Briefly, it consists of a main unit and a probe unit. The main unit consists of a one-chip central processing unit (CPU), an LED driver, an amplifier, a memory card interface, a liquid crystal display, and a power source. The probe unit, molded in elastic black silicon rubber, has a photodiode (the detector) in the center and two-wavelength (760 and 840 nm) near-infrared LEDs (illuminators) on either side. This instrument is connected to the transmitter of a wireless system by an RS-232C cable. The size of the NIRS instrument (8 x 16 x 4 cm, 340 g) is about the same size as the transmitter of the wireless. These are packed in a small bag that a subject carries (Fig. 5B). NIRS signals are sent by wireless to the receiver, which is connected to a laptop computer, on which data are displayed in real time. NIRS signals can be transferred to a place at a maximum distance of 30 m in an open field, but about 10 m inside a building. This NIRS system makes it possible to monitor brain activity of freely-moving subjects outside of laboratories.

3. Subjects and Experimental Procedures

Twenty-three children (4-7 year-old, 10 boys, 13 girls) participated in this study. All the subjects except three were right-handed. As a control group, 6 adults (21-24 year-old, 3 males, 3 females, right-handed) were also examined. Both children and adult subjects were healthy by medical interview. Prior to each measurement, written informed consent was obtained from each child's parent and adult subject.

An illuminator and a detector with a separation of 3 cm were placed on the left forehead (BA 10). Changes in oxy-Hb were measured as an indicator of changes in rCBF during 4 motor paradigms: (1) asynchronous bimanual movement (ASBM), (2) tandem gait (TG), (3) walk and stop to a command (WS), and (4) reaching and pointing. Each motor paradigm consisted of a test and a control task. The control task was assumed to require less motor control than the test task. Each set of four tasks was performed in random order. In the ASBM task, the subjects were instructed to alternately have thumb and fingers extended with one hand simultaneously with making a fist with the other hand to a 1-Hz pacing sound for 60 seconds (Fig. 5A). In the control task, they were told to alternately have thumb and fingers extended and make a fist synchronously with the bilateral hands (synchronous bimanual movement, SBM). In the TG task, they were told to go back and forth on a balance beam twice. In the control task, they went back and forth on the floor at the same distance as the balance beam twice (control gait, CG). In the WS task, they were instructed to walk about in the gymnasium to a familiar song that was randomly interrupted for a brief time (2-5 seconds), in which they were told to stop (Fig. 5B). The duration of this task was about 70 seconds. In the control task, they simply walked about in the gymnasium to the same song that was not interrupted for about 55 seconds (walk, W). The ASBM and SBM tasks were repeated twice in a counterbalanced fashion, while the TG, CG, WS, and W tasks were performed only once. The TG and W tasks were followed by the CG and WS tasks, respectively.

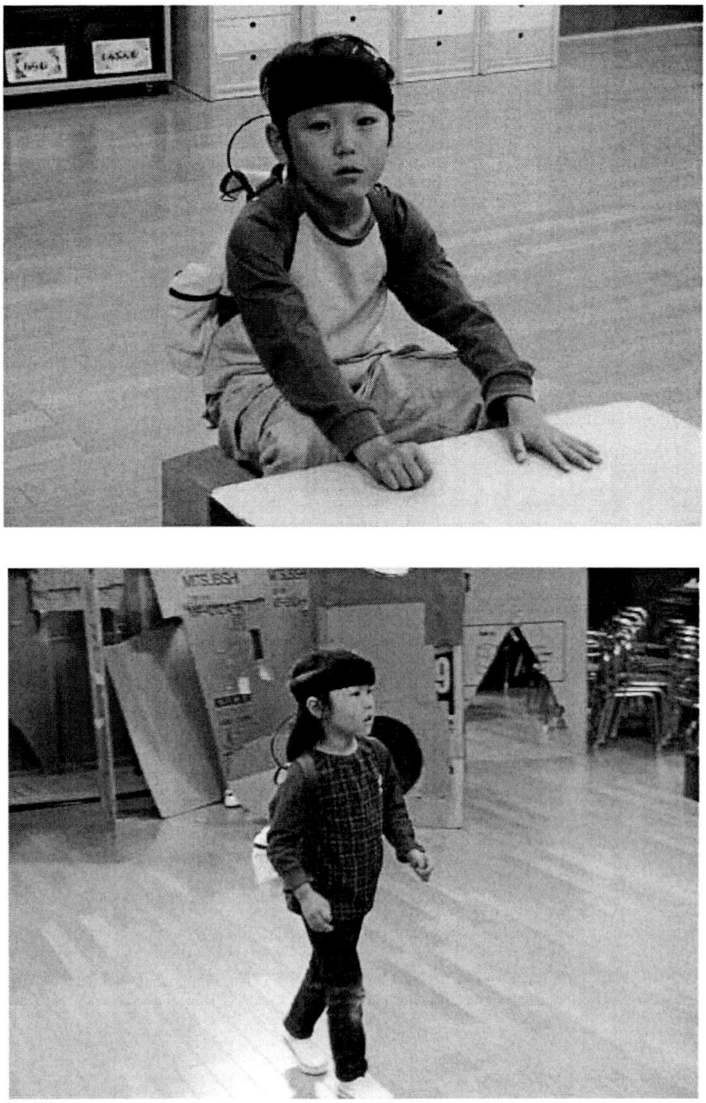

Figure 5. Measurement being performed using the wearable NIRS system. A, the boy performed the ASBM (asynchronous bimanual movement) task; B, the girl performed the WS (walk and stop) task

In the reaching and pointing task, the subjects sat on a chair in front of a 17-inch computer display, of which the center was at eye level and at an optimal distance so that a target could be easily pointed at with the arm near full extension. A target, which was a colored doughnut-shape (inner diameter, 12mm; outer diameter, 28mm; four colors, yellow, blue, pink, and green), and presented on the computer screen in a random location (Fig. 6A). The target remained on the screen for 2 seconds and then disappeared as the next target appeared. Subjects were instructed to rest their dominant index finger on their nose tip until the target appeared. Then, they were told to reach and point at the center of the target (the inner circle) and to return the hand to the resting position (reaching and pointing at a moving target, RPMT). Subjects also performed three control tasks: (1) reaching and pointing at a fixation target in the center of the screen (RPFT), which changed its color every 2 seconds (Fig. 6B), (2) looking at a moving target (LMT), (3) looking at a fixation target in the center of the screen (LFT).

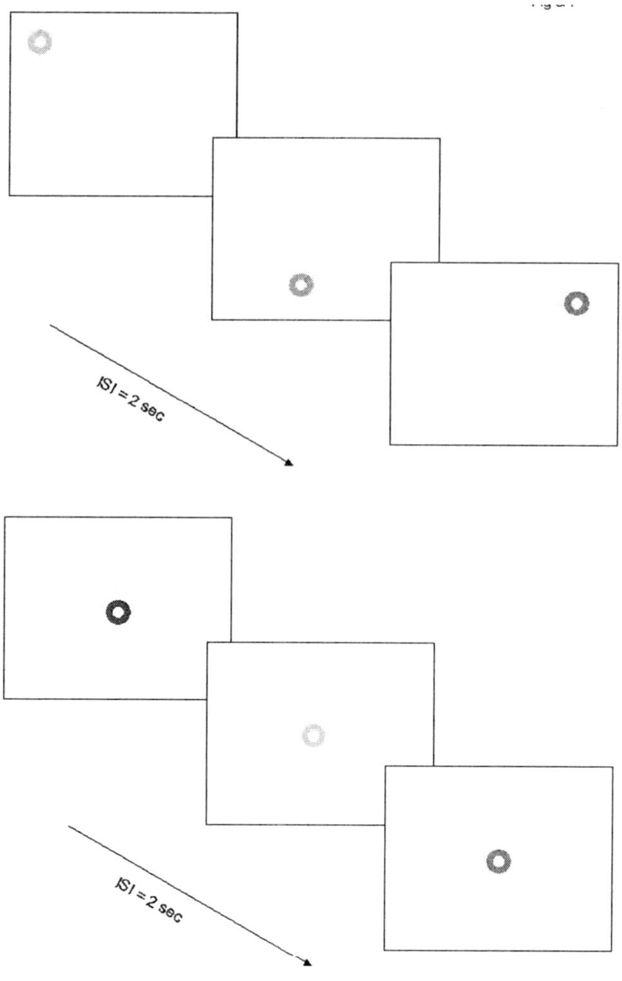

Figure 6. A The RPMT (reaching and pointing at a moving target) task; B, the RPFT (reaching and pointing at a central fixation target) task.

The target used in the control tasks was the same as that in the RPMT. In the RPFT, subjects were instructed to reach and point at the center of the target as in the RPMT when its color was changed. In the LMT and LFT tasks, they were told to simply look at the moving and fixation target, respectively. The duration of each control task was the same as that of the RPMT (60 seconds). Each task was performed once in a counterbalanced fashion. For performance measurements, the hand position was recorded by a video camera. Task performance was judged by numbers of pointing at the inner circle (IC), the colored ring (CR), and the outside of the target (O). Subjects practiced all the tasks for a couple minutes prior to the NIRS measurement.

4. Data Analysis

The value of oxy-Hb at the beginning of each task was taken as zero (the baseline) and calculated an average of changes during the task. A 20-second period just before the beginning of each task was defined as a resting state. The value at the point 20 seconds before the beginning of each task was taken as zero and calculated an average of changes in oxy-Hb during the resting state. Changes in oxy-Hb during each test task were compared with those during the corresponding control task or the resting state within subjects by paired t-test. Changes in oxy-Hb during each control task were also compared with those during the corresponding resting state. $P < 0.05$ was considered as a significant level.

5. Results and Discussion

Two children who could not perform the ASBM task and three children who fell from the balance beam were excluded from analysis. Figure 7 shows an example of NIRS trace, which was obtained from a 5-year-old boy during performing the three test and control tasks. Tables 1 and 2 summarize rCBF changes (oxy-Hb changes) during the three movement tasks (ASBM, TG, and WS) in children and adults, respectively. During the ASBM and SBM tasks, rCBF tended toward an increase in both children and adults, although such increases were not significant compared with the resting state. The degree of increases in rCBF during the SBM task was larger than that during the ASBM task in children ($P < 0,05$), while there was no difference in adults. Bimanual synchronous tasks are not difficult, since bimanual tasks are controlled as if they represented a single task and thus are controlled simultaneously by similar brain regions (Bernstein, 1967). Studies on the neural connectivity of the brain with monkeys have provided evidence for bilateral control originating from a single cortical source within the primary motor area that are active only during bimanual tasks (Aizawa et al., 1990). In contrast, bimanual asynchronous tasks, which might depend on sensory feedback to higher brain centers, require more concentration to maintain the asynchronous pattern (Wiesendanger et al., 1994). It is, thus, unexpected that the SBM tasks activated the frontopolar cortex more than the ASBM tasks in children. This might be related to the maturational processes of bimanual upper extremity control.

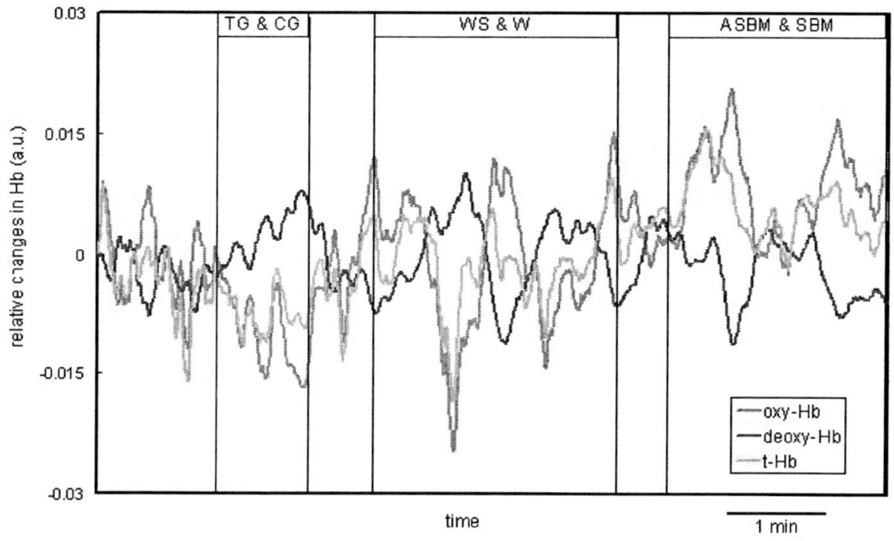

Figure 7. Changes in oxy-Hb, deoxy-Hb, and t-Hb during performing the TG (tandem gait), CG (control gait), WS (walk and stop), W (walk), ASBM (asynchronous bimanual movement), and SBM (synchronous bimanual movement) tasks in a 5-year-old boy

Table 1. Changes in CBF during each motor task in children

ASBM		TG		WS	
ASBM vs SBM	D	TG vs CG	ns	WS vs W	ns
ASBM vs Rest	ns	TG vs Rest	ns	WS vs Rest	D
SBM vs Rest	ns	CG vs Rest	ns	W vs Rest	D

ASBM, asynchronous bimanual movement; SBM, synchronous bimanual movement, TG, tandem gait; CG, control gait; WS, walk and stop; W, walk; D, decrease; ns, not significant ($p > 0.05$)

Table 2. Changes in CBF during each motor task in adults

ASBM		TG		WS	
ASBM vs SBM	ns	TG vs CG	ns	WS vs W	ns
ASBM vs Rest	ns	TG vs Rest	ns	WS vs Rest	D
SBM vs Rest	ns	CG vs Rest	ns	W vs Rest	D

ASBM, asynchronous bimanual movement; SBM, synchronous bimanual movement, TG, tandem gait; CG, control gait; WS, walk and stop; W, walk; D, decrease; ns, not significant ($p > 0.05$)

In contrast to the difference in rCBF changes between the ASBM and SBM tasks, no significant difference in rCBF changes was observed between the TG and CG tasks in either children or adults. Unlike upper extremity control, central pattern generators (CPGs), which refer to a grouping of neurons or neural circuits that can generate coordinated movements autonomously, for locomotion has been identified in the vertebrate spinal cord (Jankowska et al., 1967). Because CPGs generate coordinated locomotor movements, even in the absence of all movement-related afferent feedback (Grillner and Zangger, 1975; Grillner et al., 1976), the TG task might not require more cognitive processes than the CG task.

Since the WS task requires motor preparation, execution, and judgment, it was expected that the frontopolar cortex would be more activated during the WS task than during the W task. However, there were no significant differences in rCBF changes between the two tasks. Furthermore, rCBF during the WS and W tasks significantly decreased compared to those during the resting state. The task-related decrease in rCBF is explained by deactivation or stealing of blood flow. However, it is unlikely that deactivation of the left frontopolar cortex was required to walk about. It is rather conceivable that the illuminator-detector position in this study was adjacent to the activation area and blood flow at the NIRS sampling area was stolen to the activation area. In a series of our studies, we have often observed that the frontopolar cortex is activated during performing various cognitive tasks. Thus, another possible explanation is that mental activity arising spontaneously during the resting state, which activated the frontopolar cortex, was suppressed during performing the WS and W tasks.

Table 3. Task performance of the reaching and pointing task

No.	Age (y)	Sex	RPFT (control)			RPMT (test)		
			IC	CR	O	IC	CR	O
1	4	F	1	17	12	1	22	7
2	5	F	14	16	0	10	18	2
3	5	F	14	16	0	6	20	4
4	5	F	14	16	0	10	20	0
5	5	F	8	19	3	11	17	2
6	5	M	0	20	10	0	20	10
7	5	M	8	18	4	10	16	4
8	5	M	20	10	0	9	18	3
9	5	F	3	22	5	0	26	4
10	5	M	26	4	0	30	0	0
11	6	F	17	10	3	10	17	3
12	6	F	22	8	0	26	4	0
13	6	M	11	19	0	20	9	1
14	6	F	14	16	0	20	10	0
15	6	M	2	25	3	6	18	6
16	6	F	6	18	6	0	28	2
17	6	F	16	12	2	9	20	1
18	7	M	24	5	1	7	18	5
19	7	F	25	4	1	24	6	0
20	7	M	24	6	0	21	9	0
21	7	F	17	13	0	21	9	0

IC, inner circle; CR, colored ring; O, outside of the target; F, female: M, male

Two children who could not concentrate on the reaching and pointing task were excluded from further analysis. Table 3 shows subjects' task performance. As expected, older children showed better task performance. There were no differences in task performance between the RPMT and RPFT tasks. This explains no significant differences in rCBF changes between the RPMT and RPFT tasks (Table 4). Significant differences in rCBF changes were observed only between the RPMT and LMT tasks: the degree of increases in rCBF during the RPMT was smaller than that during the LMT task. It is likely that children were thinking of something during the LMT task, which induced increases in rCBF in the fontopoplar cortex. This also explains that the LFT task increased rCBF in several children (data not shown). In adults, directions of changes in rCBF during the three control tasks were an increase and differences in rCBF changes between the RPMT and each control task were significant (Table 5).

Increases in rCBF during the LMT and LFT tasks suggest the possibility that as in children, mental activity also occurred in the adult subjects while they were simply looking at the target. During the RPMT task, a tendency to a decrease in rCBF, which was not significant compared with the resting state, was observed. A recent multichannel NIRS study has reported that the reaching task with and without the visual feedback delay caused deactivation indicated by decreases in oxy-Hb and t-Hb at the dorsolateral prefrontal area and the degree of decreases in oxy-Hb and t-Hb was larger in the delayed conditions than in the normal condition and as the subject made more errors (Shimada et al., 2004). The decreases in oxy-Hb and t-Hb were observed extensively over the measured frontal area involving a part of the frontopolar cortex, and it was speculated that prefrontal deactivation was related to the visuomotor recalibration process to suppress visuomotor responses. We might have detected the margin of such an extended deactivated area. Since children, however, did not show the tendency to a decrease in rCBF, further investigations are required to explain the tendency to a decrease in rCBF observed in adults.

Table 4. Changes in CBF during the reaching and pointing task in children

RPMT vs RPFT	RPMT vs LMT	RPMT vs LFT
ns	D	ns

RPMT, reaching and pointing at a moving target; RPFT, reaching and pointing at a central fixation target; LMT, looking at a moving target; LFT, looking at a central fixation target

Table 5. Changes in CBF during the reaching and pointing task in adults

RPMT vs RPFT	RPMT vs LMT	RPMT vs LFT
D	D	D

RPMT, reaching and pointing at a moving target; RPFT, reaching and pointing at a central fixation target; LMT, looking at a moving target; LFT, looking at a central fixation target

6. Conclusion

These results suggest that the area of the left frontopolar cortex measured in this study does not directly participate in the motor programming. To gain further insights into the role of the prefrontal cortex in motor control, measurements in multiple regions are required.

Thus, the instrumentation and data analysis of the technique are being improved to meet a multichannel system.

Problems of NIRS

1. Quantification of Cerebral Hb Concentration

Quantification of NIRS data has been a central issue in the NIRS field. When Hb concentration changes are global within the tissue, quantification is possible with TRS and PRS. In the case that Hb concentration changes are localized, such as functional brain activation, however, those changes cannot be quantified accurately. The optical pathlength determined by TRS and PRS is the mean t-PL but not the mean p-PL in the cerebral tissue. Since the t-PL is much longer than the p-PL (Firbank et al., 1998; Fukui et al., 2003), Hb concentration changes are underestimated when t-PL is substituted in the Eq. 3 (partial volume error). However, measurement of p-PL is not feasible. To quantify NIRS data obtained from CW measurements without measuring t-PL, the assumption that the ratio of the source-detector separation to the t-PL is constant has often been made (Delpy et al., 1988). Arranging the source-detector separation for each pair at the same time, in which the t-PL can be considered a constant if the assumption is correct, multichannel CW–type instruments generate topographical images of relative concentration changes in Hb. However, this assumption is not correct. The ratio of the source-detector separation to the t-PL (DPF, differential pathlength factor) (Deply et al., 1988) varies with each position (Zhao et al., 2002). Furthermore, the ratio of the p-PL to the t-PL varies with each wavelength and each measurement position (Hoshi et al., in press). Therefore, comparing amplitudes of data obtained by CW measurements is not valid for comparison of cerebral Hb concentration changes. This should be considered in the interpretation of topographical images produced by CW instruments.

The μ_a of the head estimated by TRS represents μ_a of the cerebral tissue rather than that of the extracerebral tissue, but is not equal to the former (Patterson et al., 1989; Steinbrink et al., 2001). Theoretical analyses with two-layered head models have demonstrated that when the μ_a of the upper layer is smaller than that of the lower layer, the estimated μ_a of the head is smaller than that of the lower layer (Kienle et al., 1998). Reported optical properties indicate that the μ_a of the extracerebral tissue is smaller than that of the cerebral tissue (Bevilacqua et al., 1999; Sassaroli et al., 2000; Simpson et al. 1998). Thus, accurate quantification of concentration change in cerebral Hb remains difficult.

Elimination of the effects of hemodynamic changes in the scalp, which occur on various occasions, such as doing physical exercises and performing mental tasks, is also a challenging issue. Methods to solve the two problems simultaneously are being explored. Diffuse optical tomography (DOT), which reconstructs images of Hb concentration changes using multiple light sources and detectors, is a potential technique for quantitative detection of focal changes in cerebral hemodynamics (Arridge, 1999). DOT is not based on the modified Beer-Lambert law and can be performed with a time-domain system (Gao et al., 2002), a frequency-domain system (Pogue, et al., 1995), and a CW system (Boas et al., 2004).

However, this technique, which requires multichannel instruments, is still in the developmental stage. TRS is also a potential tool for this purpose. The temporal profile of detected light intensity carries information about depth-dependent attenuation because light that penetrates into deeper positions in the head is detected later. Several time-domain methods to determine absorption changes with depth resolution have been proposed (Hielscher et al., 1996; Steibrink et al., 2001). While these methods were successful in certain cases, further investigation must be continued in order to apply them to human head measurements.

Cross-talk between oxy-Hb and deoxy-Hb was first shown in measurements in the visible light region by Mayhew et al. (Mayhew et al., 1999). They explained that it was related to the fact wavelength-dependent changes in optical pathlength are large in the visible light region, while in the NIR region the actual difference between the pathlengths at different wavelengths is rather slight. Recently, however, cross-talk has also become an issue in NIRS measurements. Strangman et al. reported that cross-talk was estimated by a function of wavelength (D) and a difference in the ratio of the partial pathlength to the total pathlength between two wavelengths, and that D quickly grew with wavelengths greater than approximately 770nm when paired with 830nm (Strangman et al., 2003). They and some other research groups have reported that appropriate wavelengths selection (e.g., 690nm and 830nm) can minimize cross-talk and improve signal-to-noise ratio (Strangman et al., 2003; Uludağ et al., 2004; Sato et al., 2004). However, it is still unknown whether wavelength-dependent partial pathlengths within the wavelength region of 750-850 nm, which is widely used for NIRS measurements, are actually large enough to cause cross-talk. Even though it is true, the other questions arise: is the path of light at 690nm the same as that at 830nm? In modified Beer-Lambert law, it is assumed that the unknown term G, which is dependent on the measurement geometry and the scattering coefficient of the tissue interrogated, does not change during the measurement period. It has not been confirmed that this assumption holds at 690nm. Thus, further investigations are required to settle this issue.

2. Practical Issues

Except for neonates, it is not feasible for NIRS to measure deep brain structures such as the diencephalons noninvasively. It is also difficult to identify the exact brain areas that are beneath the NIRS probes, which requires 3-D MRI measurements. However, it has been reported that there is an appropriate relationship between the international 10-20 system of electrode positioning in electroencephalogram and the cortical anatomy (Okamoto et al., 2004; Towle et al., 1993). Thus, the measured brain area can be roughly deduced by using the location of the 10-20 system as a landmark.

Data in functional mapping studies with PET and fMRI are usually analyzed with some form of statistical parametric mapping that refers to the construction of spatially extended statistical processes to test hypotheses about regionally specific effects in neuroimaging data (Friston et al., 1991). However, statistical parametric mapping cannot be directly applied to NIRS studies because there are too few measurement portions compared with the voxel numbers in PET and fMRI. The fact that NIRS data is time series data makes it more difficult to develop appropriate statistical analyses. Thus, standard approaches remain to be developed for the analysis of NIRS data.

Future Prospects

As was mentioned in the previous section, there remain a number of technical issues to be explored and practical difficulties to be solved. Nevertheless, NIRS, especially multichannel wearable NIRS, is a tool distinct from other neuroimaging techniques for studies of brain functions and for the diagnosis, assessment and treatment of psychoneurological diseases. Thus, there will be a variety of novel applications of NIRS. For example, the multichannel NIRS wearable system enables us to detect hemodynamic changes associated with various unpredictable symptoms, such as hallucination, headache, and partial complex seizures.

NIRS-based brain computer interface (BCI) is another potential application of NIRS. BCI has been given much attention recently as an alternate mode of communication and control for the disabled, such as patients suffering from amyotrophic lateral sclerosis (ALS) or "locked-in" patients (Donoghue, 2002; Wolpaw et al., 2002). Most of the current BCI systems that rely on the brain electrical activity producing scalp EEG signals. Since the scalp EEG signals, however, are inherently noisy and non-linear, a more accessible interface that uses a more direct measurement of brain function to control an output device is being explored. NIRS is considered as a possible alternative to electrical signals (Ranganatha et al., 2005).

Conclusion

Although there is still plenty of room for improvement, strengths and advantages of NIRS are expected to provide a new direction for functional mapping studies that other neuroimaging techniques cannot. Thus, NIRS shows great promise for providing further insights into brain functions and for clinical tools.

References

Aizawa, H., Mushiake, H., Inase, M., and Tanji, J. (1990). An output zone of the monkey primary motor cortex specialized for bilateral hand movement. *Exp. Brain Res.*, *82*, 219-221.

Arridge, S. R., Cope, M., and Delpy, D. T. (1992). Theoretical basis for the determination of optical pathlengths in tissue: temporal and frequency analysis. *Phys. Med. Biol.*, *37*, 1531-1560.

Arridge, S. R. (1999). Optical tomography in medical imaging. *Inverse Problems*, *15*, R41-R93.

Auer, L. M., and Sayama, I. (1983). Intracranial pressure oscillations (B-waves) caused by oscillations in cerebrovascular volume. *Acta Neurochir., 68*, 93-100.

Bernstein, N. *The coordination and regulation of movements.* New York: Oxford; 1967.

Bevilacqua, F., Piguet, D., Marquet, P., Gross, J.D., Tromberg, B.J., and Depeursige, C. (1999). In vivo local determination of tissue optical properties: applications to human brain. *Appl. Opt., 38*, 4939-4950.

Boas, D. A., Culver, J. P., Stott, J. J., and Dunn, A. K. (2002). Three dimensional Monte Carlo code for photon migration through complex heterogeneous media including the adult human head. *Opt. Express, 10*, 159-170.

Boas, D. A., Chen, K., Grebert, D., and Franceschini, M. A. (2004). Improving the diffuse optical imaging spatial resolution of the cerebral hemodynamic response to brain activation in humans. *Opt. Lett., 29*, 1506-1508.

Brazy, J. E., Lewis, D. V., Mitnick, M. H., and Jöbsis, F. F. (1985). Noninvasive monitoring of cerebral oxygenation in preterm infants: preliminary observation. *Pediatrics, 75*, 217-225.

Chance, B., Leigh, J. S., Miyake, H., Smith, D. S., Nioka, S., Greenfeld, R., Finander, M., Kaufmann, K., Levy, W., Young, M., Choen, P., Yoshioka, H., and Boretsky, R. (1988). Comparison of time-resolved and –unresolved measurements of deoxyhemoglobin in brain. *Proc. Natl. Acad. Sci. USA, 85*, 4971-4975.

Colier, W. N., Quaresima, V., Oeseburug, B., and Ferrari, M. (1999). Human motor-cortex oxygenation changes induced by cyclic coupled movements of hand and foot. *Exp. Brain Res., 129*, 457-461.

Delpy, D. T., Cope, M., van der Zee, P., Arridge, S., Wray, S., and Wyatt, J. (1988). Estimation of optical pathlength through tissue from direct time of flight measurement. *Phys. Med. Biol., 33*, 1433-1442.

Donoghue, J. P. (2002). Connecting cortex to machines: recent advances in brain interfaces. *Nat. Neurosci., 5*, 1085-1088.

Duncan, A., Whitlock, T. L., Cope, M., and Deply, D. T. (1993). A multiwavelength, wideband, intensity modulated optical spectrometer for near infrared spectroscopy and imaging. *Proc. SPIE, 1888*, 248-257.

Eda, H., Oda, I., Ito, Y., Wada, Y., Oikawa, Y., Tsunazawa, Y., Takada, M., Tsuchiya, Y., Yamashita, Y., Oda, M., Sassaroli, A., Yamada, Y., and Tamura, M. (1999). Multi-channel time-resolved optical tomographic imaging system. *Rev.Sci. Instrum., 70*, 3595-3602.

Fagard, J. (1994). Manual strategies and interlimb coordination during reaching, grasping, and manipulating throughout the first year of life. In: S. P. Swinnen, H. Heuer, J. Massion, and P. Casaer (Eds.), *Interlimb Coordination: Neural, Dynamical, and Cognitive Constrains* (pp. 439-460). New York: Academic Press.

Firbank, M., Okada, E., and Delpy, D.T. (1998). A theoretical study of the signal contribution of regions of the adult head to near-infrared spectroscopy studies of visual evoked responses. *NeuroImage, 8*, 69-78.

Fox, P., and Raichle, M. E. (1986). Focal Physiological uncoupling of cerebral blood flow and oxidative metabolism during somatosensory stimulation in human subjects. *Proc. Natl. Acad. Sci. USA, 83*, 1140-1144.

Friston, K.J., Frith, C.D., Liddle, P. F., and Frackowiak, R. S. J. (1991). Comparing functional (PET) images: The assessment of significant change. *J. Cereb. Blood Flow Metab., 11*, 690-699.

Fukui, Y., Ajichi, Y., and Okada, E. (2003). Monte Carlo prediction of near-infrared light propagation in realistic adult and neonatal head models. *Appl. Opt., 42*, 2881-2887.

Gao, F., Zhao, H., and Yamada, Y. (2002). Improvement of image quality in diffuse optical tomography using full time-resolved data. *Appl. Opt., 41*, 778-791.

Gemba, H. (2002). Motor programming for hand and vocalizing movements. In: D. T. Stuss, and R.T. Knight (Eds.), *Principles of Frontal Lobe Function* (pp. 127-148). New York: Oxford.

Gratton, G., Maier, J. S., Fabiani, M., Mantulinm W. W., and Gratton, E. (1994). Feasibility of intracranial near-infrared optical scanning. *Psychophysiol., 31*, 211-215.

Grillner S., and Zangger P. (1975). How detailed is the central pattern generation for locomotion? *Brain Res., 88*, 367-371.

Grillner S., Perret C., and Zangger P. (1976). Central generation of locomotion in the spinal dogfish. *Brain Res., 109*, 255-269.

Heekeren, H. R., Obrig, H., Wenzel, R., Eberle, K., Ruben, J., Villringer, K., Kurth, R., and Villringer, A. (1997). Cerebral haemoglobin oxygenation during sustained visual stimulation – a near-infrared spectroscopy study. *Philos. Trans. R. Soc. London B Biolo. Sci., 352*, 743-750.

Hess, A., Stiller, D., Kaulisch, T., Heil, P., and Scheich, H. (2000). New insights into the hemodynamic blood oxygenation level-dependent response through combination of functional magnetic resonance imaging and optical recording in gerbil barrel cortex. *J. Neurosci., 20*, 3328-3338.

Hielscher, A. H., Liu, H., Chance, B., Tittel, F. K., and Jacques, S. L. (1996). Time-resolved photon emission from layered turbid media. *Appl. Opt., 35*, 719-728.

Hirschfeld, H., and Forssberg, H. (1994). Epigenetic development of postural responses for sitting during infancy. *Exp. Brain Res., 97*, 528-540.

Horovitz, S. G., and Gore, J. S. (2004). Simultaneous event-related potential and near-infrared spectroscopic studies of semantic processing. *Human Brain Mapp., 22*, 110-115.

Hoshi, Y., and Tamura, M. (1993a). Detection of dynamic changes in cerebral oxygenation coupled to neuronal function during mental work in man. *Neurosci. Lett., 150*, 5-8.

Hoshi, Y., and Tamura, M. (1993b). Dynamic multichannel near-infrared optical imaging of human brain activity. *J. Appl. Physiol., 75*, 1842-1846.

Hoshi, Y., Hazeki, O., Kakihana, Y., and Tamura M. (1997a). Redox behavior of cytochrome oxidase in the rat brain measured by near-infrared spectroscopy. *J. Appl. Physiol., 83*, 1842-1848.

Hoshi, Y., and Tamura, M. (1997b). Fluctuations in the cerebral oxygenation state during the resting period in functional mapping studies of the human brain. *Med. Biol. Engin.Comput., 35*, 328-330.

Hoshi, Y., Kosaka, S., Xie, Y., Kohri, S., and Tamura, M. (1998). Relationship between fluctuations in the cerebral hemoglobin oxygenation state and neuronal activity under resting conditions in man. *Neurosci. Lett., 245*, 147-150

Hoshi, Y., Kobayashi, N., and Tamura, M. (2001). Interpretation of near-infrared spectroscopy signals: a study with a newly developed perfused rat brain model. *J. Appl. Physiol., 90*, 1657-1662.

Hoshi, Y., Shimada, M., Sato, C., and Iguchi, Y. (2005) Reevaluation of near-infrared light propagation in the adult human head: implications for functional near-infrared spectroscopy. *J. Biol. Opt.* (in press).

Ishimaru, A. (1978). Diffusion of a pulse in densely distributed scatters. *J. Opt. Soc. Am., 68*, 1045 -1050.

Jankowska, E., Jukes, M. G. M., Lund S., and Lundberg A. (1967). The effect DOPA on the spinal cord. 5. Reciprocal organization of pathways transmitting excitatory action to alpha motoneurons of flexor and extensors. *Acta Physiol Scand.*, 70, 369-388.

Jöbsis, F. F. (1977). Noninvasive infrared monitoring of cerebral and myocardial oxygen sufficiency and circulatory parameters. *Science, 198*, 1264-1267.

Kato, T., Kamei, A., Takashima, S., and Ozaki, T. (1993). Human visual cortical function during photic stimulation monitoring by means of near-infrared spectroscopy. *J. Cereb. Blood Flow Metab., 13,* 516-520.

Kienle, A., Patterson, M. S., Dognitz, N., Bays, R., Wagnieres, G., and van den Bergh, H. (1998). Noninvasive determination of the optical properties of two-layered turbid media. *Appl. Opt.*, 37, 779-791.

Kleinschmidt, A., Obrig, H., Requardt, M., Merboldt. K-D., Dirnagl, U., Villringer, A., and Frahm, J. (1996). Simultaneous recording of cerebral blood oxygenation changes during human brain activation by magnetic resonance imaging and near-infrared spectroscopy. *J. Cereb. Blood Flow Metab., 16*, 817-826.

Lakowicz, J. R., and Berndt, K. (1990). Frequency domain measurement of photon migration in tissues. *Chem. Phys. Lett., 166*, 246-252.

Lindegaard, K. F., Lundar, T., Wiberg, J., Sjøberg, D., Aaslid, R., and Normes, H. (1987). Variations in middle cerebral artery blood flow investigated with noninvasive transcranial blood velocity measurements. *Stroke, 18*, 1025-1030.

Mayhew, J., Zheng, Y., Hou, Y., Vuksanovic, B., Berwick, J., Askew, S., and Coffey, P. (1999). Spectroscopic analysis of changes in remitted illumination: the response to increased neural activity in brain. *NeuroImage, 10*, 304-326.

Miyai, I., Tanabe, H. C., Sase, I., Eda, H., Oda, I., Konishi, I., Tsunazawa, Y., Suzuki, T., Yanagida, T., and Kubota, K. (2001). Cortical mapping of gait in humans: a near-infrared spectroscopic topography study. *NeuroImage, 14*, 1186-1192.

Oda, M., Yamashita, Y., Nakano, T., Suzuki, A., Shimizu, K., Hirano, I., Shimomura, F., Ohmae, E., Suzuki, T., and Tsuchiya, Y. (1999). Nearinfrared time-resolved spectroscopy system for tissue oxygenation monitor. *Proc. Society of Photo-Optical Instrumentation Engineers, 3597*, 611-617.

Okada, E., Firbank, M., Schweiger, M., Arridge, S.R., Cope, M., and Delpy, DT. (1997). Theoretical and experimental investigation of near-infrared light propagation in a model of the adult head. *Appl. Opt., 36*, 21-31.

Okamoto, M., Dan, H., Sakamoto, K., Takeo, K., Shimizu, K., Kohno, A., Oda, I., isobe, S., Suzuki, T., Kohyama, K., and Dan, I. (2004). Three-dimensional probabilistic anatomical cranio-cerebral correlation via the international 10-20 system oriented for transcranial functional brain mapping. *NeuroImage, 21*, 99-111.

Patterson, M. S., Chance, B., and Wilson, B. C. (1989). Time resolved reflectance and transmittance for the noninvasive measurement of tissue optical properties. *Appl. Opt., 28*, 2331-2336.

Pogue, B. W., Patterson, M. S., Jiang, H., and Paulsen, K.D. (1995). Initial assessment of a simple system for frequency domain diffuse optical tomography. *Phys. Med. Biol., 40*, 1709-1729.

Ranganatha, S., Hoshi, Y., and Cuntai, G. (2004). Near Infrared Spectroscopy based Brain-Computer Interface, 3rd International Conference on Experimental Mechanics (ICEM), 29 Nov – 1, Dec, 2004, Singapore.

Rea, P. A., Crowe, J., Wickramasinghe, Y., and Rolfe, P. (1985). Non-invasive optical methods for the study of cerebral metabolism in the human newborn: a technique for the future? *J. Med. Eng. Technol., 9.*, 160-165.

Sato, H., Takeuchi, T., and Sakai, K. L. (1999). Temporal cortex activation during speech recognition: an optical topography study. *Cognition, 73*, B55-B66.

Sato, H., Kiguchi, M., Kawaguchi, F., and Maki, A. (2004). Practicality of wavelength selection to improve signal-to-nosie ratio in near-infrared spectroscopy. *NeuroImage, 21*, 1554-1562.

Sassaroli, A., Martelli, F., Tanikawa, Y., Tanaka, K., Araki, R., Onodera Y., and Yamada, Y. (2000). Time-resolved measurement of in vivo optical properties of piglet brain. *Opt. Rev., 7*, 420-425.

Schroeter, M. L., Zysset, S., Kupka, T., Kruggel, F., and Yves von Cramon, D. (2002). Near-infrared spectroscopy can detect brain activity during a color-word matching Stroop task in an event-related design. *Human Brain Map.,17*, 61-71.

Sevick, E. M., Frisoli, J. K., Burch, C. L., and Lakowickz, J. R. (1994). Localisation of absorbers in scattering media by use of frequency domain measurements of time dependent photon migration. *Appl. Opt., 33*, 3562-3570.

Shiga, T., Yamamoto, K., Tanabe, K., Nakase, Y., and Chance, B. (1997). Study of an algorithm based on Model experiments and diffusion theory for a portable tissue oximeter. *J. Biomed. Opt., 2,* 154-161.

Shimada, S., Hiraki, K., Matsuda, G., and Oda, I. (2004). Decrease in prefrontal hemoglobin oxygenation during reaching tasks with delayed visual feedback: a near-infrared spectroscopy study. *Cogn. Brain Res., 20*, 480-490.

Simpson, C. R., Kohl, M., Essenpreis, M., and Cope, M. (1998). Near-infrared optical properties of ex vivo human skin and subcutaneous tissues measured using the Monte Carlo inversion technique. *Phys. Med. Biol., 43*, 2465-2478.

Steinbrink, J., Wabnitz, H., Obrig, H., Villringer, A., and Rinneberg, H. (2001). Determining changes in NIR absorption using a layered model of the human head. *Phys. Med. Biol., 46*, 879-896.

Strangman, G., Franceschini, M. A., and Boas, D. A. (2003). Factors affecting the accuracy of near-infrared spectroscopy concentration calculations for focal changes in oxygenation parameters. *NeuroImage, 18*, 865-879.

Tanosaki, M., Hoshi, Y., Iguchi, Y., Oikawa, Y., Oda, I., and Oda, M. (2001). Variation of temporal characteristics in human cerebral hemodynamic responses to electric median nerve stimulation: a near-infra-red spectroscopic study. *Neurosci. Lett., 316*, 75-78.

Toronov, V., Francecshini, M. A., Filiaci, M., Fantini, S., Wolf. M., Michalos, A., and Gratton, E. (2000). Near-infrared study of fluctuations in cerebral hemodynamics during rest and motor stimulation: temporal analysis and spatial mapping. *Med. Phys., 27*, 801-815.

Toronov, V., Webb, A., Choi, J. H., Wolf, M., Michalos, A., Gratton, E., and Hueber, D. (2001). Investigation of human brain hemodynamics by simultaneous near-infrared spectroscopy and functional magnetic resonance imaging. *Med. Phys., 28*, 521-527.

Towle, V. L., Bolanos, J., Suarez, D., Tan, K., Grzeszczuk, R., Levin, D. N., Cakmur, R., Frank, S. A., and Spire, J. (1993). The spatial location of EEG electrodes: locating the best-fitting sphere relative to cortical anatomy. *Electroencephalogr. Clin. Neurophysiol., 86*, 1-6.

Uludağ, K., Steinbrink, J., Villringer, A., and Obrig, H. (2004). Separability and cross talk: optimizing dual wavelength combinations for near-infrared spectroscopy of the adult head. *NeuroImage, 22*, 583-589.

Villringer, A., Plank, J., Hock, C., Schleikofer, L., and Dirnagl, U. (1993). Near-infrared spectroscopy (NIRS): a new tool to study hemodynamic changes during activation of brain function in human adults. *Neurosci. Lett., 154*, 101-104.

Wiesendanger M., Wicki U., and Rouiller E. (1994). Are there unifying structures in the brain responsible for interlimb coordination? In: S. P. Swinnen, H. Heuer, J. Massion, and P. Casaer (Eds.), *Interlimb Coordination: Neural, Dynamical, and Cognitive Constrains*. (pp.179-207). New York, Academic Press.

Wolpaw, J. R., Birbaumer, N., McFarland, D. J., Pfurtscheller, G., and Vaughan, T. M. (2002). Brain-computer interface for communication and control, *Cin. Neurophysiol., 11*, 767-791.

Wyatt, J. S., Cope, M., Delpy, D. T., Wray, S., and Raynolds, E. O. R. (1986). Quantification of cerebral oxygenation and haemodynamics in sick newborn infants by near infrared spectrophotometry. *Lancet, ii,* 1063-1066.

Zhao, H., Tanikawa, Y., Gao, F., Onodera, Y., Sassaroli, A., Tanaka, K., and Yamada, Y. (2002). Maps of optical differential pathlength factor of human adult forehead, somatosensory motor, occipital regions at multi-wavelengths in NIR. *Phys. Med. Biol., 47*, 1-18.

In: Progress in Brain Mapping Research
Editor: F. J. Chen, pp. 231-246
ISBN 1-59454-580-4

Chapter 7

Integration of fMRI and ERP Information in Parametric Designs

***Silvina G. Horovitz*[8,2], *Pawel Skudlarski*[3] *and John C. Gore*[2]**
[1]EAS- Yale University
[2]Vanderbilt University Institute of Imaging Science
[3]MRRC- Yale University School of Medicine

Abstract

Neuroimaging studies seek to determine 'when' and/or 'where' activation occurs in the brain. Different techniques have the ability to adequately measure either one or the other type of information. Electrophysiological recordings have excellent time resolution (i.e., they can accurately assess the 'when'), of the order of milliseconds, but the information on localization is poor. Conversely, using metabolic or hemodynamic measurements, such as PET or fMRI, accurate localization (i.e., the 'where') is possible but the time resolution of such measurements is intrinsically limited. Thus, in order to better understand brain function, integration of these different modalities is desirable. We have developed an approach to integration that uses parametric studies wherein the amplitude of a particular ERP is modulated by varying some aspect of a task. These varying amplitudes are then applied as regressors to find activations in a corresponding fMRI data set. The resultant data reveal regions whose activities covary with the ERP. In recent studies, we have applied this method to an oddball (P300) paradigm and a face-detection (N170) paradigm, obtaining a more refined set of activations than with traditional fMRI analyses alone. These are examples of how ERP information may be used synergistically in fMRI analyses, and vice versa. fMRI parametric designs with correlational analysis may provide some timing information on fMRI activity and help identify the generators of ERP signals.

---

[8] Contact information: Silvina G. Horovitz, PhD. Advanced MRI, LFMI, NINDS, NIH. 9000 Rockville Pk, Building 10, Room B1D722, Bethesda, MD. 20892-1065, Phone: 301 451 9915 Fax: 301 480 1981; e-mail: silvina.horovitz@aya.yale.edu

Introduction

Neuroimaging techniques are commonly used to obtain information to help understand some aspect of how the brain works, and how brain functions are affected by various pathologies or as a result of different treatments. Non-invasive techniques for probing brain function are based on the observation of time-varying electrophysiological and/or metabolic changes that occur in the brain in different conditions. Different techniques have different abilities to measure different aspects of function. Electrophysiological recordings, such as electroencephalograpy (EEG), magnetoencephalography (MEG) or event related potentials (ERPs) possess excellent time resolution (and thus may measure the 'when' of functional events), of the order of milliseconds, and have been used for decades in psychology, psychiatry and the cognitive sciences to study timing differences in brain activation among tasks or populations. The localization of activation in these modalities is relatively poor, and the magnitudes of the signals measured are not usually quantified. The improvement of EEG systems and their associated computational power make it possible now to estimate the locations of activations which generate electrical signals based on recordings collected from the scalp. However, these estimates of the activation are based on assumed and approximate models of the head and the conductances of different tissues. Source localization from EEG or MEG data is an ill-posed inverse problem because the head is a volume conductor.

On the contrary, metabolic or hemodynamic measurements such as those obtained from PET (positron emission tomography) or functional magnetic resonance imaging (fMRI), can provide accurate localization of activations (i.e., the 'where' of neural events), but the temporal resolution is limited by the physiological time courses of the phenomena measured. Metabolic changes are indirect reflections of changes in neuronal activity; an increase in neuronal activity is followed by an increase in metabolism, which is associated with a change in cerebral blood flow and oxygenation. These changes affect the fMRI BOLD (blood oxygenation level dependant) signal and PET or MRI measurements of blood flow based on the transit time of an intravascular label. The metabolic changes may be related to changes in the frequency of electrical spikes (Rees, 2000) or changes at the postsynaptic level. Data from simultaneous measurements of single and multi-unit spike activity, local field potentials (LFP) and BOLD signals (Logothetis, 2001) suggest BOLD is a better indicator of changes in LFP's than of spiking activity (Logothetis, 2003). However, when measuring from the scalp, the LFP's are farther away from the sensor, and affected by brain tissue and skull, which act as a low-pass filter. Thus not all LFP's contribute to the signal measured at the scalp, they may add to or cancel each other depending on their orientations and locations, so that direct comparisons of BOLD and EEG are non-trivial.

It seems plausible that strategies which combine modalities in a synergistic manner are likely to be of useful in practical applications. In this chapter, we present two studies in which EEG and fMRI measurements were combined in a novel manner to shed light both on the locations of neural activations as well as the connection between electrical and metabolic indices of activity.

Experimental Paradigm

Many ERP and fMRI experiments incorporate comparisons of at least two conditions, selected by the experimenter. These two conditions are often presented in block designs (e.g. Kwong, 1992; Ogawa, 1992; Blamire, 1992; Bandettini, 1992) or as event related designs (Buncker, 1996; McCarthy, 1997). However, when combining different modalities, the relationship among the different techniques is unknown, so comparisons between more than two conditions are desirable. Parametric designs, which may use either event related or block presentation of stimuli, offer the possibility of comparing multiple conditions. In such experiments, one dimension of the stimulus is changed across conditions, thereby modulating the response (see figure 1). Parametric designs allow measurements of brain activation across a continuum of conditions rather than in any single condition, and are more suited for the types of regression analyses we used in our studies.

The two studies described in this chapter take advantage of parametric paradigms and combine them with regression analysis as a novel approach to the integration of ERP and fMRI data. ERP and fMRI have complementary abilities, with different temporal and spatial resolutions. Comparing parallel changes in ERP and fMRI data in parametric designs provides a novel method for connecting these two different modalities.

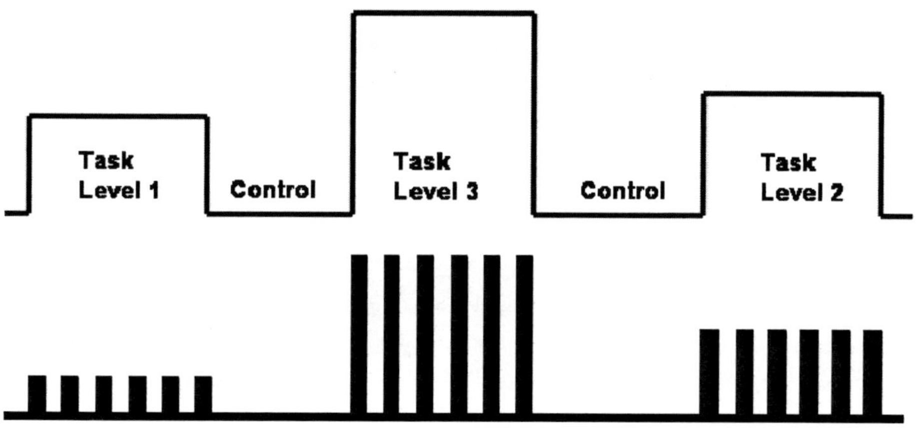

Figure 1. Parametric design. One dimension of the stimulus is changed during the experiment; as a result, changes in intensity of the response are expected

The first experiments consisted of an event related 'oddball' task that is commonly used to elicit an electrophysiological P300 response, in which we kept constant the intensity of the stimuli but varied frequency of occurrence of the oddball stimuli. This allowed us to explore which brain regions were affected by the experimental manipulation in the same way in the fMRI and the ERP[9]. In the second study, we aimed to clarify the sources of the N170 evoked

---

[9] Reprinted from Magnetic Resonance Imaging, Vol 20, Silvina G. Horovitz, Pawel Skudlarski and John C. Gore, Correlations and dissociation between BOLD signal and P300 amplitude in an auditory oddball task: a parametric approach to combining fMRI and ERP , Pages 319-325., Copyright (2002), with permission from Elsevier.

response during face and object processing using a parametric design for both fMRI and ERP measurements[10]. These parameter manipulations were based on previous ERP studies (Sutton, 1965; Tueting, 1971; Duncan-Johnson, 1977; Jemel, 2003).

Materials and Methods

Subjects

All subjects provided their informed consent in accordance with a protocol reviewed and approved by the Human Investigation Committee of Yale University School of Medicine. Each subject was studied on two different days, once for the fMRI experiment and secondly for the ERP experiment. The same paradigm was used in both sessions. Seven healthy subjects (range= 21-37 years, 2 females) participated in the oddball task and five (range= 21-35 years, 3 females) in the face processing paradigm.

The oddball paradigm: The oddball paradigm has been in common use for about four decades (Sutton, 1965), and consists of the presentation of a series of repetitive stimuli at regular intervals, in which is interspersed, infrequently and at random, a target stimulus. A main characteristic in the electrophysiological recordings is the P300 wave which arises between 260 and 500 milliseconds after the onset of the stimulus. The latency and amplitude of P300's are affected by physiological and experimental manipulations. This paradigm was appealing for our purpose because it has been well known for many years (e.g. Tueting and co-workers (1971)) that the probability of the target affects the amplitude of the P300 wave. The version used here consisted of audio tones, of different frequencies (1000 Hz for the common one, 1500 Hz for the target) presented for 100 ms and at intervals of 1.5 s. Target tones were separated by 19.5±1.5, 25.5±1.5, 37.5±1.5 and 75.0±1.5 seconds, representing local probabilities of 8, 6, 4, or 2% respectively. In each session, a total of 438 tones were presented in each of six runs, thereby incorporating up to 96 targets (24 at each probability). Subjects were asked to press a button when the target tone was presented.

Face processing paradigm: Pictures of faces or objects (cars) with different noise levels and different colors were presented. Using Matlab (Mathworks, Inc), a set of pictures of faces and cars was modified by changing the color to grey or magenta, and by adding Gaussian noise with standard deviation of 0, 0.025, 0.075, 0.1, 0.2 or 5 (figure 2). A total of 216 pictures were presented in each run. Each picture was presented for 500 ms and was followed by a blank screen that was shown for 1150 ms. Blocks of six of the same object and noise level with different colors pseudo-randomly intermixed were presented in order to obtain a sustained hemodynamic response (figure 3). Subjects were naïve to the actual task, since they were asked to make a response based on the color of the picture. Six to eight runs of fMRI and 4 runs of ERP were collected for each of the five subjects.

[10] Reprinted from Neuroimage, Vol 22, Silvina G. Horovitz, Bruno Rossion, Pawel Skudlarski and John C. Gore, Parametric design and correlational analyses help integrating fMRI and electrophysiological data during face processing, Pages 1587-1595., Copyright (2004), with permission from Elsevier

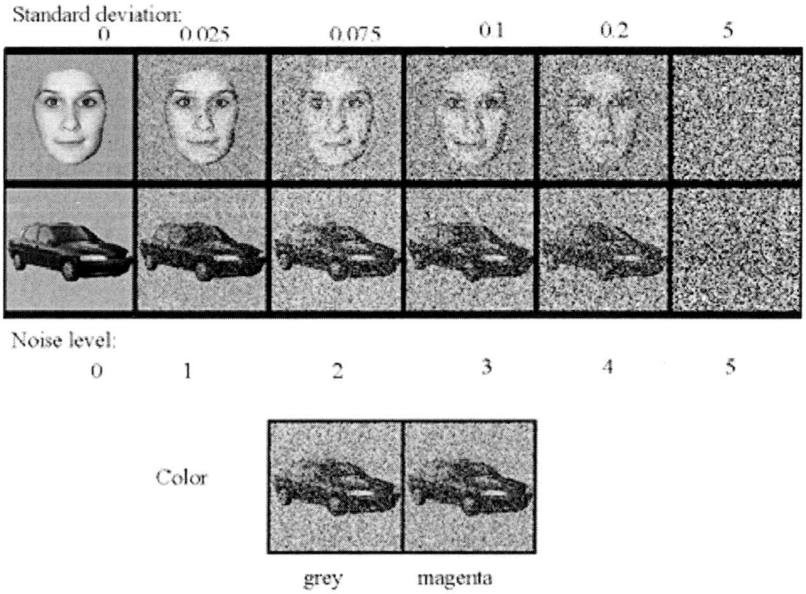

Figure 2. Sample of the stimuli used in the face processing paradigm. Shown are two pictures at each level of noise presented. Pictures at noise level 1 to 5 were created by adding Gaussian noise of standard deviation 0.025, 0.075, 0.1, 0.5 or 5 to the images at noise 0. Images were presented either in grey or magenta.

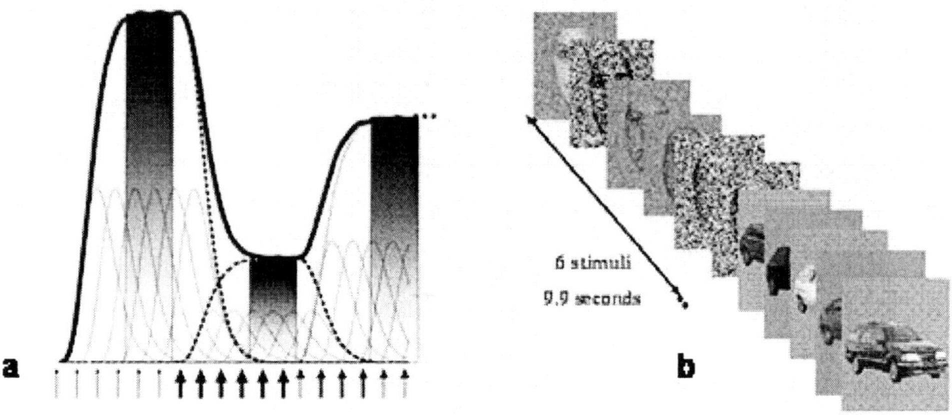

Figure 3.a. Simulated time series, representing three blocks of six responses each. Each block represents a different noise level. Bars indicate image 4-6 at each level, and it can be observed that the simulated hemodynamic response has reached a plateau. Those images are used to construct maps at each noise level. b. a series of 6 pictures with the same noise level are presented consecutively.

EEG Recording and Processing

ERP Recordings

The ERPs were collected on a computer running Scan 4.1 software (NeuroScan, Inc, El Paso, Tx) and controlling SynAmp amplifiers (NeuroScan, Inc). For the oddball task, data were collected from 11 locations of the 10-20 System (F3, F4, C3, C4, T3, T4, P3, P4, Fz, Cz and Pz) using an electro-cap (Electrocap International Inc., Eaton, Ohio) with tin electrodes. Crossed earlobes were used as a reference and forehead as ground. Impedances were kept below 5 kΩ using an electrode gel. Additional electrodes were used to monitor eye movements. The acquisition was performed continuously at 500 Hz (2 ms time resolution). A band pass filter was set to 0.05 - 100 Hz, and an additional filter was used for rejection of 60 Hz. Gain was set to 500 for all channels.

For the face processing paradigm, ERP's were collected with the same system, but using a modified cap with 32 tin electrodes and common earlobe reference. Ground was placed on the forehead. Gain was set to 2500, sample rate to 500 Hz and acquisition bandwidth was between 0.01 and 70 Hz.

ERP Data Analysis - Oddball Task

Data processing was performed using Scan 4.1 software. The signal was divided into epochs of 1024 ms (including 200 ms pre-stimulus and 824 ms after stimulus presentation). Ocular artifacts were removed using the method proposed by Semlitsch (1986). The resulting data were then baseline-corrected for each subject and low pass filtered to 30 Hz. Finally, an average wave was obtained for each condition and each subject, and the amplitude of the ERP of interest (P300) was measured for each average. For each probability of oddball and for each subject, the P300 amplitude was assessed as the difference between the baseline and the more prominent positive peak occurring between 260 and 500 ms after stimulus onset. A repeated-measures analysis of variance (ANOVA) (within subject factor: target probability and electrode location) was performed to study the effect of target probability on the amplitude of the P300. The effect of probability on the amplitude of the N100 peak was also studied.

ERP Data Analysis: Face Processing Paradigm

Data processing was performed using Scan 4.2 software. First, data were filtered (1-30 Hz), then ocular artifacts were removed. Data were then referenced to a common ground and divided into epochs, starting 200 ms before the object presentation and lasting for 998 ms after the onset of the stimulus, and these were then baseline-corrected. Finally, for each subject, an average wave was obtained for each object and noise level (total of twelve conditions). N170 amplitudes and latencies were measured for each averaged waveform as the largest negativity in the interval 100 to 200 ms at occipito-temporal electrodes in right and left hemispheres. P1 was also measured, as the positive peak prior to the N170. Repeated measures ANOVAs were computed on the amplitude and latency of N170 and P1. The model included 4 factors (Noise level (0-5), object (face/car), electrode (P/PO) and side (right/left). All reported statistical values are Greenhouse-Geisser corrected, unless otherwise noted.

fMRI Recording and Processing

fMRI Recordings

Images were acquired using a 1.5 T Signa LX scanner (General Electric, Milwaukee, WI). First, T1-weighted anatomical images were collected in the same location as the desired functional data. In the oddball paradigm, ten slices, parallel to AC-PC were selected with a slice thickness of 7.0 mm and inter slice interval of 2.0 mm. For the face processing paradigm, eighteen slices (9.0 mm thickness, 1.0 mm inter slice interval), perpendicular to AC-PC were defined. Functional data were then collected in the same planes, using a single shot gradient echo-planar imaging sequence (TE=60, flip angle = 60°, FOV=20 x 20 cm^2 and matrix size = 64 x 64, achieving an in-plane resolution of 3.125 x 3.125 mm^2). For the oddball paradigm TR was set to 1500 ms and for the face perception paradigm to 1650 ms.

fMRI Data Analysis

fMRI data were first motion-corrected using SPM96 software [Wellcome Department of Cognitive Neurology, University College, London, *http://www.fil.ion.ucl.ac.uk/spm*)]. The remaining analyses, including the calculation of statistical maps, were performed using the Yale fMRI Analysis Package (*http://mri.med.yale.edu/individual/pawel/fMRIpackage.html*) running under MATLAB (The MathWorks Inc., Natick, MA).

Functional images were realigned and registered with the corresponding anatomical images. Pixels with signal smaller than 5% of the maximum value for each run were masked in order to reduce noise. Images were smoothed in the space domain using a Gaussian filter (6.25 mm FWHM) and high-pass filtered (0.006 Hz) in the time domain to reduce effects of time drifts (Skudlarski, 1999). Data were then converted into Talaraich space (Talairach, 1988).

For the oddball paradigm, the analysis was divided in three steps. First, we performed an event related fMRI analysis for all oddballs, regardless of the target probability. This was done mainly to verify if the results we obtained were in agreement with previous studies. Second, we looked for correlations between predefined regions of interest (ROIs) and the ERP data. Finally, we created correlation maps to look at the correlations between BOLD signal change and ERP amplitudes on a voxel by voxel basis. For the face processing paradigm, ROI analysis and voxel by voxel correlation analyses between BOLD signals and N170 amplitudes were performed.

Event Related fMRI

For each subject, we identified the images corresponding to the presentation of the target tone. We considered the baseline signal to be the average of the five images prior to the target presentation, and the activated signal to be the average of images numbered 3, 4 and 5 after the target presentation (this corresponds to 3 to 6 seconds after onset of the stimulus). We computed a t-statistic between the activated signal and the baseline signal (see figure 4.b) for each voxel in each run and then averaged the results across runs. This procedure reduces the effects of global intensity changes between separate runs (Skudlarski, 1999).

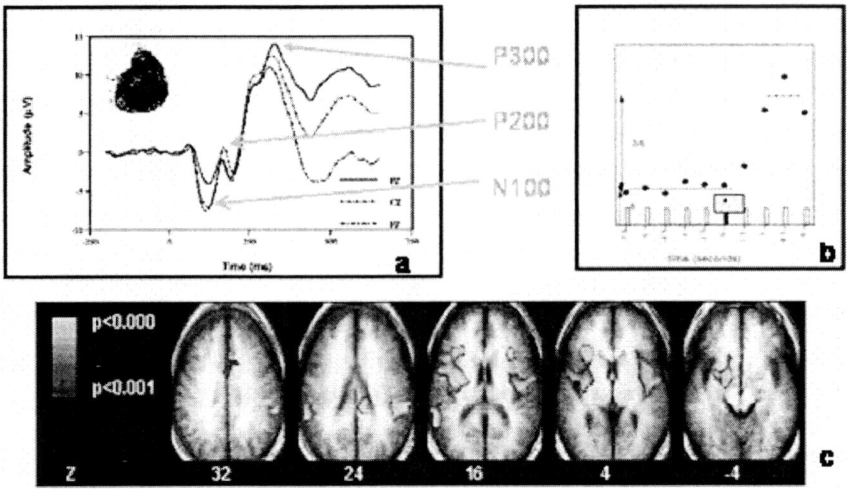

Figure 4. Response to the event related oddball task. a. timecourse of the ERPs at central electrodes. b. timecourse of the hemodynamic response. The insert shown at onset of the stimulus is the ERP timecourse at the same scale as the fMRI. Notice that all the peaks indicated in a. occur before the onset of the hemodynamic response, therefore making difficult to identify to which peak the fMRI activation corresponds to. c. fMRI activation maps

ROI Analysis

For the oddball paradigm, ROIs were defined prior to the fMRI data analysis in anterior cingulate, posterior cingulate, superior-middle frontal gyrus, superior temporal gyrus, supramarginal gyrus, insula, hippocampus and thalamus. These regions were defined anatomically and their selection was based upon previously reported oddball experiments (Menon, 1997; Stevens, 2000). Targets were then sorted into four probability groups and the mean percentage BOLD signal change for each interval and each subject for each region was computed as the ratio between the activation signal increase and the baseline (see figure 4.b). Values for each ROI were correlated with ERP P300 peak at the most significant electrode and the correlations were then combined across subjects.

For the face perception paradigm the midfusiform region was functionally defined for each subject as the result of the statistical (t-test) map obtained by comparing faces versus cars. This was performed after collapsing data across noise levels 1 to 3 (see figure 2). Once identified, BOLD signal changes for the ROI were measured at each noise level and these values were then correlated with the amplitude of the N170 peak measured at electrode PO8. Since face paradigms usually generate several ERP components, we performed a post-hoc correlation analysis on the amplitude of peaks measured in 100 ms windows in the range 0 to 800 ms at electrode PO8 and BOLD signal changes in the midfusiform area. For each subject, ERP values were normalized by subtracting the mean and dividing by the standard deviation.

Correlation Maps

Activation maps were obtained for each subject and each experimental level. These maps were used for a voxel-by-voxel combination of fMRI and ERP data for each subject and then averaged across subjects.

In the oddball paradigm, the statistical maps were constructed as in the ROI analysis. For the face perception paradigm, the statistical maps where constructed comparing images 4, 5 and 6 after presentation of the face (active task) with images 4, 5 and 6 after presentation of noise (baseline) for each subject (see figure 3.a).

Results

Oddball Paradigm

All subjects showed a P300 response to the oddball stimulus, with the most prominent response over the centro-parietal area (figure 4.a). There was a significant effect of probability of oddball ($p<0.046$) and also a significant linear contrast effect (within subject, probability level: $p<0.030$; electrode: $p<0.013$). The probability effect was more significant at electrode Fz ($p<0.030$) and at this electrode the linear contrast within subject was also significant ($p<0.015$). In order to ensure that the P300 wave was specifically affected by our paradigm, we performed the same analysis using the N100 amplitude as parameter. The observed differences across probabilities were not statistically significant. Figure 5.a shows the ERP averaged over all subjects at electrode Fz for the four probabilities.

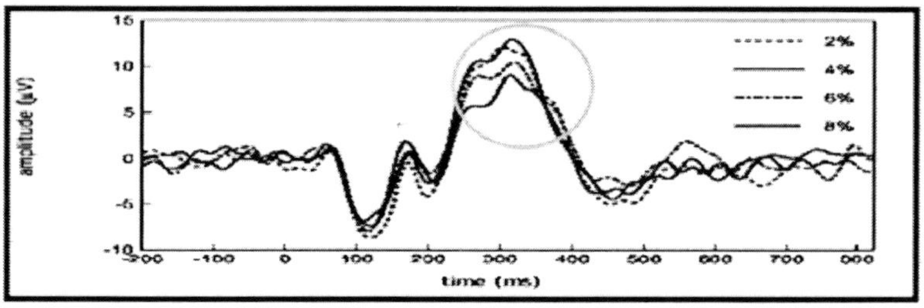

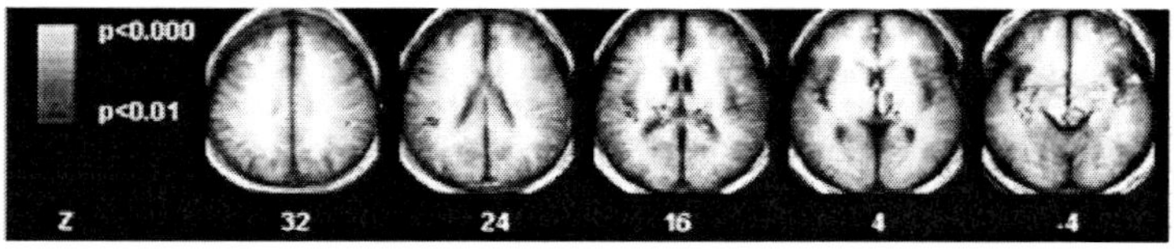

Figure 5.a. Group average ERP timecourse at electrode Fz for each of the four target probabilities. Note that the differences among the traces are significant at the P300 peak. b. fMRI activation maps.

In the traditional fMRI analysis, activations were observed in bilateral insula, supramarginal gyri, superior temporal gyri and anterior and posterior cingulate. Figure 4.c shows maps of t-values ($p<0.001$ uncorrected) for the group average. The results of the voxel by voxel correlation analysis are shown in figure 5.b. At a significance level of $p<0.01$, activations modulated by oddball probability in similar fashion to the P300 amplitude were observed bilaterally in supramarginal gyri, insula, thalamus and right medial frontal gyrus.

ROIs values were correlated with the amplitude at electrode Fz for each subject and average across subjects. Significant correlations were observed in right supramarginal gyrus and left insula ($p<0.05$ corrected).

Face Perception Paradigm

N170 waves were observed in all subjects for both cars and faces, in all conditions, (see figure 6a); however, amplitudes were larger for faces than for cars ($p=0.019$). The decrease (in absolute value) of the N170 was significant for noise level ($p = 0.022$) (see figure 6.b). There was also a significant linear contrast effect for noise level ($p=0.007$). The latency showed a significant effect for electrode ($p=0.012$) and size ($p=0.044$). The amplitude of the P1 did not show any significant effect.

For all subjects the fusiform face area was identified (mean center of activation $x = 34.7 \pm 3.5$; $y = -53.0 \pm 5.3$; $z=-12.7 \pm 4.8$). Figure 7.a shows the average time courses for the fusiform area indicated in figure 7.b. The mean activation in these regions showed a significant correlation with the ERP data ($r = -0.728$, FFA defined as maps of faces-cars, on the right hemisphere); figure 7.d shows the data as a scatter plot. The post-hoc analysis of the windows between 0 and 800 ms indicated that the N170 is the wave that has the largest correlation between changes in both modalities.

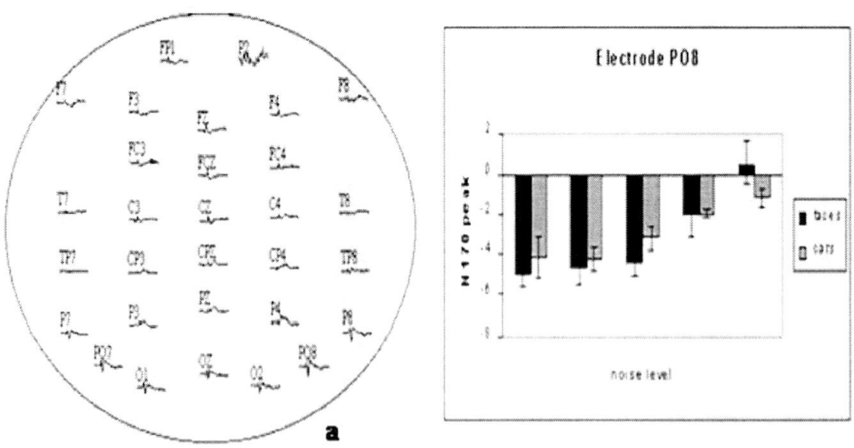

Figure 6.a. Scalp distribution of response to faces. b. Bar plot of N170 amplitude for faces (in dark) and cars (in light) for each noise level. Peaks are larger for faces than cars at each noise level, and peaks are larger in absolute values for pictures with lower level of noise.

Correlations between N170 amplitude for faces at electrode PO8 and voxel by voxel fMRI data were most significant ($p<0.001$) in bilateral fusiform gyri, right middle frontal gyrus and caudate body and antrerior cingulate (8.a). When using values from electrode P7 instead, correlations of highest significance ($p<0.001$) were found in the right superior temporal gyrus. For cars, no significant correlations were observed at the threshold used for faces. When decreasing the threshold to 0.005, significant correlations were observed at left inferior temporal gyrus, parahippocampal region, posterior cingulate (see figure 8.b) for electrode PO8 and the strongest correlations between ERP amplitude at electrode P7 and fMRI data were observed in superior temporal gyrus (p<0.001).

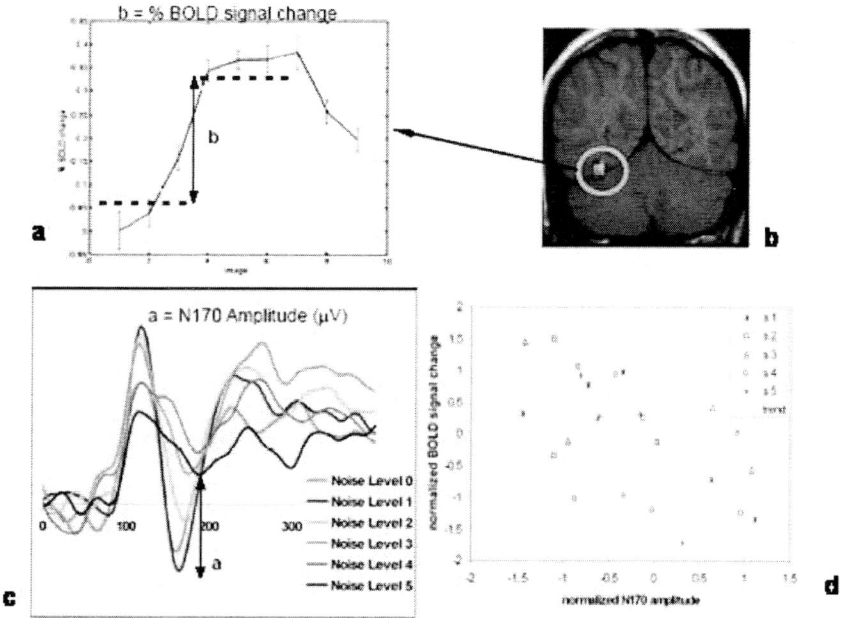

Figure 7.a. Time course of hemodynamic response of the right fusirorm area, functionally defined as activation of faces minus cars, and shown in b. c. Timecourse of the ERP response to face presentation at each of the noise levels. d. scatter plot of the N170 amplitude (a) versus the BOLD signal change(b)

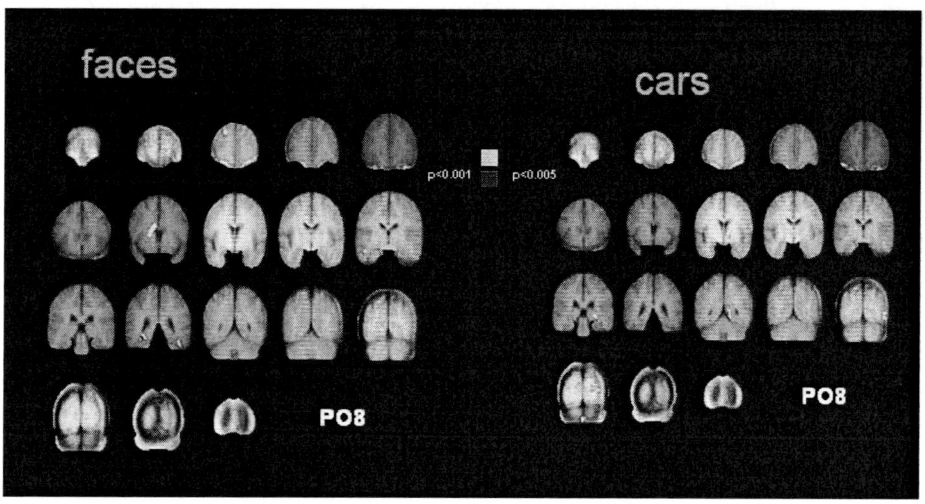

Figure 8. Activation maps observed for the correlation between N170 amplitude at electrode PO8 and BOLD signal change (left). for faces (threshold = 0.001) and (right) for cars (threshold = 0.005). In both cases cluster size was set to 20. Maps are composite of all 5 subjects

Discussion

Oddball Paradigm

After data pre-processing, which included filtering, artifact removal and averaging, we obtained ERP waveforms containing the characteristic peaks (the auditory specific N100; the P200 associated with the biological significance of the event and finally the P300 that reflects the cognitive processing). This is in agreement with findings by Duncan-Johnson (1977) and others. Picton reviewed the probability effect as reported in the literature (Picton, 1992) and showed a small increase in amplitude as the time elapsed between targets increased for the ranges we explored in this work (18 s to 75 s). However, the rationale to use these intervals was to allow the hemodynamic response to fully evolve before the presentation of the next target. As shown by Robson et al. (1997) this time is about 18 seconds. Faster event related paradigms can be used in fMRI, but we wished to avoid any assumptions about the linearity of the response. It is worth noting that in recent years efforts have been made to overcome this limitation; for example, paradigms have been implemented in fMRI in recent studies (Kellman, 2003) allowing separation of linear and non linear responses.

The fMRI analysis collapsing across probabilities show regions of activations that agree with regions activated in previous oddball studies (including insula, supramarginal gyrus, anterior cingulate (Menon, 1997; Stevens, 2000)). However, while these regions are activated by the stimulus, not all of them reflect the activity of the P300. As shown in figures 4 and 5, when separating the ERP data into 4 groups, the amplitude of the P300 increases as probability decreases depending on the target probability while N100 and P200 are not affected by the target manipulation. The correlations between the ROIs and P300 amplitudes were significant for insula and supramarginal gyrus. The voxel by voxel analysis explores the whole brain, without predefined regions or boundaries. By looking at these results (figure 5.b) and comparing the activated regions with those in the traditional analysis (figure 4.c) it is clear that not all the same regions are activated. It is not straightforward to do a direct statistical analysis to compare maps, since they are constructed using different statistics. Nonetheless, for a given threshold the observed maps show different areas of activation. Our data suggest that not all regions activated in a single implementation of the task respond to those manipulations of the probability that affect the ERP data. While activity within the supramarginal gyri and insulae are highly correlated with the P300 amplitude, the activity within the anterior cingulate is not. Therefore, these regions presumably do not contribute to the changes in P300 that occur when the oddball frequency is changed. We have shown that for auditory stimuli the amplitude of the hemodynamic responses in supramarginal gyri, thalami, insulae and right medial frontal gyrus follow the amplitude of the ERP as the probability varies. We therefore postulate that these regions contribute to the variations in the ERP amplitude.

Even though the time scales of fMRI and ERP are different, and though they measure different physiological events, the BOLD response seems to be modulated in part by the same factors that affect the amplitude of the evoked electrical response. The ROI analysis indicated that BOLD signals from left insula have the highest correlation with the amplitude of the P300, followed by right supramarginal gyrus. Supramarginal gyrus has been largely accepted as one of the sources of the P300 (Menon, 1997; Linden, 1999). The voxel by voxel correlation analysis provided a bilateral source distribution, with activations in supramarginal gyri, insula, thalamus, and right medial frontal gyrus. Since the ERP is more prominent in the scalp electrodes located over the longitudinal fissure, it was expected that generators of the P300 would be located bilaterally, as found here.

Supramarginal gyrus was also found to respond to oddball experiments in studies using intracranial recordings of P300-like responses (Halgren, 1995). In these studies, Halgren distinguished three processing levels for each auditory oddball. The earlier one, automatic, with no attention involved, induced activation at the superior temporal pole. This is followed by activity corresponding to a rapid evaluation of stimulus significance, with sources in anterior cingulate, and parietal and dorsal frontal areas. Finally, there is a cognitive stage with activity originating in limbic structures, medial temporal lobule and association cortex. In this model, there are several circuits activated by the oddball paradigm and the temporal resolution of the fMRI does not allow us to separate them.

However, by correlating BOLD changes to ERP changes we identify more accurately which regions contribute to features of the electrical response. By using a parametrical design we were able to measure changes in BOLD signal that correlated with changes in the amplitude of the P300.

Face Processing Paradigm

Our ERP results agree with previous studies: N170 showed more prominently in occipito-parietal electrodes (Bentin, 1996; Bötzel, 1995) and was larger for faces than for objects (Bentin, 1996; Bötzel, 1995; Eimer, 2000; Rossion, 2000, 2003). The origin of the N170 is largely debated in the literature. Recent studies, using source localization analysis, have pointed toward bilateral dipolar sources in the posterior part of fusiform gyri or inferior occipital cortices (Halgren, 2000; Iter, 2002; Rossion, 2003; Schweinberger, 2002, Watanabe, 2003), and some studies have shown a right hemisphere dominance (Halgren, 2000; Rossion, 2003). We performed the ROI analysis using the fusiform area (defined as activation for faces minus activation for cars) and observed a strong correlation between the activation in this area and the amplitude of the N170 component. The post-hoc analysis over a larger timeframe indicated that the interval including the N170 was the most significant. The correlations performed on a voxel by voxel basis showed a very significant correlation of ERP to fusiform area for faces and to parahippocampal regions for cars. These regions are involved in face processing according to single cell recording studies, patient and neuroimaging studies (Haxby, 2000).

Conclusion

Through the two presented studies, it has been shown that fMRI and ERP parametric studies, when combined with correlation analysis, may allow for detection of a more specific net of activations than single condition subtractions. The inclusion of ERP data as the parameter to follow in the fMRI analysis enhanced the detection of hemodynamic responses that follow neurological activation. The networks studied showed hemodynamic responses that followed the neuronal response in a linear fashion. Through such parametric fMRI-ERP studies, we have shown it is possible to enhance the fMRI analysis by adding ERP information. This is an example of how ERP information may be used synergistically in fMRI analyses. fMRI parametric designs of this type may provide some timing information about fMRI measurements and help identify the generators of ERP signals.

References

Bandettini PA, Wong EC, Hinks RS, Tikofsky RS, Hyde JS. (1992). "Time course EPI of human brain function during task activation." *Magnetic Resonance in Medicine* 25: 390-397.

Bentin S, Allison T, Puce A, Perez E, McCarthy G. (1996). "Electrophysiological studies of face perception in humans." *Journal of Cognitive Neuroscience*, 8, 551-565.

Bötzel K, Schulze S, Stodieck SRG, (1995). "Scalp topography and analysis of intracranial sources of face-evoked potentials." *Experimental Brain Research*, 104, 134-143.

Blamire AM, Ogawa S, Ugurbil K, Rothman D, McCarthy G, Ellermann JM, Hyder F, Rattner Z, Shulman RG, (1992) " Dynamic mapping of the human visual cortex by high-speed magnetic resonance imaging." *Proceedings of the National Academy of Sciences of the United States of America.* 89(22):11069-73.

Buckner RL, Bandettini PA, O'Craven KM, Savoy RL, Petersen SE, Raichle ME, Rosen BR, (1996). "Detection of the cortical activation during averaged single trials of a cognitive task using functional magnetic resonance imaging" *Proc Natl. Acad. Sci USA* 93 (25)14878-14883.

Duncan-Johnson C, Donchin E. (1977) "On quantifying surprise: the variations of event-related potentials with subjective probability." *Psychophysiology* 14:5:456-67.

Eimer, M. (2000). "The face-specific N170 component reflects late stages in the structural encoding of faces." *Neuroreport*, 11, 2319-2324.

Halgren E, Baudena P, Clarke JM, Heit G, Liégeois C, Chauvel P, Musolino A. (1995) "Intracerebral potentials to rare target and distractor auditory and visual stimuli. I. Superior temporal plane and parietal lobe." *Electroencephalography and Clinical Neurophysiology* 94:191-220.

Halgren, E., Raij, T., Marinkovic, K., Jousmaki, V., Hari R. (2000). Cognitive response profile of the human fusiform face area as determined by MEG. *Cerebral Cortex*, 10 69-81.

Haxby JV, Hoffman EA, Gobbini MI (2000). "The distributed human neural system for face perception." *Trends in Cognitive Science,* 4, 223–233.

Horovitz SG, Skudlarski P, Gore JC (2002)." Correlations and dissociations between BOLD signal and P300 amplitude in an auditory oddball task: a parametric approach to combining fMRI and ERP." *Magnetic Resonance Imaging*, 20,(4) 319-325.

Horovitz SG, Rossion B, Skudlarski P, Gore JC (2004)." Parametric design and correlational analyses help integrating fMRI and electrophysiological data during face processing." *NeuroImage*, 22, 1587-1595.

Itier RJ, Taylor M.J. (2002). "Inversion and contrast polarity reversal affect both encoding and recognition processes of unfamiliar faces: a repetition study using ERPs." *NeuroImage*, 15, 353-72.

Jemel B, Schuller AM, Cheref-Khan Y, Goffaus V, Crommelinck M, Bruyer R. (2003), Stepwise emergence of the face-sensitive N170 component in a gradual presentation procedure. *NeuroReport*, 14, 2035-2039.

Kellman P., Gelderen, P., de Zwart, J.A., Duyn, J.H., (2003). " Method for functional MRI mapping of nonlinear response." *NeuroImage*, 19, 190-199.

Kwoung KK, Belliveau JW, Chesler DA, Goldberg IE, Weisskoff RM, Poncelet BP, *et at.* (1992) "Dynamic magnetic resonance imaging of human brain activity during primary sensory stimulation." *Proc Natl. Acad. Sci USA* 89:5675-5679.

Linden DEJ, Prvulovic D, Formisano E, Völlinger M, Zanella FE, Goebel R, Dierks T. (1999) "The functional neuroanatomy of target detection: an fMRI study of visual and auditory oddball tasks." *Cerebral Cortex* 9: 815-23.

Logothetis, N.K., J. Pauls, M.A. Augath, T. Trinath and A. Oeltermann. (2001) "Neurophysiological Investigation of the Basis of the fMRI signal." *Nature*, 412, 150-157.

Logothetis, N.K. (2003). "The Underspinnings of the BOLD Functional Magnetic Resonance Imaging Signal." *The Journal of Neuroscience* 23(10), 3963-3971.

McCarthy G, Luby M, Gore JC, Goldman-Rakic P. (1997) "Infrequent events transiently active human prefrontal and parietal cortex as measured by functional MRI." *J of Neurophysiology* 77: 1630-4.

Menon V, Ford JM, Lim KO, Glover GH, Pfefferbaum (1997) "A. Combined event-related fMRI and EEG evidence for temporal-parietal cortex activation during target detection." *NeuroReport* 8:14: 3029-37.

Ogawa S, Tank DW, Menon R, Ellermnn JM, Kim S-G, Merkle H, *et al.* (1992). "Intrinsic signal changes accompanying sensory stimulation: functional brain mapping with magnetic resonance imaging." *Proc Natl. Acad. Sci. USA* 89:5951-5955.

Picton TW. (1992) "The P300 wave of the human event-related potential." *J. Clinical Neurophysiology* 9:2:456-79.

Polich J, Kok A. (1995) "Cognitive and biological determinants of P300: an integrative review." *Biological Psychology* 41:103-46.

Rees G, Friston K, Koch C. (2000) "A direct quantitative relationship between the functional properties of human and macaque V5." *Nat Neurosci.* Jul;3(7):716-23.

Robson MD, Dorosz JL, Gore JC. (1998) "Measurements of the temporal fMRI response of the human auditory cortex to train of tones." *NeuroImage* 7:185-98.

Rossion, B., Joyce, C., Cottrell, G, Tarr, M.J. (2003). Early lateralization and orientation tuning for face, word and object processing in the visual cortex. *NeuroImage*, vol. 20, 1609-1624.

Rossion, B. Curran, T., Gauthier, I. (2002). A defense of the subordinate-expertise account for the N170 component. *Cognition,* 85 189-96.

Schweinberger, S.R., Pickering, E.C, Jentzsch, I., Burton, A.M., Kaufmann, J.M. (2002). Event-related brain potential evidence for a response of inferior temporal cortex to familiar face repetitions. *Cognitive Brain Research.* 14, 398-409.

Semlitsch HV, Anderer P, Schuster P, Presslich O (1986). "A solution for reliable and valid reduction of ocular artifacts, applied to the P300 ERP." *Psychophysiology* 23:6:695-703.

Skudlarski P, Constable RT, Gore JC. (1999) "ROC analysis of statistical methods used in functional MRI: individual subjects." *NeuroImage* 9:3:311-329.

Stevens AA, Skudlarski P, Gatenby JC, Gore, JC. (2000) "Event-related fMRI of auditory and visual oddball tasks." *Magnetic Resonance Imaging* 18:5:495-502.

Sutton S, Baren M, Zubin J, John ER. (1965) "Evoked potential correlates of stimulus uncertainty." *Science* 150:1187-8.

Talairach J, Tournoux P. (1988) Co-Planar stereotaxic atlas of the human brain. 3-Dimensional proportional system: an approach to cerebral imaging. New York, NY, Georg Thieme Verlag.

Tueting P, Sutton S, Zubin J.(1971) "Quantitative evoked potential correlates of the probability of events." *Psychophysiology* 7:3:385-94.

Watanabe S, Kakigi R, Puce A (2003) "The spatio-temporal dynamics of the face inversion effect: a magneto- and electro- encephalographic study". *Neuroscience* 116, 879-895.

Index

A

B

C

D

E

F

G

H

I

J

K

L

M

N

R

S

T